T0358166

Representing Argentinian Mothers

Clio Medica: Perspectives in Medical Humanities

92

Representing Argentinian Mothers

Medicine, Ideas and Culture
in the Modern Era, 1900-1946

Yolanda Eraso

Amsterdam - New York, NY 2013

Cover illustration: Detail of the fresco *Elogio al Sentimiento*
by Guido Buffo, Chapel Buffo. Courtesy of the Casa Museo y
Capilla Buffo, Unquillo, Córdoba.
This image depicts the journalist and writer Leonor Allende
with her daughter. It was painted by her husband, Guido
Buffo, who erected a chapel in their memory in which the
fresco was painted.

The paper on which this book is printed meets the
requirements of "ISO 9706:1994, Information and
documentation - Paper for
documents - Requirements for permanence".

ISBN: 978-90-420-3704-5
E-Book ISBN: 978-94-012-0961-8
© Editions Rodopi B.V., Amsterdam – New York, NY 2013
Printed in The Netherlands

Contents

Abbreviations

IICAOyG	II Congreso Argentino de Obstetricia y Ginecología
IVCAOyG	IV Congreso Argentino de Obstetricia y Ginecología
VCAOyG	V Congreso Argentino de Obstetricia y Ginecología
IICNM	II Congreso Nacional de Medicina
IVCNM	IV Congreso Nacional de Medicina
VCNM	V Congreso Nacional de Medicina
VICNM	VI Congreso Nacional de Medicina
CCD	Consortium of Catholic Doctors
NDMI	National Direction of Maternity and Infancy
PACC	Pan-American Child Congress
RCMC	Revista del Círculo Médico de Córdoba

List of Illustrations

Acknowledgements

In the writing of this book I am indebted to a large number of institutions and individuals, lecturers, colleagues and friends on both sides of the Atlantic for their help and support to whom I extend my sincere thanks in the lines that follows.

In the earlier stages of the research for this book whilst I was in Argentina, Dora Barrancos provided mentoring, intellectual nurturing and enthusiastic support for the project. Also I am indebted to María Teresa Dalmasso and my colleagues of the programme of studies on Social Discourse and Gender Studies at the Centro de Estudios Avanzados, Universidad Nacional de Córdoba, for providing a forum for discussion as well as constructive criticism for which I have benefited greatly.

In England, my sincere thanks go to the erstwhile Director of the Centre for Health, Medicine and Society at Oxford Brookes University, Steve King, for his trust, esteem and encouragement during my time spent as a doctoral student. I am also very grateful to John Stewart who offered perceptive comments and practical help during the preparation of this work, as well as friendship and enjoyable talks about gender and welfare, which convinced me to transform what was originally a chapter of this project into a chapter for a volume I edited exclusively dedicated to women and welfare in Latin America. Most of all, I must thank Anne Digby for her mentoring throughout the research and writing process, for her generous support, for being a continuous source of challenge to my ideas, and above all, for her extraordinary sense of dialectics and flair in asking valuable questions. I am also grateful to the valuable suggestions and comments of Hilary Marland, Alberto Mira, and more recently, the anonymous referees who read the first draft of the book.

I have also learnt a great deal from discussions with the history of medicine group at Oxford Brookes and the Seminar Series at the Centre for Health, Medicine and Society, where in 2004, I also had the chance of delivering a paper and discuss the same issues of eugenics that I present in Chapter 2. Participants at the conferences organised by the Society for Latin American Studies at the universities of Nottingham (2004) and Cambridge (2005) also provided interesting questions and comments to my preliminary chapters, which have undoubtedly helped in making my analysis stronger.

This project was made possible through the financial support of various funding bodies: the Secretaría de Ciencia y Técnica of the Universidad Nacional de Córdoba granted a Doctoral Studentship that allowed me to initiate work on a fundamental section of this book, entitled 'the medical record'. In England, the Overseas Research Students Awards Scheme contributed a vital grant for my studies, and especially the Wellcome Trust provided the core of my funding through a doctoral studentship held at Oxford Brookes University, for which I am most grateful.

At the core of this book and part of what I hope is valuable about *Representing Argentinian Mothers* rests a wide range of sources of diverse nature that are scattered in so many places and whose access I have so often (almost literally) celebrated. Therefore, I extend a sincere gratitude and appreciation to the librarians and archivists who have generously provided their expertise in locating many of the demanding and unfamiliar sources that made up my study, and who patiently and kindly granted access to special sections of libraries, archives and collections considering the time constrains of my travels to Argentina. Without their proficiency and unhesitant wiliness to help us, we, as researchers, will surely draw on less varied, less rich and less stimulating materials. I would like to thank in Argentina: the staff of the 'Hemeroteca de la Legislatura de Córdoba' who patiently helped me with the location of newspapers; Susana Luna and Romina Otero from the Museo Provincial de Bellas Artes 'Emilio A. Caraffa'; Jorge González and Marcela Santanera of the 'Museo Municipal de Bellas Artes Dr. Genaro Pérez', to María Celina Audisio del Archivo del Arzobispado de Córdoba, to the staff of the following libraries of the Universidad Nacional de Córdoba: Facultad de Ciencias Médicas, Biblioteca Mayor, Instituto de la Maternidad Nacional, Facultad de Filosofía y Humanidades. In England, I am indebted to the librarians at the Bodleian Library, the Radcliffe Science Library and the Taylor Institution Library of the University of Oxford, and the Wellcome Library in London.

I am particularly grateful to the copyright holders of many of the images that appear in this book, mainly institutions and family members of the artists who have generously provided authorisation to reprint: Family Berni, Spilimbergo Foundation, Gabriela Antonowicz, and the directors of the Museo Provincial de Bellas Artes 'Emilio A. Caraffa', Museo Municipal de Bellas Artes 'Dr. Genaro Pérez', Museo Nacional de Bellas Artes, and newspaper *La Voz del Interior*. On the other hand, I should state that attempts to locate the copyright owners for the newspaper *Los Principios* and the painting *Figura* by Batlle Planas were not fruitful.

Parts of Chapter 2 of this book have appeared before, although in different forms. It draws on two previously published pieces: first, I offer a revised version of my article, 'Biotypology, Endocrinology and Sterilization: The Practice of Eugenics in the Treatment of Argentinian Women during the 1930s', first published in *Bulletin of the History of Medicine* 81.4 (2007), 793-822 (copyright © 2007 The Johns Hopkins University Press, reprinted with permission by The Johns Hopkins University Press); and second, I incorporate some concepts developed in my chapter in Spanish, 'Género y Eugenesia: Hacia una Taxonomía Médico-Social de las Mujeres-Madres en la Década de 1930' in Bravo, Gil Lozano, and Pita (eds). *Historias de Luchas, Resistencias y Representaciones. Mujeres en la Argentina, siglos XIX y XX*. Tucumán: Editorial de la Universidad Nacional de Tucumán, 2007, 361-90.

My deep appreciation also extends to Brian Dolan, Executive Editor of *Clio Medica: Perspectives in Medical Humanities* series for efficiently providing all kind of editorial support as I prepared the final manuscript, to Carina Bartleet for taking the time to read and help with editing the book, and to the editorial staff at Rodopi, Esther Roth and Christa Stevens.

Finally I should like to thank the loving support of my friends, in particular Leonardo, Marcela, the late Dorothy Wheeler, Gabriela, Carina and Oscar, my family, and especially, my parents, who have unfailingly provided love and moral support during all these years in Oxford. In a book entirely dedicated to the significance of motherhood in Argentinian culture I would be no exception and so I especially acknowledge my mum, Yolanda, whose immense love continues to surprise me. I dedicate this book to her.

For mum

Introduction

Motherhood holds a special place in Argentinian culture. Mothers have occupied a central place within the family structure, have been emissaries of human piety, mediators between the state and the poor, venerated by Catholic (Italian and Spanish) and Jewish cultures, and have, among other things, been traditionally responsible for their children's traumas and fortune, including that of their biological endowment. Such a ubiquitous presence is even reflected and transmitted through the colloquial language where the maternal is able to communicate, in equal terms, sympathy and kindness as much as spiteful, violent insults. An improvised account of mother-images that are deeply embedded in Argentinian culture would return a polysemic figure: In 1977 the 'Mothers of Plaza de Mayo', a women's movement created by the mothers of the political dissidents that were disappeared during the brutal military dictatorship (1976-83), gave rise – in their claim for justice for the human rights violations – to the idea of a political motherhood that inverted the order of the biological one, as encapsulated in their famous slogan: 'Our children gave birth to us'. In the 1950s, Eva Perón, the iconic First Lady, was famously worshiped as 'the mother of the poor'. Eva, ironically a childless woman, became a political mother too, of the working classes and the underclass. Folk religion had in the mythological figure of *Difunta Correa*, a woman who around the 1840s 'miraculously' breast fed her baby after she died in the deserted roads of San Juan province, a popular saint mother who is still venerated by truck drivers in the countless little shrines improvised all over the country's roads. Another example of the densely interwoven meanings associated with the maternal is found in the leading maternity hospital of the country, the Institute of Maternity in Buenos Aires, which opened to the public in 1928. Inside the building there is a main portico with a slogan sculpted on its arch that says, 'the mother is mother, and that is all'. Yet for all its multiple meanings and extolled figures constantly struggling to embody the essence of the mother, Argentinians have a legendary popular adage that belies the notion of a plural location, 'mother there is only one'. In fact the wide variety of forms, often contradictory, in which motherhood and the maternal have been used in Argentinian culture, the subjects of its enunciation and the public to which they were geared suggest the multiple purposes which various representations has served.

During the period of nation-building, towards the end of the nineteenth century and until the first decades of the twentieth century, notions of maternity in Argentina were intertwined with medical ideas of maternal virtue that were variously associated with mother's responsibility in rearing healthy citizens, with growing concerns on infant mortality, and with providing a healthy pregnancy and delivery. Discussions of the maternal-biological process were frequently connected with matters of national relevance, perceived as a sign of civilisation and often associated metaphorically with the idea of a 'gestating' state. I would contend, however, that the overloaded meaning attributed to 'the medical' in many scholarly studies has tended to obscure the responses that culture may have formulated on the maternal in this particular period. This book is concerned with the way in which medical representations of maternity have been implicated, echoed and/or contested in certain areas of the social and cultural field. At the same time, it evaluates the new representations those areas have built. In this sense, the ubiquitous nature of motherhood in Argentinian culture offers us a particularly fruitful ground for examining the intensity, impact and penetration of medical ideas in society at large. To this aim the study adopts an interdisciplinary approach. While engaging critically with the existing literature (literary criticism, feminist studies, cultural studies and medical history), it proposes a different interpretation provided by an innovative framework based on categories and notions drawn from the history of ideas and cultural history.

My interest in exploring the representations of motherhood in an interdisciplinary way has not been exclusively inspired by motherhood's pervasive presence, rather it has been informed by different perceptions, criticism, and recommendations often observed in surveys of medical history and women and science. In my research an important motivation has been induced by the term 'medicalisation' which in the topic of maternity has had overarching connotations as a widely encompassing, micro-controlled medical power exerted over women's bodies. Another incentive has been the very existence of a significant body of international scholarly studies that made it bluntly evident that new research on the history of maternity needed a fresh look and not merely a new case study of a less explored context. My approach has been motivated by an attempt of 'altering' the *status quaestionis* rather than of 'confirming' its main hypothesis in different scenarios.

There is plainly a consensus in scholars of women and science on the need, as Marina Benjamin has proposed, of 'overstepping the territorial boundaries established by any one discipline' and 'the need to consult a wide diversity of historical sources from all areas of cultural activity'.[1] Yet it seems that there is still much to enquire about those interrelated areas. A diversification of sources to explore should necessarily be accompanied by a revision of the questions that orient the investigation. Studies that have scrutinised various sources have tended to look at visual images, novels, advertisements, and other forms of cultural production *only* in those works that have served to convey and spread specific medical ideas, without assessing the wide range of circulating texts and cultural products at a given moment. Although they add richness to the empirical evidence, they risk emphasising the penetration or pervasiveness of medical knowledge in culture, thus offering a less balanced perspective. Representations on the maternal, as I propose in this book, should abandon a unidirectional perspective of influence, i.e. from medicine to culture, and adopt instead a more open, multi-layered flux of interactions in each disciplinary context. In this sense, *Representing Argentinian Mothers* seeks to analyse the main determinants (medical, social, cultural, religious) that have influenced the representations of motherhood from 1900 to 1946, through a reconstruction of medical discourse and its articulation (appropriation, re-signification) in other significant socio-cultural spheres (Catholic beliefs, literature, press, and fine arts).

Locating the scene

The topic of motherhood during this period of Argentinian history offers a privileged viewpoint to explore the tensions and conflicts underlying the country's unequal modernisation process. In order to highlight the importance of the context in framing different representations, the book seeks to draw attention to the contrasting developments observed at the provincial level, taking the case of Córdoba as a main example, alongside examples of the Federal Capital and, to a lesser extent, of other locales representative of the national level. Two main reasons underpin this selection of places. The first one is related to the interdisciplinary nature that informs this book whereby the resort to local case studies may provide, despite their always limited representativeness, the best strategy against sweeping generalisations in a country that differs considerably between its provinces and capital. It has long been argued that the local case study has the ability of amending encompassing assumptions in the historiography. To which we can add that by stressing differences and similarities among settings lays an opportunity to tease out broader implications. The second reason for this spatial selection is related to the relevance and particularities that Córdoba offers within the Argentinian context.

The city of Córdoba, capital of the homonymous province and located some 790 km south-east from Buenos Aires, is the second city of Argentina. During the colonial period, the city occupied a central position as a commercial route connecting Buenos Aires and the western territories with the administrative centre of the Spanish Viceroyalty situated in Peru. Location gave Córdoba an identity much closer to Spain and Catholicism in comparison to the outward looking port cities of Rosario, Paraná and Buenos Aires. Between 1895 and 1914, Argentina witnessed an unprecedented growth of European immigration, mostly from Italy and Spain, which was stimulated by the government to boost the country's economic development. The immigrant population soon spread around the towns and cities close to the richest agricultural region of *la pampa* (the central plain), yet concentration varied amongst places, having a different impact in the composition of the population and in shaping the future character of cities. Thus, the percentage of foreigners in Córdoba and Buenos Aires, although important in the former, were notoriously high in the federal capital (Córdoba, 1895:11.25; 1914:22.50; 1947:10.40; Buenos Aires, 1895:52; 1914:49.3; 1947:27.5).[2]

Immigrant populations played the protagonists in the modern transformation of Córdoba's economy and society. Spanish immigrants, for example, constituted a powerful group of importer traders, financiers and industrialists who concentrated the commercial activities with the Northern provinces and the coastal city-ports of Buenos Aires and Rosario. Spaniards became easily integrated into Córdoba's society through matrimony and a shared Catholic-Spanish tradition, which in turn strengthened the economic position of the existing elite. The traditional ruling class in Córdoba had the particularity of being a professional caste, whose power, unlike the one of Buenos Aires, was not primarily based in landed property. Their prestige and economic power was founded in the exercise of liberal professions, mostly in the judiciary, medical, and the university sectors, and to a lesser extent in land ownership and business.[3]

The unprecedented influx of a transatlantic immigration also revealed important undesirable consequences in the rapidly expanding urban areas: growing levels of poverty, housing problems (overcrowding and poor hygiene); a deficient structure of sanitary services – that favoured the spread of diseases related to the environment; high maternal and infant mortality rates together with a weak hospital and welfare structure. As a result, a strong interrelation between statesmen, hygienists and physicians took place, oriented to the interpretation and search for social solutions, transforming medical specialists into legitimate figures of the state order. Yet the assumption of the 'social question' precipitated an important ideological debate amongst leading political groups and intellectuals[4] about the destiny of the Nation. In this context, Positivist ideas constituted the main discourse of the period in terms of the interpretation of reality and of the nation's destiny, as well as, in practice, by influencing the development of several institutions (educational, medical, and legal).[5] The devotion to science, rationality and progressive knowledge consciously grew as a new foundation for a national intellectual order set in sharp contrast to a colonial past, grounded in scholasticism, doctrinal knowledge, and Catholic values. This implied a somewhat contradictory yet enduring process, whereby nation building was envisioned by social reformers against its colonial and pre-hispanic past, as Tulio Halperín Donghi has noted, rather than on its foundations.[6] As a consequence, the Church's former ideological influence declined considerably, most notably in the federal capital and in the passing of secular national legislation, although with a differentiated impact in the rest of the territory.

Córdoba provides a case in point and hence an interesting place for discussion. The 'city of bells', as it is commonly referred to in allusion to the numerous churches and known pious devotion, was a place where the influence of the Church was never completely undermined, and where the process of modernisation would operate differently, especially at a sociocultural level. A modern and laicised society was the driving force for the liberal, national government, and to which a 'restrictive global project, governed by exclusive values'[7] was opposed by those who defined themselves under the identity of 'Catholics'. Inside these forces, there was a battle for the definition of the social order, including the educational system, the economic model of integration, the political form of citizen participation, and the delineation of a family model. At its heart lay the Catholic opposition to the laicisation of society undertaken by the national government from 1880 up until the 1930s, and whose most conspicuous materialisation were the laws of lay education (1884) and civil matrimony (1888). In the medical field, for example, parallel to the conformation of an elite of liberal, Positivist hygienists in the national state, there was an elite of Catholic hygienists who attempted to imbue Cordoban state policy with the stamp of Catholicism. Still more remarkably, the so-called 'battle for ideas' in education – staged

5

by secular and Catholic forces – would experience in the university space the most hectic and resonant conflict. The University of Córdoba, founded by the Jesuits in 1613, is the oldest in the country, giving the city its most prestigious symbol, expressed in its slogan, *Córdoba la docta* ('Córdoba the learned'). Despite its nationalisation in 1854, the University epitomised the Church's traditional role in education. Ideological tensions, however, reached their peak in 1918 when the University was the site of the first student rebellion leading to the University Reform of that year that revolutionised university education and inspired student politics well into the 1960s. Indeed, the students' rebellion soon spread, affecting first Buenos Aires and later most Latin-American universities, and although in its dissemination the Reform movement was informed by different sources of thought (Marxism-Leninism, Nietzsche and Greek philosophy), what made it triumphant in Córdoba was precisely its profound anticlericalism. If the Reform of 1918 marked the triumph of the liberal forces against the Catholics ones, it also spurred on a rapid and effective backlash from the faithful, initiating what historians have termed a process of 'clericalisation of public life'.[8] Disputes between University and Church, liberals and Catholics, would have a profound impact not only in the delineation of state policies and medical ideas concerning mother and child issues, but more broadly in the cultural life of the city, including the press, artistic tendencies, and literary expressions, as I will discuss in the chapters that follow. Maternity played a significant role in these debates as the biological and spiritual processes associated with mothering became matters of paramount importance not just for the nation's future citizens, but for the place of religion in modern society, and the role of the family in shaping that future.

While in Córdoba Catholic forces were active from the consolidation of the Argentinian state in 1880, at the national level it was not until the military *coup d'état* of September 1930 that Catholics intervened directly in the government of the nation. The new military rule, in alliance with the Church, proposed to regenerate society's moral values and Argentinian national cohesion through the restoration of Catholic spirituality and a corporate social order organised along fascist lines. This unprecedented amalgamation of church and armed forces, known as 'Catholic integralism', positioned Catholicism as the 'true' cultural matrix of the Argentine nation. On the one hand, the alternation in power of military and conservative governments elected in fraudulent elections was notorious for its corruption and economic scandals leading historians to dub this period 'the infamous decade' (1930-1943). On the other, conservative and militant Catholics embarked in an 'anti-liberal crusade' stimulated by the creation of the Catholic Action in 1931, the local chapter of the worldwide movement backed by Pius XI to coordinate lay activities under the strict guidance of the ecclesiastic hierarchy. The Catholic Action movement pursued nothing less than the 're-Christianisation of society' and its dogged presence resonated in the political, social, and cultural life of the country as demonstrated by its multiple interventions in spheres such as the army, unions, education, and professions. Moreover, a renewed cultural project grounded in nationalism and Hispanism, with an ample insertion in both the intellectual and popular field, soon disseminated through a myriad of institutions and publications underpinning a Catholic ideology whose various strands and internal differences remain largely unexplored.

The 1930s and 1940s constitute a fruitful period to examine the maternal, firstly for their medical institutionalisation and biological, eugenic inscriptions, and secondly, for their ideological tensions, in particular, the spiritual one through the re-elaboration of the Marian cult, both with formulations in the journalistic, fictional, and visual registers. The arrival of Juan Domingo Perón to the presidency of the nation in 1946 marks the chronological scope of this study – although some references to his government will be noted – for *peronismo* inaugurated a new era in Argentinian history with radical transformative consequences. The first four decades of the twentieth century thus appears to be constituted by fragmented scenarios, with Buenos Aires as the capital that connects the country with the economic and cultural European centres where the city itself aspires to be integrated, and Córdoba, the provincial city, with its own system of European references, and less ready to disown its Spanish-Catholic past. The attempt to build a 'Catholic nation' in the 1930s relocates these debates at the national level giving room to new formulations as they became articulated with a different set of problems. It is the divergent, fragmented and asynchronic nature of these developments as well as the very contingency (in the making) of the modernising process, what makes them privileged spaces for a study that attempts to account for the shaping of motherhood and its representations.

Themes and perspectives

Historical approaches to maternity have become an exciting and sophisticated field of research that in the last three decades has grown mainly within the area of gender and women's studies and their numerous disciplinary fields. Concentrating in the area of medical history, much work has focused around midwifery, the professionalisation and conformation of medical specialties, such as obstetrics, gynaecology, paediatrics, the organisation of maternal services, and the medicalisation of childbirth amongst others, where studies became enriched from the articulation of specific settings.[9] The proliferation of these surveys observed within the European and Anglo-Saxon contexts has also been accompanied by an increasing body of literature in the Latin American context, although more in the article format than in monograph studies, whose contribution would be impossible to recount in this section but will be commented on throughout the book.[10] One feature of the studies that have focused on the Argentinian context has been a tendency to concentrate on medical aspects of maternity more through the lenses of state welfare policies, feminist movements, female charity and philanthropy, or legislation concerning working women, than through a systematic analysis of medical ideas, institutions, and practices related to women's health or women and science more broadly.

The pioneer works of Marcela Nari for the case of Buenos Aires in the 1990s constitute a valuable starting point to interpret how maternity and the maternal became a primary medical concern, including such related issues as the country's low birth-rate, infanticide and child abandonment, the rise of puericulture and maternal education, and the changing perspectives of medical specialists as they addressed the maternal under different constraints. Most of Nari's works were posthumously published in the volume, *Políticas de Maternidad y Maternalismo Político en Buenos Aires (1890-1940)*[11] where it is possible to observe the articulation between medical ideas and state policies in relation to the so-called 'political maternalism' that identified Argentinian feminists during the first decades of the twentieth century. This perspective has had an enduring influence in that many of the works that followed added depth and detail to the interface of state physicians, female organisations, and the feminist movement in delineating a mother and child agenda, most notably studied by Donna Guy's *Women Build the Welfare State: Performing Charity and Creating Rights in Argentina, 1880–1955*.[12] At the same time, this perspective has also been instrumental in bringing attention to female voluntarism and welfare state-building, especially charities and beneficent societies, thus revising the role that women have played as agents in this process. Until recently, Argentinian female charities and beneficent societies have been depicted as pre-state, traditional and conservative models of assistance and above all, as institutions run by the elite and the Catholic Church with the aim of controlling the poorer sectors of society. The latter has been contested by a perspective that offers a more complex picture of the role and motivations of women's welfare activism, including a reappraisal of their activities as welfare providers, their 'political conduct' and 'creativity',[13] and taken together, their provision of 'a blueprint of social policies for the subsequent formation of a Peronist welfare state based upon concerns for children and mothers'.[14]

This book is not primarily concerned with maternal policies nor with the role of female voluntarism in the shaping of welfare policies, although they constitute an important backdrop as they frame discussions and serve to support representations of the maternal by different social and cultural registers. In this sense, I propose two different dimensions to elucidate 'the maternal' as representations emerging from, on the one hand, the development of mother and child welfare policies, and on the other, the role women played as agents in this process. Firstly, I am interested in exploring both medical concepts and practices. This book will argue that it is in maternal institutions, more than in the analysis of the laws and the debates they generated, where we can gain a different insight into the implementation of medical ideas in Argentina. This is particularly the case for eugenically-oriented ideas during the 1930s when, as Nancy Stepan[15] and others have observed, eugenics became more vigorously debated and some important laws (prenuptial certificate, maternity leave and insurance) were passed. I am particularly interested in reviewing the eugenic tendencies that defined treatments, concepts and representations of the female body from the point of view of fertility. In so doing, I contend that, until recently, the prevailing historiographical perception of a soft, sanitary-oriented, positive eugenics in Argentina have tended to consider eugenic ideas as a set of interventions on the environment rather than in the physical contrition of individuals.[16] Secondly, in relation to the broader topic of women as agents of welfare, I am only concerned with the perceptions and representations of the figure of the charitable lady or the matron, as she embodies a political figure of the maternal given her central role in the provision of welfare to mothers and children during the period. Here, I am more interested in the political uses of motherhood through representations elaborated over its most prominent public figure, rather than in analysing women's political maternalism or charitable motivations, in order to reveal the politicisation of the matron by other discourses, i.e. medical, Catholic, liberal, fictional, etc.

The Catholic doctrine maintained that the family was society's most important institution, so that women's role as mothers was 'naturalised' but in ways that differed from that of the medical perspective. Gender historians have signalled that Catholic discourses emphasised a representational image of the mother, as nurturing, kind, virginal, and sacrificed. Yet those images require an historical contextualisation, not because they were absent, but because the timing of their appearance, as well as their changing nature, reveal a Catholic cultural project that, as I mentioned earlier, has been little explored. Catholic rhetoric worked in varied ways, through exhortatory writings, the press, rituals (street parades, virgin's enthronements), novels and artistic production, thus encompassing text and images whilst intervening both in the spiritual and secular realms. Through the examination of a range of Catholic sources I argue that maternal representations did not embody immutable doctrinal values, but were the result of particular contexts that shaped their ideological and symbolic content at particular times. Luisa Accati's perceptive analysis of motherhood through Catholic symbology and iconography will provide a useful framework to analyse representations on the maternal in the Catholic order, especially in her interpretation of Marian sacred iconography as illuminating 'a logic of the power of the son (in the shape of unmarried priests) over the mother, instead of one wherein the husband has power over the wife'.[17]

Against the pervasive Catholic culture lay liberal and secular forces, which encompassed a varied range of ideas, and whose public identity was defined as 'anti-clerical', 'liberal' or 'anti-Catholic'. The utility of this conventional division, 'Catholic vs. anti-Catholic, liberal', etc. does not attempt to undermine the internal differences that both terms implied, but instead to signal a horizon of ideas that deeply divided societies like Córdoba during this time. Secular culture, like the Catholic one, found expression through an ample area of cultural production, including the press, artistic and literary movements, which I will examine with the aim of reconstructing their own particular representation of the maternal together with its relation to those produced in the medical context. The latter connect us with another important mainstream area of scholarly work, the so-called 'cultural studies of science and women'. A central topic in this approach has been the dialectical relationship between nature and culture, which has led to a series of gendered dichotomies, mostly conveyed through sexual metaphors, where masculine science unveils, penetrate and dominates a female nature portrayed as secret, mysterious, and unruly. Reading and interpreting medical images of the female and the maternal body, for instance, has almost become mandatory for

Women's Studies in the past decades. Much feminist criticism of visualisation technologies, especially those concerned with images of the foetus, has concentrated upon the ways in which these visual languages have exposed the most intimate parts of the female body to the 'objective' medical male gaze, which, in turn, has led to the disembodiment of the pregnant woman and the divestment of ownership of her body.[18] As discussed at the beginning of this introduction, these studies have been dominated by a somewhat exclusive focus on the power of medicine to objectify women in varied cultural representations. On the other hand, scholarly work on the topic of the representation of motherhood has concentrated around certain areas within cultural studies, mainly literature, film, and media culture, and has used specific perspectives, primarily psychoanalytic theory, feminist studies, and literary criticism.[19] Yet despite their different approaches there is no study that seeks to illuminate the inter-connectedness between these areas and the medical field. This book proposes to fill this gap in the literature by using wider empirical evidence in the sources consulted, from national and Cordoban repositories, along with a new interpretative framework. My interpretation engages with the perspective of intellectual history or the history of ideas in order to develop a more complex theoretical understanding of how social representations of motherhood came to be elaborated, stabilised, and mobilised. In doing so, my perspective is not supported by a particular study whether of motherhood or any other social, historical object, it is a perspective built upon *directions*, since there is no methodology as such that defines the history of ideas. Indeed, authors have been reluctant to specify either a particular methodology or obligatory concepts but rather *directions* from which to conduct the research. In this sense, the directions that I have chosen to orientate my work could be formulated, as Roger Chartier has posed it, as two-dimensional,

> which permits simultaneous conceptualization of an intellectual or artistic product within the specifity of the history of its genre or discipline, within its relation to other contemporaneous cultural products, and within its relation with various referents situated in other fields, socio-economic or political, of the whole of society.[20]

In my analysis, the 'first dimension' (conceptual) will characterise the medical discourse on maternity, which involves the analysis of practices, concepts and metaphors that have been elaborated within the medical field. Whilst the 'second dimension' (socio-cultural) will enquire into the appropriation and

11

re-signification of medical ideas in and through journalism, literature, and visual images that have circulated during the period under investigation while revealing the representations generated within each of these fields. My aim is twofold. Firstly, to understand social representations of motherhood as an object constructed in the interplay of, at the very least, all the above-mentioned variables. Secondly, to explore the extent and scope of medical ideas in other significant social spheres in order to have a better approach to its penetration in the realm of 'notions', 'ideas', 'beliefs' and 'images' at a given moment. Working at the intersection of these two spaces of signification, historian Hugo Vezzetti has proposed that, 'an intellectual history would be characterised by a plural location, prepared to displace itself so long as its 'objects' are configurated in 'constructions' that could be differentiated in two spheres: sociocultural and conceptual'.[21] In this sense, it is the dual model of questioning what elaborates the object of study which otherwise would remain invisible as such.[22] 'Elaboration' does not mean an object invented *ex nihilo* – as another historian of ideas has aptly put it[23] – but a way of surfacing and making intelligible links that are empirically implicated with the object of study and that are *only* observable in the object's displacement.

Part I, 'The Medical Record', analyses the medical discourse in two main periods. The first one focuses on the main medical concepts and representations of maternity from the beginning of the century until 1930, during the time of professional consolidation of obstetrics and paediatrics as medical specialties. Doctors' changing perceptions of the maternal figure in the light of perceived social 'deviations' (infanticide, abortion and child abandonment) are explored along with the medical language that stemmed from the medicalisation of childbirth and the resulting metaphors utilised to refer to maternal bodies. The second period (1930-1946) draws attention to the construction of an eugenically-oriented 'biotype' of the fertile woman that promoted a new corporal representation of motherhood adjusted to desirable social values (abnegation, sacrifice, physical strength, and multiparity). Sterilisation practices and debates are also discussed to demonstrate that, contrary to historians' assumptions, negative measures of eugenics, although legally banned, still found a subtle application in Argentina.

The following two parts of this research are directed to demonstrate that however powerful medical discourses may seem, the socio-cultural representations on maternity or the construction of a maternal ideal need to be explored in other social spheres. Is it possible to assign to medical discourse a fundamental role? Which other discourses had intervened in that process of representing maternity and how had they done this? What kind of relationship had they sustained with medical ideas? If we are to consider to what extent medical discourses have penetrated into society at one particular time, these issues and assumptions need to be disclosed. In Part II, 'The Textual Record', Chapters 3-4 offer insight into motherhood's representations in the journalistic field, and it does so through the main circulating newspapers that represented the ideological divide that characterised Cordoban society at the time. Thus, Chapter 3 focuses on the Catholic newspaper *Los Principios*, and provides a close examination of the changing nature of the figure of the Catholic mother and its associations with the Marian cult, in view of the problems posed by the 'woman question', feminism and the modern women. The newspaper *La Voz del Interior* is analysed in Chapter 4 to consider the elaborations of the maternal in liberal thought, and draws attention to the political uses of motherhood through an analysis of a 'maternal campaign' organised by the paper. For both newspapers, and whenever possible, I used a sample of two months per year. The section is completed with a study of the fictional representation of motherhood which reveals a rather neglected aspect of Argentinian literature, especially in the first half of the twentieth century. Chapter 5 focuses on a corpus of six novels that are representative of the circulating visions of motherhood, from a range of acclaimed as well as little known authors, thus showing the variety of literature available at the time. The texts account for a broad range of topics where the mother's presence resulted in competing images and representations: Between the mainstream, essentialised forms of representation and the modern, emerging ones, the chapter shows how the mother, as social subject, was acquiring a segmented identity.

Part III, 'The Visual Record' moves the enquiry of social representations of motherhood to the realm of visual images through a survey of photojournalism, and the artistic field. The analysis of photojournalism in Chapter 6 operates as a continuation of the case study offered by the previous chapters focusing on the press, but seen from the particularities introduced by visual language. In its relationship to news and information, photojournalism emerged to support the 'truth', in order to make written words visually irrefutable. It is this particular commitment to 'real facts' and the status of 'truth' that photojournalism has since enjoyed, that prompted me to look in newspapers, rather than in other type of photographic records, images of the maternal. I enquire if mothers, whose existence was explored in texts produced by medical, journalistic and literary discourses, were worthy of being visualised, and if so, how did visualisation accommodate motherhood's paradoxical meanings.

Both artistic production and literature have been traditionally assessed as privileged sites where gendered identities can be evaluated. As such, I argue that they could be sites of consolidation as well as of contestation for prevailing discourses on motherhood. Chapter 7 explores this in more detail through a repertoire of nearly a dozen artistic works. I propose that some of these productions have mobilised a female subjectivity that not only contested the medically constructed, but somehow evidenced what was socially intelligible in other areas of mothers' lives: a tendency towards family planning, a growing participation in public activities (welfare and politics), and an inclination to expose the anxieties or discontentment of sexual life introduced by the dissemination of psychoanalysis in mass culture.

In the chapters that follow, the trajectory that I set out for this book will take us from a medically-defined motherhood (as an object of study) to its reconfiguration by each of the socio-cultural intersecting areas or disciplines with which it engages, with the particularity that those reconfigurations are only perceptible through the object's displacements.

Notes

1   M. Benjamin, 'Introduction', in M. Benjamin (ed.), *Science and Sensibility: Gender and Scientific Enquiry, 1780-1945* (Oxford: Basil Blackwell, 1991), 1-23: 15.

2   *Población 1869-1960* (Córdoba: Dirección General de Estadística, Censos e Investigaciones, 1961); 'El aporte de la migración internacional en el crecimiento de la ciudad de Buenos Aires. Años censales, 1855/2010' (Buenos Aires: Dirección General de Estadística y Censos, Ministerio de Hacienda, 2011) Online at: http://www.estadistica.buenosaires.gov.ar/areas/hacienda/sis_estadistico/ir_2011_471.pdf (consulted 22.08.2011).

3   J. C. Agulla, *Eclipse of an Aristocracy: An Investigation of the Ruling Elites of the City of Córdoba* (Alabama and London: University of Alabama Press, 1976), Ch. 5.

4   Cfr. E. Zimmermann, *Los Liberales Reformistas. La Cuestión Social en la*

Argentina, 1890-1916 (Buenos Aires: Sudamericana y Universidad de San Andrés, 1994).

5   See the thought-provoking study of J. Rodriguez, *Civilizing Argentina: Science, Medicine, and the Modern State* (Chapel Hill: The University of North Carolina Press: 2006).

6   T. Halperín Donghi, *El Espejo de la Historia. Problemas Argentinos y Perspectivas Latinoamericanas* (Buenos Aires: Sudamericana, 1998), 147.

7   S. Roitemburd, *Nacionalismo Católico Cordobés. Educación en los Dogmas para un Proyecto Global.* PhD Thesis. Universidad Nacional de Córdoba, 1998, 4.

8   See G. Vidal, 'El Avance del Poder Clerical y el Conservadorismo Político en Córdoba Durante la Década del 20'. Paper presented at the *Latin American Studies Association* (Miami, March 2000), 5.

9   Some of the classic works on the topics enumerated in the text, are: H. Marland (ed.), *The Art of Midwifery: Early Modern Midwives in Europe* (London and New York: Routledge, 1993); and H. Marland and A. M. Rafferty (eds.), *Midwives, Society and Childbirth: Debates and Controversies in the Modern Period* (London and New York: Routledge, 1997); L. Schiebinger, *The Mind has no Sex?: Women in the Origins of Modern Science* (London, Massachusetts: Harvard University Press, 1989). O. Moscucci, *The Science of Woman: Gynaecology and Gender in England, 1800-1929* (Cambridge: Cambridge University Press, 1990); A. Oakley, The Captured Womb: A History of the Medical Care of Pregnant Women (Oxford: Basil Blackwell, 1984). J. Lewis, *The Politics of Motherhood: Child and Maternal Welfare in England, 1900-1939* (London: Croom Helm, 1980); S. Williams, *Women and Childbirth in the Twentieth Century: A History of the National Birthday Trust Fund, 1928-93* (Stroud: Sutton, 1997).

10   A thorough historiographical account on Latin America can be found in A.E. Birn, 'Child Health in Latin America: Historiographic Perspectives and Challenges. *História, Ciências, Saúde –Manguinhos*, 14, 3 (2007), 677-708. For the Argentinian case, some of the chapters and articles that have tackled a range of topics, such as, the medicalisation of childbirth, abortion, contraceptive practices, child abandonment, and infanticide, are: A. Correa, 'Parir es Morir un Poco. Partos en el Siglo XIX', in F. Gil Lozano, V. Pita and G. Ini (eds.), *Historia de las Mujeres en la Argentina. Tomo I, Colonia y Siglo XIX* (Buenos Aires: Taurus, 2000), 193-213; Y. Eraso, 'Ni Parteras, ni Médicos: Obstetras. Especialización Médica y Medicalización del Parto en la Primera

Mitad del Siglo XX', *Anuario de la Escuela de Historia, Universidad Nacional de Córdoba*, 1 (2001), 109-124, and 'Los Sucesores de Ilitía. La Construcción de la Identidad Femenina desde el Parto', in A. Boria and M. T. Dalmasso (eds.), *Discurso Social y Construcción de Identidades: Mujer y Género* (Córdoba: Ferreira Editor, 2003), 61-70; D. Barrancos, 'Contracepcionalidad y Aborto en la Década de 1920: Problema Privado y Cuestión Pública', *Estudios Sociales*, 1 (1991), 75-86; M. Nari, 'Las Prácticas Anticonceptivas, la Disminución de la Natalidad y el Debate Médico, 1890-1940', in M. Lobato (ed.), *Política, Médicos y Enfermedades. Lecturas de Historia de la Salud en la Argentina* (Buenos Aires: Biblos, 1996), 154-89; M.J. Billorou, 'Madres y Médicos en Torno a la Cuna. Ideas y Prácticas sobre el Cuidado Infantil (Buenos Aires, 1930-1945)', *La Aljaba*, Segunda Época, XI (2007), 167-192. K. Ruggiero, 'Honour, Maternity and the Disciplining of Women: Infanticide in Late Nineteenth-Century Buenos Aires', *Hispanic American Historical Review*, 72 (1992), 353-73; D. Guy, 'Niños Abandonados en Buenos Aires (1880-1914) y el Desarrollo del Concepto de la Madre', in L. Fletcher (ed.), *Mujeres y Cultura en la Argentina del siglo XIX* (Buenos Aires: Feminaria, 1994), 217-26 and G. Ini, 'Infanticidios, Construcción de la Verdad y Control de Género en el Discurso Judicial', in F. Gil Lozano, V. Pita and G. Ini (eds.), *Historia de las Mujeres en la Argentina. Tomo I, Colonia y Siglo XIX* (Buenos Aires: Taurus, 2000), 235-51. M.S. Di Liscia, 'Hijos Sanos y Legítimos: Sobre Matrimonio y Asistencia Social en Argentina (1935-1948)', *História, Ciências, Saúde-Manguinhos*, 9, suppl. (2002), 209-32.

11   M. Nari, *Políticas de Maternidad y Maternalismo Político en Buenos Aires (1890-1940)* (Buenos Aires: Biblos, 2005).

12   D. Guy, *Women Build the Welfare State: Performing Charity and Creating Rights in Argentina, 1880–1955* (Durham and London: Duke University Press, 2009).

13   *Cfr.* K. Mead, 'Beneficent Maternalism: Argentine Motherhood in Comparative Perspective, 1880-1920', *Journal of Women's History*, 12 (2000), 120-45; and 'Gender, Welfare and the Catholic Church in Argentina: Conferencias de Señoras de San Vicente de Paul, 1890-1916', *The Americas*, 58 (2001), 91-119; M. Bonaudo, 'Cuando las Tuteladas Tutelan y Participan. La Sociedad Damas de Caridad (1869-1894)', *Signos Históricos*, 15 (2006), 70-97; M.J. Billorou, M.S. Di Liscia, and A.M. Rodríguez, 'La Disputa en la Construcción

de la Cuestión Social en el Interior Argentino. Tensiones entre el Estado y las Mujeres (1900-1940)', in C. Bravo, F. Gil Lozano and V. Pita (eds.), *Historia de Luchas, Resistencias y Representaciones. Mujeres en la Argentina, Siglos XIX y XX* (Tucumán: Universidad Nacional de Tucumán, 2007), 123-49; G. Dalla Corte and P. Piacenza, *A las Puertas del Hogar: Madres, Niños y Damas de Caridad en el Hogar del Huérfano de Rosario, 1870-1920* (Rosario: Prohistoria Ediciones, 2006); B. Moreyra, *Cuestión Social y Políticas Sociales en la Argentina. La Modernidad Periférica. Córdoba, 1900-1930* (Bernal: Universidad Nacional de Quilmes, 2009); Y. Eraso, 'Introducción: Mujeres y Asistencia Social, Problemáticas y Perspectivas Históricas', in Y. Eraso (ed.) *Mujeres y Asistencia Social en Latinoamérica, siglos XIX y XX* (Córdoba: Alción Editora, 2009), 1-14.

14 Guy, *Women Build the Welfare State*, 58.

15 N. Stepan, *"The Hour of Eugenics": Race, Gender and Nation in Latin America* (Ithaca and London: Cornwell University Press, 1991).

16 For a perspective that have questioned the very existence of a 'positive eugenics' in Argentina, see M. Miranda, 'La Antorcha de Cupido: Eugenesia, Biotipología y Eugamia en Argentina, 1930-1970', *Asclepio*, 55, 2 (2003), 231-55; Y. Eraso, 'Biotypology, Endocrinology, and Sterilization: The Practice of Eugenics in the Treatment of Argentinian Women during the 1930s', *Bulletin of the History of Medicine* 81, 4 (2007), 792–822; A. Reggiani, 'Depopulation, Fascism, and Eugenics in 1930s Argentina', *Hispanic American Historical Review* 90, 2 (2010), 283-318. For a historiographical discussion in the Latin American context, see J. Rodriguez, 'A Complex Fabric: Intersecting Histories of Race, Gender, and Science in Latin America', *Hispanic American Historical Review*, 91, 3 (2011), 409-28; and for a discussion of international eugenic perspectives, see P. Levine and A. Bashford, 'Introduction: Eugenics and the Modern World', in A. Bashford and P. Levine, *The Oxford Handbook of the History of Eugenics* (New York: Oxford University Press, 2010), 3-24.

17 L. Accati, 'Explicit Meanings: Catholicism, Matriarchy and the Distinctive Problems of Italian Feminism', *Gender and History*, 7 (1995), 241-59: 244.

18 As an example of those works considered now classic on this subject Cfr. L. Jordanova, *Sexual Visions: Images of Gender in Science and Medicine Between the Eighteenth and Twentieth Centuries* (London: Harvester Wheatsheaf, 1989); P. Treichler, L. Cartwright and C. Penley (eds.), *The*

Visible Woman: Imaging Technologies, Gender, and Science (New York: NYU Press, 1998); B. Duden, *Disembodying Women: Perspectives on Pregnancy and the Unborn* (Massachusetts and London: Harvard University Press, 1993); A. Balsamo, *Technologies of the Gendered Body: Reading Cyborg Women* (Durham: Duke University Press, 1996).

19 A. Kaplan, *Motherhood* and *Representation: The Mother in Popular Culture and Melodrama* (New York: Routledge, 1992); and D. Bassin, M. Honey, and M. Kaplan, *Representations of Motherhood* (New Haven and London: Yale University Press, 1994); A. Hall and M. Bishop (eds.), *Momy Angst: Mothers in American Popular Culture* (California: Praeger, 2009). In Argentina, an excellent literary analysis of motherhood post-1950s has been done by N. Domínguez, *De Donde Vienen los Niños. Maternidad y Escritura en la Cultura Argentina* (Rosario: Beatriz Viterbo, 2007).

20 R. Chartier, *Cultural History* (Oxford: Polity Press, 1988), 46. The two-dimensional perspective oriented, according to Chartier, much of the analysis of French historians of ideas at the end of the 1980s. It also informed the works of Hayden White and Carl Schorske (Cfr. H. White, 'The Task of Intellectual History', *The Monist*, 53 (1969), 606-26 and C. Schorske, *Fin-de-Siècle Vienna: Politics and Culture* (New York: Knopf, 1980). In Argentina, this perspective has particularly influenced a group of historians working from the 1990s until today in the in the area of Intellectual History at the *Centro de Historia Intelectual, Departamento de Ciencias Sociales, Universidad Nacional de Quilmes* (Buenos Aires), whose works have been published in the Centre's journal, *Prismas. Revista de Historia Intelectual.*

21 H. Vezzetti, 'Historia del Freudismo e Historia de la Sexualidad: El Género Sexológico en Buenos Aires en los Treinta', *Prismas. Revista de Historia Intelectual,* 1 (1997), 211-18: 213.

22 To express it in Chartier's words once again, 'To read a text or decode a system of thought means, then, to embrace all the different questions which, when they are fitted together, make up what can be considered to be the actual object of study of intellectual history'. In Chartier, *Cultural History*, 46.

23 J. Myers, 'Historia de las Ideas e Historia Disciplinares. Comentario a la Ponencia de Hugo Vezzetti', *Prismas. Revista de Historia Intelectual,* 1 (1997), 219-26: 220.

PART I: THE MEDICAL RECORD

1

Mothers and the First Medical Concerns

In 1890, the Mayor of Buenos Aires ordered a special research on the causes of infant mortality and child abandonment in the city from a commission of prominent hygienists headed by Dr Emilio Coni (1855-1928), and with the aim of outlining a programme relating to children's health and welfare. The *Patronato de la Infancia* (1892) was the semi-public institution created as a result of the report, which became instrumental in subsequent years in the advocacy of child protection laws, as well as in the creation of child institutions, such as medical consulting rooms, *Sala Cuna* (nursery), and schools for urban and rural children. The report also suggested a series of measures directed towards mothers, including the teaching of puericulture, the sanitary control of wet nurses, and the creation of a range of dispensaries to assist mother and child.[1] Although the plan was only partially implemented, the main lines of intervention allow us to have an idea of hygienists' priorities at the time: first, the healthcare of children had to be done scientifically, that is, through the French principles of puericulture; second, welfare provision had to be shared by private philanthropy and the state; third, the main efforts in the provision of assistance had to concentrate on infants rather than mothers. These types of measures spread rapidly, although unevenly, in the main cities of the country, especially in those where a professional structure, like a Faculty of Medicine, was able to provide the specialist's view to influence governments' health priorities and initiatives.

At the same time that Coni was preparing the report for Buenos Aires, in the city of Córdoba, Dr José M. Álvarez (1859-1916), a hygienist and national senator, was preparing a tract (published in 1896) on the 'advantages of public hygiene', the available means, and the sanitary challenges ahead.[2] The report also addressed the causes of high infant mortality (-2 years), assessed the existing institutions, and suggested policies that contemplated social rather than technical aspects of the problem. Álvarez proposed to 'complement and perfect' a system that had already started to be developed in childcare services. He put emphasis on the inspection of wet nurses, and in the control of the quality of milk supplied and milk depots available in the city, since sullied milk was thought to cause gastroenteritis, the disease that ranked highest in infant mortality rates. If those measures implied a 'direct protection' of infancy, Álvarez also urged the government to concentrate on the 'indirect protection', that is, the one exerted on the mother, including: the protection of pregnant, poor women; the health of working women; the teaching of child rearing; the battle against illegitimacy; and the control of syphilis.[3] Álvarez, like others before him, considered female private charity as an indispensable ally in the provision of child welfare, so he supported the work of a well-established, nineteenth-century network of charitable female organisations acting in the province, many of which also existing at national level, such as the Society of Ladies of Beneficence, the Society of Ladies of Saint Vincent de Paul, and the Ladies of Providence, which, at the time of his report, run most of the available maternal and child institutions.

Female charitable involvement in maternal and child institutions was ubiquitous in Argentina as it was in most Latin-American countries after they initiated a process of nation-building, where women were directly or indirectly entrusted by state officials with running welfare institutions.[4] Elite, upper and middle-class women, conservative, Catholic and liberal shared a language of motherhood to justify their public activities and advance a mother and child welfare agenda, which soon revealed differences in approaches, initiatives and implementation. Within this ample spectrum, there was a group of leading liberal feminists, the so-called 'maternalist feminists', mainly composed by university women, who at the beginning of the twentieth century, played a prominent role in bringing child and maternal issues to the fore of the international agenda, when in 1916 they organised the First Pan American Child Congress in Buenos Aires. Between 1916 and 1948, nine Pan American congresses took place across the Americas, becoming a forum for paediatricians, educationists, criminologists, feminists of different strands, and policy makers to discuss their views on welfare strategy.[5] As we shall see later in this chapter, disagreement amongst these key actors (male hygienists and paediatricians, feminists and powerful female organisations like the Society of Beneficence) resulted in a fragmented agenda, however, this did not hinder the development of child policies that, in the long term, became embraced by the international community as demonstrated by the sanction of the Children's Sanitary Code in 1948.[6] Thus, the process that started with Argentinian hygienists compiling statistics on infant mortality rates and child abandonment soon took national and international stage through, although not exclusively, vigorous female participation. And, although it is not the task of this book to situate the nature of maternal policies that those actors generated during the period, I will focus on some of their underlying concepts in as much as they configured specific representations of the maternal that will be later challenged in non-medical scenarios.

A second aspect of interest is related to what Álvarez perceived as infancy's 'indirect protection', that, is, the attention to mothers. In order to explore this, I will turn to obstetricians, who became perhaps less visible – in comparison to paediatricians – although not less active in developing mother and child welfare initiatives. Indeed, mothers' health and welfare was the main concern of obstetricians, who played a key role in advancing medical notions of maternity and the maternal body from both a sociological and a biological point of view. Yet obstetrics did not develop as a medical specialty in an uncharted territory. Midwives and general practitioners were already practising 'the art of delivery' with uneven success, while the social aspects of maternal welfare were the focus of different women's organisations. In addition, this sort of dual space of medical intervention, on the one hand, mother and child healthcare, on the other, prenatal care and childbirth, led to the elaboration of different types of representation. In the first one, is possible to trace doctors' changing perceptions of the maternal figure in the light of perceived social 'deviations', i.e. infanticide, abortion and child abandonment. In the second one, it is the medical language that emerges as an unprecedented source of representation, one that stems from childbirth's medicalisation and its associated metaphors introduced to nominate the maternal body.

An overcrowded field: Midwives, general practitioners and feminists

At the First National Child Congress (1913) organised by feminist doctor Julieta Lantieri Renshaw, Dr Eliseo Cantón (1861-1931), who was the chair of Clinical Obstetrics at the University of Buenos Aires while serving as deputy for the capital district at the national parliament (1904-1912), presented his views to one of the congress' sessions entitled, 'Protection to mothers and children'. Venerated at the time as the 'Father of Argentinian Obstetrics', Cantón was a strong advocate for French puericulture, the scientific rearing of children devised by Adolphe Pinard (1844-1934) that implied the integral caring of the mother since conception until puerperium, or as Pinard denominated them, *puériculture intra-utérine* and *puériculture extra-utérine*. Imbued by French innovative ideas, especially those devoted to offer medical caring to destitute pregnant women, Cantón made a plea to the state for the building of a 'maternity shelter' to protect poor and single mothers. The idea was to offer assistance from the seventh month of pregnancy until three months after delivery, when the mother would abandon the place once she recovered her strength, and provided her child was healthy, and she had secured sufficient means to earn a leaving.[7] Cantón showed to the audience the architectural lay-out of the maternity, with its different three main areas (for pregnant women, childbearing, and convalescent mothers), and their respective services and dependencies. The idea, he insisted, was to centralise the administration of medical and Social Services by concentrating them in only one institution, thus differing from European maternities at the time which normally offered them separately. Cantón's maternity would materialise some years later, but under one of his disciples, Dr Alberto Peralta Ramos, who in 1921 started the building of the future Institute of Maternity in the capital city. A year later, Peralta Ramos and prominent paediatrician, Dr Juan Garrahan, asserted, 'In the past ten years, the campaign against infant mortality has intensified, especially in Buenos Aires. The general hygiene and culture of the population has evidently progressed, and the centres of puericulture have multiplied.'[8] Indeed, puericulture, in particular the one oriented to infants, caught on rapidly in Buenos Aires. With the support of hygienists and obstetricians, the Public Assistance created a special office in 1908 named 'Protection to Infancy', which by 1921 had eighteen infant dispensaries (outpatients), and five institutes of puericulture (where children could be hospitalised along with their mothers), as well as a section for the sanitary inspection of wet nurses. Statistics, on the other hand, favourably accompanied such institutional improvements: between 1901 and 1921 infant motility rate dropped from 95-100 to 80 per 1,000 live births.[9] However, the mother's social and medical care before and after delivery was deemed deficient, and progress was only restricted to establishing maternity wards within Buenos Aires's general hospitals, where women were obliged to leave soon after delivery. Yet lack of institutional development was not the only problem that obstetricians encountered as they mobilised to improve maternal health conditions. The competitive presence of midwives became a priority for many specialists, who soon sought to coordinate efforts with the state in an attempt to bring midwifery intervention on childbirth under control.

The first School of Midwives in Buenos Aires was created by President Rivadavia in 1822, but the practice of delivery by *comadronas* and 'healer woman' predominated in the city, a situation that would start to change in the 1890s when hygienists and social reformers tackled infant mortality more seriously as part of their broader nation-building concerns. A differentiated education between medical students and midwives, as well as the subordination of midwives' teaching programmes to the Faculty of Medicine was a first strategic step taken by obstetricians in 1882, when the School of Midwives became annexed to the university Obstetrics Department. At the same time, graduated midwives also took measures that reflected the changing perception towards their trade, as well as the need of becoming involved in a process to which midwives have barely been invited to contribute. A clear example is given by the foundation of the National Obstetrics Association (1901) by feminist doctor Cecilia Grierson, with the aim of professionalising the field and securing uniform rules that would grant the licence to practise to those graduates from the School. On the other hand, the need of separating 'legal' from 'illegal' midwives was strongly advocated by obstetricians, who became disappointed by the authorities' lack of initiative at the National Department of Hygiene, who despite existing legislation, did not efficiently chase or prosecute those practising without the required registration.[10]

A similar situation was found in Córdoba. In 1916 the Provincial Council of Hygiene decided to examine 'those women who, without a degree, have practiced the art of delivery with some competence'.[11] The measure was triggered by accusations against the number of active 'healer women' posed by the local newspaper *La Voz del Interior*, which endorsed the doctors' association between *comadronas* and high rates of maternal mortality and puerperal infections. However, the government's weak and sporadic campaigns to control and examine non-professional midwives were also reflected in the parliament, as the latter remained reluctant to increase the penalties contained in existing laws. Yet differentiating legal from illegal midwives was only part of obstetricians' concern. As the urban presence of professional midwives rose, after the creation of the School of Midwives in 1890, they too became a direct target for medical specialists. Certainly, the sensitive topic of the 'criminal abortion' provided obstetricians with a source of stigmatisation and distrust towards a female profession that was striving for a legitimate recognition. In 1921, Dr Galíndez stated, 'We all know that today the main focus of the perpetration of abortion resides in the midwives' profession; it is fair, then, that to them should be addressed the consequent prophylaxis'.[12] Apart from abortions, the high incidence of puerperal infections, which constituted almost half of maternal deaths for the period 1913-1927,[13] encouraged hostility against *comadronas* and healers, but also against the techniques

25

used by professional midwives during childbirth's complications. Control over midwifery was strengthened in 1925 when the School of Midwives was separated from the School of Medicine, through the management (by obstetricians) of their educational programmes, thus ensuring that midwives' learning and practices were limited to the attendance of normal deliveries. Legislation passed in that year further reinforced this perspective by licensing midwives only in the faculty of prescribing medicines and materials needed for the assistance of 'normal deliveries', while preserving the complicated cases only for the obstetricians. Such division of labour in the assistance of childbirth, however, will not loom large as the definition of what constituted a 'normal delivery' will be narrowly redefined not only to limit even more midwives' competence, but to anticipate parturients that a 'normal childbirth' was a rather rare physiological event, whose degree of normality, in any case, will be always better judged by a specialist.

It is also interesting to observe that the dispute for the monopoly of women's assistance also led obstetricians to openly battle within their own professional milieu. Obstetricians seemed to be more preoccupied in distancing themselves from the role of the general practitioner, who assisted normal births, rather than that of the surgeon. In fact, it was due to the development of surgical techniques that obstetricians could later profess and claim skills and achievements as their own. Probably the first occasion where these ideas were openly debated was at the Second National Congress of Medicine in 1922. There, Dr Peralta Ramos reviewed the latest and most complex surgical interventions that the discipline had attained, to conclude with the following plea, 'such surgical operations . . . should be practiced at the clinic and not at home, and therefore should not be available to the non-specialist general practitioner'.[14] He also went as far as posing ethical questions in defence of the authority of the new medical experts, demanding the general practitioner 'to surrender to the specialist with a clear conscience and a sense of honest self-criticism'.[15]

While the struggle against midwives and general practitioners for childbirth's intervention was acquiring a rapid legitimacy in medical circles, its success in society at large would depend much on the creation of maternal institutes and centres, where obstetricians could exert the authority that, they insisted, corresponded to their specialist knowledge. And this revealed problems of a different kind, given the reluctance of national and provincial governments to regularly invest in health and welfare, something that particularly affected the provision of maternity services. Welfare policy, however, did not discourage professionals from systematically claiming government funding by framing the maternal question as a national concern, in a language that merged the provision of institutions with ongoing discourses of progress, civilisation and nationhood. As most significant changes to the welfare system were only introduced after the rise of the welfare state post-1946, in the meanwhile, doctors had to adapt, with strategic vision and uneven sympathy, to work within a regime (mixed economy of welfare) that relied heavily on private beneficence and charity. This, in turn, introduces us to another social actor that obstetricians and paediatricians had to deal with in their consolidating path as specialists, the feminist movement.

The involvement of Argentinian feminists in mother and child issues can be traced to the very beginning of the movement in 1900. Feminists found in maternal and child welfare advocacy a reforming agenda from which to achieve women's rights in the civic and civil arena. This was especially the case for the most radical members of the movement, congregated around the Argentine Association of University Women (1902), an organisation integrated by a group of Socialists and professionals, mostly doctors and specialists in the diseases of women and children.[16] Having integrated the National Women Council of the Republic (1900), alongside various associations and women's groups, including the powerful sector of 'matrons', the group of 'university' women separated from the Council in 1910 revealing irreconcilable principles and goals in relation to the group of beneficent women. The former became later identified with the 'maternalist' or 'relational' side of the feminist movement, where maternity notions emphasised the value of sexual difference and complementary role of women in society, thus constituting a springboard for their political and civil demands of women's equality and social justice. Their views in relation to mother and child advocacy were, at the beginning, most notably played at the international stage.

In 1911, Dr Julieta Lantieri Renshaw (1873-1932) launched the League for the Rights of Mothers and Children that organised the above-mentioned first National Child Congress in the capital of the Republic. This first meeting was the prelude of the first international Pan-American Child Congress (PACC) gathered in Buenos Aires in 1916, of which Lantieri Renshaw also served as president. Both congresses included prestigious male specialists who were also seeking to set up important reforms in the provision of child welfare. Their visions, however, differed markedly from the one posed by feminists. In those congresses, paediatricians and obstetricians emphasised the need for mothers' education in the notions of puericulture to improve

27

their maternal skills, since the mother's ignorance, more than poverty and lack of assistance, was considered to be the underlying cause of infant mortality and morbidity.

At the Second PACC Congress of 1919, Cordoban paediatrician, Dr Benito Soria,[17] justified the setting up of a 'School for Mothers' at the Orphan House (administered by the Ladies of Providence) by arguing that, 'the majority of young mothers in this time of poverty in which we live, know absolutely nothing of what they should in respect of their children's care'.[18] According to Donna Guy, feminists presented plans to close down orphan institutions like the one mentioned by Soria, in order to replace it with a system whereby orphaned children would be placed in foster families.[19] This illustrates another point of discussion between male physicians and feminists, namely, the role that female charitable organisations should play as welfare providers. The group of 'University Women' held long-standing confrontations, especially with women of the elite in charge of these institutions, championing instead for state agencies to be involved in the provision of services. Male physicians, on the other hand, had no inconvenience in working with charitable ladies, as long as, as some cases have illustrated, they were able to do so in their own institutions. In Córdoba, the activity of female charities was very important at both medical and social levels: Under their auspices the first Children's Hospital (1894), the Orphan House (1884), and many maternal asylums for the protection of infancy and single mothers were created.

More importantly, male physicians' stress on the mother's ignorance differed largely from the vision of feminists, who assumed a more comprehensive approach towards the mother's needs and their living conditions, which accounted for the elaboration of a more reforming agenda. Unlike their male colleagues, feminists claimed that in the creation of 'maternal homes' mothers could work and look after their children. In addition, they proposed a series of reforms in the Civil Codes that included children's custody rights for married women, legal equality for legitimate and illegitimate children, and the judicial investigation of paternity for single mothers. They also sought to improve labour legislation for working mothers and the need to set up a programme of school sexual education. As the decade of the 1920s progressed, male specialists dominated the policy of the PACC, while feminists, as Guy has noted, left international efforts to concentrate locally in various activities related to woman's enfranchisement, education and welfare programmes.[20] After the feminists' withdrawal, the PACC took an orientation completely alien to their reformist view. As we have seen through the proposals of Soria, this policy had an overriding purpose to assist children rather than mothers, and this was the dominant tendency once female voices, at least those representative of the maternalist feminism, disappeared from the Pan American congresses. As we will see later in the book, feminist ideas during this period had a profound impact on Argentinian society in that they framed discussion on women's role, including their maternalist reforming agenda, whose implications within Catholic and liberal ideas will inspire and produce other uses and representations of the maternal.

Meanwhile, the 1920s were productive years in terms of child welfare initiatives and debates, both internationally and nationally. Amongst them, the Inter-American Institute for the Protection of Children (1927) based in Montevideo and presided by prominent Argentinian hygienist Gregorio Aráoz Alfaro (1870-1955) concentrated the research and compiled statistics for Latin American countries on child welfare, infant mortality, and childhood diseases. With the support of the League of Nations' Health Organisation and the exceptional advocacy of Uruguayan feminist Dr Paulina Luisi (1875-1950) – delegate to the League of Nations – the Institute's activities held an international reputation while pioneering legislation (notably the sanction of Children's Code and the creation of *ad hoc* child offices) and advancing polices into the international agenda.[21] Focus on maternal welfare, however, never fully reached the international health agenda, although initiatives were discussed by feminists in different forums, amongst which, it is worth mentioning the Third International Feminist Congress gathered in Buenos Aires in 1928, and organised by Argentinian doctor Elvira Rawson de Dellepiane. The congress' 'Sociology section', as Dora Barrancos has noted, 'could not elude the obsessive frame of "the protection of maternity"'.[22] The topics discussed revealed the social emphasis of the feminist perspective which continued developing proposals that claimed from the state the integral protection of working-class mothers and reforms to the civil code. Special discussion was given to the creation of the maternity insurance, which ended in one of the most significant votes of the meeting. Another proposal insisted on the creation of 'maternal homes' as a way of preventing suicide, infanticide and child abandonment. This type of institution attempted to keep together mother and child, and it was thought as a better solution to the one offered by the orphan house that, in feminists' views, only sought a solution for the child.

This platform, in turn, differed from the one launched in 1927 by Dr Soria in Córdoba, entitled, 'Committee for the Defence of Infancy', which he

29

presented in a conference-festival in the city's main theatre. Soria's speech evidenced the child defence-focus of the specialists that integrated the PACC to the detriment of the mother *and* child perspective of the feminists. Although he spoke about the need to recognise the mother's role 'to exalt and stimulate the defence and protection of maternity', he did not back this formulation with initiatives or legislative proposals. The need for maternal education, on the contrary, proved to be the main paradigm in relation to infant and child care.[23] Soria also remarked on the importance of co-operation with female charitable organisations and private philanthropy, when he considered that, 'the state should not be more than an auxiliary in the work of charity and humanity', 'the cold and impersonal state', 'wants the *woman* of all social classes and the *citizen* of all social spheres to contribute with their alms and efforts'.[24]

The introduction into the international health agenda of innovative policies (proposed by hygienists, paediatricians, and feminists) in child welfare rights some of which were subsequently adopted at national level, has justifiably drawn the attention of Latin American historians. In this sense, obstetricians, however, appear as less-studied actors, not least because what started out as a 'mother and child' agenda soon reoriented its focus towards infancy and child healthcare. As I will argue here, initiatives on maternal healthcare, in the form of puericulture, took the 'mother and child binomial' to put it in obstetricians' terms, as the focus of specific initiatives which also materialised in the design of special institutions that achieved recognition at national and international level. In other words, the obstetricians' ideas during this time went beyond the construction of maternity wards. In the 1920s Buenos Aires' obstetricians rapidly materialised and to some extent anticipated the functionality of the French principles of puericulture through a comprehensive social and medical system of three-stage assistance: prenatal, natal, and postnatal.

Maternities and puericulture institutions

A review of modern maternity services in Buenos Aires takes us back to 1887, when the Society of Beneficence inaugurated the new women's hospital, the Hospital Rivadavia. There, the old Women's Hospital was moved alongside its precarious maternity service, which in the new building occupied one of the five pavilions that made up the brand-new hospital. This maternity clinic along with the one at the Hospital San Roque, site of the university Obstetric Clinic, were the first specialised maternity services in the city, although many more were to be opened in a relatively short period of time. Between 1900 and 1915 maternity wards and clinics were inaugurated within the following general hospitals: Tornú, Fernández, Alvarez, Rawson, Pirovano, Argerich and Durán. Yet the rapid expansion of maternity services in the capital of the Republic did not entirely satisfy obstetricians. As we have seen earlier in this chapter, Cantón was amongst those who anticipated the need to integrate maternity institutes with the simultaneous provision of medical and social assistance. It was obstetrician Alberto Peralta Ramos (1886-1954) who better articulated the continuum of mother and child assistance, when he proposed that infant services should form part of a unique maternity institute considering that, as he explained,

> [I]t is more likely that mothers would return to the place that had provided them assistance during pregnancy and childbirth, than to attend to other [infant] dispensaries or institutes whose existence often they ignore.[25]

At this time, Peralta Ramos had already acquired institutional experience on the workings of maternity services something for which he became absolutely passionate about, devoting years studiously analysing architectural designs and drawing service's distribution, an effort that became a fundamental part of his professional legacy. In 1915 he organised and directed the maternity service of the Durán Hospital, a position he left to become director of the most prestigious maternity service at the Hospital Rivadavia in 1919. In that year, he was also appointed to the Chair of Obstetrics by the Faculty of Medicine, a post he held until 1946 when he was made redundant, along with other academics and institute directors, during the first government of President Perón.[26] Peralta Ramos was arguably the most important figure in Argentinian obstetrics of the period, and the one who contributed most to the discipline's consolidation. An active protagonist in the process of professionalisation of obstetrics, he was one of the founder members of the *Sociedad de Obstetricia y Ginecología de Buenos Aires* (1908), presided over various scientific committees, acted as delegate for his specialty at the national parliament and at international scientific meetings (PACC, and the Pan American conferences of eugenics), and founded renowned specialised journals (*Boletín del Instituto de Maternidad*) and the most influential region-wide journal of obstetrics and gynaecology, *Obstetricia y Ginecología Latino-Americanas* (1942).

His medical techniques and institutional achievements, as we will see later in more detail, shaped the identity of the 'Buenos Aires Obstetric School', whose reputation in Latin America attracted many students across the region, an international recognition also evidenced by the numerous obstetric societies that conferred honorary membership upon him.

While working at the Hospital Rivadavia, Peralta Ramos managed to persuade the ladies of the Society of Beneficence about the necessity of building a new integral maternity that would be part of the extended network of women and child institutes, hospitals and asylums that the Society administered on behalf of the national government. Although much has been written about the Society of Beneficence, and in particular of its numerous children's institutions, very little is known about its maternity institutes, whose multiple developments in areas so diverse as laboratory and experimental research, social services and policy-design, to its more conspicuous one as centres for women's reproductive health, turned them into leading institutes of medical research and assistance. Most historical analysis of the Ladies of Beneficence has tended to portrayed them as agents in the promotion of Catholic, conservative, and class-ridden values to the poor, yet little has been explored in their role as skilful negotiators between church values and the liberal state, as Karen Mead and Donna Guy have suggested.[27] Working closely with religious orders, to whom the Society traditionally trusted the education and caring of those assisted in their institutions, the ladies also did so with the state, from which they received important subsides, and to which they supported in its liberal economic policies that constituted the very foundations of the charitable system where they excelled. Maternities, I would contend, became spaces where *damas* dovetailed Catholic values and expectations in maternal assistance with obstetricians' medical and social views, many of which were informed by eugenic principles. Peralta Ramos commended to the administrative capacity of the Society a maternity project because, in his words, ladies,

> understood that the proposed initiative implied the most modern maternal and infant medical assistance, the social protection not only against the misfortune of poverty, but also against the moral misfortune of the repudiated, forgotten, shameful maternity.[28]

Remarks that attempted to eradicate, from the outset, the social and religious stigma attached to single mothers and illegitimate children, to embrace them too, into the modern and 'civilised' principles of obstetric science. The association between civilisation and standards of maternity provision was actually a plea for women's reproductive function, regardless of her civil status or class, a good that only scientific obstetrics, unlike empirical midwifery, could effectively secure: 'The first duty of all civilised society is to offer the mother the best guaranties for her to fulfil without risks the sublime function of maternity'.[29]

In 1928 Peralta Ramos inaugurated the Institute of Maternity of the Society of Beneficence of the Capital. The maternity became a model institute in Latin America, and as it was probably the first of its kind in Western countries, its design might well have inspired other maternities beyond the continent, judging from the frequent visits of foreign doctors who came to work on medical research or to train as obstetricians. His mentor wrote extensively on the principles that guided the architecture, service organisation, and the purpose of each of its areas, a building that stands out for its innovation and originality with respect to existing European maternities. Indeed, as early as 1921 Peralta Ramos published a detailed description of the maternity's complex service organisation along with the architectural plans of the building. He did not mention any particular source of inspiration for its design, although he constantly referred to Pinard's puericulture ideas as a guiding inspiration. In this sense, and given the professional devotion that Peralta Ramos demonstrated from early in his career, it is surprising that he did not complete his medical training in Paris or Berlin, as was common for Latin American medical students at the time. Obstetrical ideas, however, circulated on both sides of the Atlantic. All seems to indicate that the rationale and organisational conception of the Buenos Aires model maternity preceded the modernisation of the Parisian Baudelocque maternity that took place between 1922 and 1929. The remodelling of the 1890 Baudelocque clinic, that Pinard directed, was initiated by his son-in-law and successor to the chair of Obstetrics, Alexandre Couvelaire. Grounded, as expected, in puericulture principles, the organisation of the modern and soon-to-become Parisian 'model maternity' was published on a pamphlet in 1930.[30] The new maternity incorporated a range of services (Social Services, milk station, prenuptial, prenatal and postnatal services, plus a separated section for tubercular mothers), and it introduced individual rooms for delivery, and small rooms for postpartum women for recovery along with her child. According to Françoise Thébaud, the latter innovations gave notoriety to the maternity across the country.[31] Yet compared with the Argentinian project, we can argue that its value as the first French maternity in capturing the essence of puericulture seems to have been subsumed by a remodelling architectural project that took place within the constraints of pre-existing premises. In addition, services were distributed around other nearby maternity units, hospitals and infant institutes of the *Assistance Publique*, which were in turn, administratively independent.[32]

The maternity of Buenos Aires, on the other hand, was conceived as an integral and autonomous institute, whose provision included practically all the maternal and child services known at the time. With an area of 5,000 sq.mts., and an initial capacity of 220 adult beds and 126 infant beds (later increased to 460 and 320 respectively in the 1930s), the institute was made up of three distinctive sectors: pre-natal care, maternity, and post natal care which altogether formed part of twelve sections of medical and social assistance, medical research and professional education.[33] Women's assistance was offered from the beginning of the reproductive years (gynaecological and prenuptial consulting rooms), and until a child reached eighteen months, thus housing in the same building the three clinics (gynaecology, obstetric and puericulture). A centralisation that must have generated professional rivalries amongst paediatricians, who were more prone to have separate infant institutes, as Peralta Ramos himself recalled the 'disagreements, selfishness and clashes due to individual interests' that he had to overcome in persuading the state on the need of such a unifying, monumental institute.[34]

Peralta Ramos' all-encompassing criteria of maternal assistance was heavily concerned with the problems associated with the so-called 'illegitimate motherhood', as shown by the explanation he gave when justifying the famous slogan engraved in the internal arch of the edifice's main entrance, he commented: 'We must make the single mother participate of all the advantages that motherhood generates. "The mother is mother, and that is all" such is the motto I have chosen for our Institute of Maternity'.[35] As we shall see later, not everybody at the time agreed, especially in certain provinces where, for example, the creation of a maternity shelter for single or abandoned mothers was much more contested.

While Buenos Aires, by the 1930, had attained with its brand-new majestic institute and other maternal clinics a significant improvement and an acceptable provision of services, 'in the interior of the country the situation is different', warned Dr José Bello, who by 1940 reported that although obstetric wards existed in almost all provincial capitals, they were part of general hospitals, and lacked the specialist services that constituted modern maternities.[36] This view was shared by the officials of the Pan-American Sanitary Office, when some years earlier, they reported that, 'with the exception of the United States and cities like Buenos Aires, there was a need of maternity beds everywhere in America'.[37] Apart from the ten maternity institutes existing in Buenos Aires' province, and one in Córdoba, there were eighteen obstetric services working in general hospitals across the country. As maternity services multiplied in Buenos Aires, the hospitalisation of childbirth significantly grew to 60 per cent of the total newborns in 1940.[38] But given the scarcity of services in the rest of the provinces, including the capitals of important provinces like Córdoba and Santa Fe, which had better medical facilitates in comparison to that of the Northern provinces, it is possible to assert that the medicalisation of childbirth was not ubiquitous in Argentina. Nor were the rates of maternal mortality considerably reduced due to pregnancy and childbirth complications. At the time that infant mortality was making remarkable progress in Buenos Aires, maternal mortality was hardly mentioned, at least statistically. International child congresses similarly lacked focussed discussion on maternal mortality, and this has been linked to the general failure in improving mortality rates due to hospitalised childbirth (sepsis), and to the thorny topic of deaths caused by abortions.[39] International statistics on maternal mortality, as Irving Loudon has argued, showed a tendency to remain stagnant between 1870 and 1935, and only began to decline in the period 1935-40, when sulphonamide drugs were introduced into the clinic.[40] In Argentina, with the exception of a handful of reports, statistics started to appear in the medical press in the mid-1950s and were usually reported by individual maternity services and institutes. A similar pattern of decline seems to have occurred following the introduction of sulpha drugs in 1941. But deaths due to obstetric interventions or 'obstetric traumatism' in the nomenclature (including uterine rupture, surgical shock, etc.) remained high as showed by one statistic of the 'Maternity J. F. Moreno' in Mendoza, for the decade 1947-56 where those causes represented still a quarter of the total of maternal deaths.[41]

Córdoba's maternity services, whose development occupied a second place in the perspective of the Pan-American Sanitary Office, kept however a remarkable distance from the ones I have commented on for Buenos Aires. It is instructive to see in more detail how maternal and child services expanded there following international, national and local ideas of assistance. The creation of obstetric services in Córdoba was closely related to the teaching of obstetrics at the University, where courses started in 1882, just five years after the creation of the Faculty of Medical Sciences. The National University of Córdoba financed the first teaching ward (a small room with 6 beds) for students' medical training, situated at the courtyard of the San Roque Hospital, then the only general hospital existing in the city. The provision of new wards improved at a very slow pace in the next decades.[42] Progress in this area was inextricably linked to the initiatives of Dr José C. Lascano (1885-?), the most outstanding Cordoban obstetrician in the first half of the century, who became instrumental in developing obstetrics into a specialty. After receiving his MD from the University of Córdoba, he followed the growing tendency of completing postgraduate training in European clinics, and spent two years in Paris at two of the most prestigious clinics of the time, the Tarnier and Baudelocque Hospitals, under the supervision of Drs Pinard, Bar, and Fabre.[43] When Lascano returned to Córdoba in 1909, he was appointed to the department of Clinical Obstetrics, and by 1913 he became head of department, a position he held until 1945. The opening of the first teaching hospital by the University in 1913, the *Hospital de Clínicas*, hardly satisfied the institutional expectations of local obstetricians. There, Lascano moved the Obstetrics Department to a pavilion with a capacity for 28 beds for pregnant and puerperal women. These beds, added to those from the San Roque Hospital (11 beds) and a few provided by the Public Assistance, totalled approximately 45 maternity beds for 140,000 inhabitants in 1916. Poor obstetric facilities led Lascano to organise in 1919 the medical provision for home deliveries within the Public Assistance, as a way of ensuring medical intervention in cases that could not be hospitalised. Yet the scarcity of hospital beds was not only a problem for maternal care, it was heavily felt across the city's whole health infrastructure, which was deemed as chaotic at the time.[44]

Not until 1932, and after near two decades of relentless negotiations at different government levels, could Lascano inaugurate the National Maternity Institute, an establishment of the University of Córdoba especially dedicated to the social and medical assistance of mother and child, and to serve as obstetrics' main teaching hospital. The maternity was opened to the public with only a third of its building capacity (60 beds and 40 cots), which, according to its mentor, scarcely met the city's real needs. The organisation of services at the maternity loyally contemplated the three phases of puericulture assistance as proposed by Pinard: before procreation, prenatal, and postnatal.

As mentioned earlier, the influence of French obstetrics had an early foothold in Córdoba, ever since Paris, Lyon and Strasburg provided the specialist training for many influential doctors in the local scenario. Moreover, academic exchanges facilitated the reception of eugenic ideas, particularly in the form of puericulture, which stressed the mother's role in determining the health of her children.[45] As Nancy Stepan has shown in her study of eugenics in Latin American countries,[46] one of its distinctive features was that Latin American eugenists supported a particular neo-Lamarckian set of ideas rather than the more racist and 'hard' Mendelian ideology that dominated in Germany, Britain, and the United States. The theory of the inheritance of acquired characteristics emphasised reform of the social environment through a series of sanitation policies destined to improve the health of the population, rather than the setting of strict reproductive regulations. This seemed, for many reasons, a more compelling idea to face the so-called 'racial poisons', i.e. those diseases transmitted to the offspring directly by parents causing permanent hereditary degenerations such as syphilis, alcoholism, tuberculosis and infections. In the next chapter, however, I shall argue that this was particularly the case for the decades of 1910-1920, but not for the decade of 1930 onwards when eugenic ideas gave room to more negative practices.

Under neo-Lamarckian principles Argentinian obstetricians defined puericulture as the 'science of the well-development of the new being', through services interacting within the already mentioned three puericulture phases, yet most initiatives started, like in Buenos Aires, predominantly focussing on infant care.[47] Thus, Córdoba's Public Assistance created in 1904 a 'Consulting Room for Infant Protection', an institution later called *Gota de Leche* – inspired in the French *Gouttes de Lait* (milk station) – with the broad aim of securing early infant medical assistance, the education of mothers, and the improvement of infant mortality rates.[48] In 1911, the provincial government turned to Paris' infant health system when it commissioned Dr Lanza Castelli to find there a potential solution to the high infant mortality rate affecting the province. After his report, two *Gotas de Leche* were set up in the city, under the Provincial Council of Hygiene.[49] Maternal welfare, on the contrary, lacked infrastructure and initiatives, and when sanitary measures involved mothers, they had a clear purpose of curbing infant mortality. That was the case of a 1919 bill creating *Cantinas Maternales* (maternal canteens) attached to the *Gota de Leche,* to nurture mothers whose children were assisted in the latter, and a *Sala cuna* (nursery), to secure the sanitary inspection of wet nurses and the medical assistance of their children.[50]

It was not until the 1930s that the health of the mother started to be considered from the perspective of prenatal care. The *Gota de Leche,* for example, was modernised with the aim of delivering a preventive role, with

37

activities such as public campaigns (on puericulture notions, and the prophylaxis of venereal diseases), and the intensification of mother's education
and surveillance (social services). In this way, the *Cantina Maternal* extended
its activities to prenatal assistance for mothers in their final month of pregnancy, and postnatal assistance for which small rooms were installed so that
mothers could be hospitalised with their child 'becoming her wet nurse and
nurse'; while visiting nurses were appointed to supervise the fulfilment of
medical prescriptions at home.[51] But the promotion of the scientific rearing
of children inspired by eugenic puericulture, including that of the healthcare
of pregnant women, still constituted isolated and uncoordinated provincial
endeavours, something that was reflected in the city's poor statistical performance. In 1935 Argentina still had, according to international criteria, a 'very
high' infant mortality rate: 102/1000.[52] Amongst the higher rates, Córdoba
figured with 156/1000 (aged 0–1). It compared unfavourably with the city
of Buenos Aires, which had the country's lowest rate (52/1000), a difference
that was broadened when infants reached 1 year of age (12 and 50/1000)
respectively.[53] Accordingly, physicians believed that the second semester of
the child's life was the one that should concentrate all medical and welfare
efforts, which stimulated, in turn, renewed accusations on mothers' incom-
petence or deliberate negligence in childrearing practices. So in addition to
claiming for service improvements,[54] experts also insisted that two major
problems should be prioritised: the prophylaxis of digestive and nutritive illness, and the protection of illegitimate and abandoned children.[55] The latter,
however, was a longstanding concern not only for specialists. Throughout
the decades, medical attitudes towards illegitimacy and child abandonment
underwent changing conceptions and inspired contrasting approaches alongside practical measures, and to which corresponded different representations
of the mother figure and her associated maternal spirit.

Illegitimacy, abortion, and infanticide:
The medical representations of the maternal figure

Women did not constitute a unitary condition for male medical discourse,
and concerns on reproduction reflected conspicuous gender and class dis-
tinctions. Early in the century, Argentinian hygienists emphasised the defence
of the family unit, which largely relied on the distinctive and complementary character of gender roles: the father was thought to be responsible for
the household income, while the mother was liable for the raising of chil-

dren, and the moral and healthy conditions of the house. As Donna Guy has observed, if a woman 'left the household to perform labour, especially for wages, she became potentially contagious [syphilis] and therefore a public menace'.[56] Undoubtedly, working-class mothers were the ones whom doctors were more concerned with because of their double condition of multiparity and poor living conditions. However, though to a lesser extent, upper-class mothers also represented a menace for a responsible childrearing for their frequent reluctance to breastfeed. Affluent mothers and poor wet nurses were thus described by the first director of Córdoba's *Gota de Leche* during the first decade of the century,

> We have, then, two types of mothers, but equally culpable of the violation of an unavoidable duty, of the delegation of maternal functions that cannot be delegated. One that resists breastfeeding for her own and better beauty; and the other one, for the attraction of a lucrative industry.[57]

This initial reproachful tone in the case of the poor mother will give way to a more conciliating interpretation of the attitudes and habits that surrounded her maternal experience as the mother became identified as a necessary actor in the battle against infant mortality. Arguably, through the decades of 1910s and 1920s the medical representation of the poor mother started to change towards a more positive one that attempted to enhance the attributes of motherhood, particularly in those for whom maternity arrived under unfavourable circumstances. After acknowledging a situation where working-class women had to work outside the home – provided they did so to contribute to the family's sustenance – doctors articulated a stance that aimed to discourage women from resorting to abortion, infanticide or child abandonment. As Dora Barrancos[58] has analysed, during the 1920s, 'criminal abortion' was the most extended female method of birth control. This was corroborated by the persistent decline of Argentina's fertility and birth rates that evidenced a clear intention of family planning among the population.[59] Notwithstanding the lack of statistics for this period, physicians viewed the number of abortions with alarm[60] for which they often blamed midwives' activities, as we have seen earlier in this chapter.

Yet the practices of abortion, infanticide, child abandonment, and contraception needed to be re-signified in the light of prevailing concepts of maternity as a woman's natural mission. In other words, how should one interpret deviations from the norm when the maternal biological instinct was thought to be an attribute ordered by natural law? Doctors managed to re-signify those practices as 'definitive' or 'temporary' lack of natural instinct, therefore placing them out of nature. Whilst the 'most aberrant crimes', such as infanticide, were put under the heading of 'degeneration', or 'puerperal madness', other transgressions of the maternal instinct were interpreted as temporary mental disorders triggered by a series of economic, familiar and social difficulties.[61] On the one hand, the 'brutal [child] abandonment by the unconscious or denaturalised mother . . . supposes in the mother a perversion of feelings that we would not say of maternity, but of humanity'.[62] On the other, misery, economic difficulties and/or the social dishonour attached to single motherhood, especially in Catholic countries, were acknowledged as the main causes of mothers' 'irrational' behaviours. To this aim doctors sought 'to stimulate by all means the strengthening of the bond between mother and child', and,

> to guarantee the abandoned mother, moral and material support to help her in her misfortune, and to make her understand that the fact of being a mother redeems her of sin if she devotes herself to her child's care.[63]

The judicial frame, on the other hand, offered doctors a slightly different perspective which, as we shall see in the next chapter, disturbed, in particular, Catholic ones. The liberal-positivist ideology of the Penal Code (1921) penalised the practice of abortion, but allowed doctors to perform the so-called 'therapeutic abortion' in order to save the mother's life. For many doctors, the penalisation of the 'criminal abortion' was not enough punishment (1 to 4 years), but less so was the level of its prosecution, including women, midwives and quacks. The figure of 'infanticide', on the other hand, received a reduced punishment compared to the perpetual imprisonment established for the typified 'homicide aggravated by familial bond'. The rationale behind such disparity lay in the fact that, in the case of infanticide, 'dishonour' was considered a mitigating factor, a mercy that even benefited other members of the family that have been ashamed.[64] As the law stressed dishonour as a juridical value, it is not surprising that it encompassed relatives of the dishonoured mother, provided they murdered the baby to cover the shame inflicted upon the family. In the case of the mother, the 'puerperal state' was understood as a temporary psycho-physiological predisposing factor concomitant with the one of dishonour. The temporary disorder was attributed to the existence of a puerperal organic disequilibrium, but not as a permanent state of insanity, which if proved, converted the mother into a non-imputable subject. However, this was less a decision of judges and obstetricians than of legal psychiatric experts, who would observe this type of female mental disorder in a more pathological way. In the largest asylum of Argentina, the *Asilo Colonia Regional Mixto de Alienados en Oliva*, a mixed colony asylum placed in the province of Córdoba, 'puerperal madness' was a nosology commonly used during the first years after the asylum's opening in 1914 only to disappear later on under the label of other affective disorders.[65] As Hilary Marland has observed for the British case, with the reception of Kraepelin's classification and the hereditary and organic causal interpretation of psychiatry more broadly, 'puerperal madness' ceased to be considered a separate pathological entity to become included within the general framework of manic-depressive illness.[66] While the mental state that led women to commit infanticide was being transformed by psychiatrists into a degenerative and hereditary disease, for obstetricians such notions reinforced the view and confirmed the rule that the maternal instinct was *within* the natural law.

Under a general concern for improving rates of infant mortality, the prevention of abortion, infanticide and child abandonment was, for many doctors, not found in the use of contraceptive methods but in the creation of maternity shelters. For others, it was in the re-establishment of the *torno* (desertion tower), that is, in places that could hide the mother's dishonour and so guarantee the birth of her child. The *torno* was the system implemented in European orphanage and hospices of the eighteenth century with the aim of reducing infanticide. It also existed in Argentina for more than a century until it was forbidden in 1891, under the initiatives of hygienists like Emilio Coni, who thought it was 'a shameful machine for a cultured society'. In Córdoba, it was installed in the outer wall of the *Casa Cuna* (foundling house) and it worked like a revolving door whereby mothers opened the front door and placed the baby inside a compartment that was on a turntable. The nuns could then rotate the turntable and remove the newborn inside the building without seeing the mother. However, it was the increasing number of abandoned children deposited through the *torno* that led physicians to propose its closure and to campaign instead for the strengthening of the mother-child bond. But not all doctors agreed with its suppression. In 1922 the reinstallation of the *torno* was vigorously discussed in the Second National Congress of Medicine, and in the context of a national law that supported its running.

41

In Córdoba, the newspaper *La Voz del Interior* commented on the Congress's resolution criticising the social rather than scientific ideas that informed many physicians, especially those 'influenced by Catholic ideas with ramifications to politics'. The Congress opposed the *torno* on the following grounds, 'Its implantation only protects the mother, who liberates herself from her child, which is deemed as a disaster for infancy.' On the other hand, the newspaper bitterly reflected, 'it is a step back. [Science] prefers the mother destroying the fruit of her entrails before letting the baby live "abandoned"'.[67]

Thus by the 1920s the 'unfortunate mother' became an ideal-type carefully supported in order to stir social compassion rather than condemnation. The 'poor mother' and the 'abandoned single mother', as an obstetrician expressed, were,

> lonely, without means, without a single voice of stimulus, these unfortunate mothers end up abandoning their newborns with the hope that a charitable soul would take them in and would provide them with the care that, because of their misfortune, they could not give.[68]

Both obstetricians and paediatricians expressed great concern about the number of illegitimates in the country, although this could be related to their comparisons with European rates, where illegitimacy was considerably lower, rather than to the rates doctors observed in the regions they represented. In Argentina, illegitimacy rates increased between 1915 and 1940 when it reached around 30 per cent of all births.[69] However, disparities amongst regions were remarkable. While the coastal, urban area, including the city of Buenos Aires where the majority of specialists came from, had percentages that oscillated around 13 and 11 per cent; the rural areas, especially in the Northern provinces, rates soared up to 40 per cent and above, showing a pattern of both high number of births and high illegitimacy rates.[70] Aware of these regional differences or not, or simply concerned with emulating the rates of European capitals, obstetricians from Buenos Aires came to the mother's defence, and supported the assistance of 'illegitimate motherhood' while aware that such a protection implied opposing entrenched values and mores: 'However much religious, political, philosophical and moral ideas disagree, all civilised people tend to channel their beneficent action in this way', said Peralta Ramos in his advocacy of a moral and material support to single mothers.[71] They voiced this too in the Parliament and in medical meetings at national level. Needless to say that they did so not because they agreed that being a single mother was a woman's decision, but for the safeguard of her children, as Peralta Ramos went on to say, 'the protection of the unfortunate mother is imperative, more than for her herself, for the salvation of her child'.[72] The 'unfortunate mother' constitutes an example of how medical representation on maternity during this particular period of nation-building was cut across by specific temporalities and contexts. On its elaboration, this representation constantly refers to tensions between practices of the past and the future (on the one hand, the *torno*, religious condemnation of illegitimate motherhood, and on the other, maternity shelter, and socio-medical protection of the 'defenceless motherhood'), and at the same time articulates those perceived tensions with cultural elements of social progress (civilisation) and patriotic zeal. It also indicates that social representations of motherhood were not fixed but elaborated in response to specific circumstances, and consequently, were often contested too from multiple perspectives. A glance at the countrywide context, will remind us that the above mentioned tensions, although present in the perspective of those obstetricians that embraced puericulture, were unevenly resolved in practice.

Thus, in spite of specialists' proclaimed protection of the defenceless, illegitimate mother, they advanced little in terms of concrete institutional support, especially if we consider that the *torno* was eradicated and maternity shelters or maternal homes to care for dishonoured mothers only provided a small number of beds in charitable institutions.[73] The most notorious exception was, as already mentioned, the Institute of Maternity of Buenos Aires, where Peralta Ramos set up a 'maternity shelter' that secured mothers' honour by keeping their identities secret inside the institution, while a group of female professional visitors, from the much valued area of Social Services, was in charge of their assistance and support. The situation in the Córdoba maternity was, however, different. Although its director insisted on the protection of illegitimate mothers, he did not plan or supply them with a dedicated space to cater for their needs. The Social Services, on the other hand, were entrusted to the Spanish Catholic congregation of nuns, *Hermanas Carmelitas Descalzas de la Tercera Orden*. If the maternity's director, who was permanently searching for funding to fully fit out the maternity's capacity, decided to sacrifice a space equivalent to 30 beds to accommodate the Sisters, in addition to a chapel, it was because he considered their contribution 'irreplaceable'. And nuns were so for different reasons. Firstly, the Sisters' availability represented a way of saving resources in personnel more than a

43

'profession of faith' in the case of Lascano, who never integrated Catholic medical circles. Moreover, nuns were especially praised for having a strict economic sense, a quality that was much needed to run health institutions with permanent deficits in funding.[74] Equally important was their role in the observance of discipline, order and morality both among the personnel, and especially amongst mothers, becoming instrumental in the provision of the maternity's Social Services, whose delicate activities were entrusted to the Mother Superior. This section was of vital importance for obstetricians, if we consider that most of them associated illegitimacy with an increased risk of infant mortality.

It is, therefore, interesting to compare the so-called 'moral results' obtained by Social Services of the maternity in Buenos Aires, run by professional visitors, with the one in Córdoba, because one encounters remarkable differences. While the former enumerated its results in: 'solved abandonment'; 'marriages'; 'legitimisations'; 'recognitions'; and 'reconciliations'; the latter did it as follows: 'civil marriages'; 'civil and church marriages'; 'church marriages' and 'child baptism'.[75] As these labels conspicuously show, in the capital district considerable efforts went into the secular, legal and social aspects that assured mother and child a better wellbeing, i.e. those that the Civil Code acknowledged but were difficult to pursue (legitimisation) or did not grant mothers with rights, like the investigation for paternity (recognition). In Córdoba, on the contrary, the efforts of Social Services seem to have been put in ensuring respect for the sacraments. Such disparity in an otherwise similarly conceived maternity institute, induces us to reflect on the paradoxes of the welfare system that I have commented earlier in this chapter, in that it led to the overlap of old and new ideas in sometimes incoherent ways. Buenos Aires developed a unique maternity institute, conceived under the most advanced medical principles of mother and child assistance, under the administration of the ladies of the Society of Beneficence; while Córdoba set up a maternity institute dependant on the national university, with Social Services run by sisters of a religious congregation.

The general consensus of doctors on the need of society to support the poor working mother and 'illegitimate motherhood' ambiguously conflated with the idea of women's motherly love. In fact, one of the challenges opened by the debates on the deviations of the maternal role was whether maternity was a matter of instinctive forces or something to be taught. Although contradictory, physicians managed to make use of both the biological idea of 'the ancestral instinct' and the cultural necessity of educating mothers to improve their maternal tasks. Puericulture became the science that would fulfil what instinct alone had proved to be insufficient. 'Where was taught to woman the essentially moral and humanistic science of learning how to be a mother?' asked a paediatrician from Córdoba in 1913 to the would-be teachers of the 'Normal School'.[76] This early series of puericulture lessons for secondary school girls, organised by the government, had the purpose 'to disseminate the indispensable knowledge to convert them [the feminine youth] into rational and conscious mothers of families or into wise directors and teachers of other future mothers of families'.[77] Fuelling the idea of maternity as a 'social function', the consequences of such an education were directly linked with the nation's destiny, as the paediatrician went on to say, 'the development of the physical and psychic character of children assures the perpetuity of men at home, the perpetuity of home in the homeland, and the perpetuity of the homeland in humanity'.[78] Naturally, the success of this social end depended much on the degree to which women individually were imbued with maternal feelings. And maternal love became, too, something to be reinforced and cultivated through puericulture, because, 'The woman that learns to know her child closely, providing him with solicitous care, learns, too, to love him more'.[79]

The organisation of puericulture lessons also sheds light on other aspects of the way in which maternity was perceived by male doctors, in that this education, and its corresponding teaching, was strictly delimited and organised on gender lines. As new disciplines emerged related to women's perceived skills and role in society, one of them in particular was paradigmatic in showing how the feminisation of specific disciplines operated: it is the so-called 'Domestic Science or Domestic Economy'. The education and professionalisation of women in this discipline relied on the assumption that education should prepare them to be 'more womanly', not just in an empirical way, but in a 'scientific' one, as they were trained in the domestic command of the house. Hygiene, economy, chemistry and the infant's first care were the skills that women should learn in the public space in order to apply them in the private world. As Marcela Nari has observed, 'a new ideal of housewife was imposed, the one emotionally and intellectually engaged with her tasks'.[80] The way in which the mother's domestic skills should be taught reveals yet more gender biases when comparing the different trajectories that Domestic Economy and Puericulture underwent at the time. If middle-class women found in the former a professional opportunity as teachers[81] (the discipline was entirely taught by women and formed part of the curricula at schools), they occupied a place in education as schoolmistresses that state and society had already trusted to them. The scientific rearing of children, on the other hand, was something absolutely entrusted to male specialists, both in the development of the programme's contents and to a large extent, in the professional practice. On the one hand, the disagreements between Argentinian feminist doctors and paediatricians during the Pan-American child congresses meant that feminists failed in imposing their reforming agenda, on the other, they were also excluded from holding chief positions in university departments throughout the period under investigation. It is true that some male doctors were, to some extent, receptive of feminist ideas, especially in relation to the social aspects of motherhood, although they differed with them in the way that such policies should be implemented. In any case, this receptiveness was favoured by the perception that male specialists had about the need of a change in attitude for society at large, for which they were prepared to publicly discuss social values, and prejudices in particular. If all these aspects framed the discussion and supported the configuration of the social representations of the maternal figure (culture), a different situation would inform the one that configured the representations of the maternal body (biology), where medical aspects of childbirth were built inside the medical field and *without* social mediation.

The obstetric schools and the medical representations of the maternal body

Medical representations of the maternal body resemble closed dialogues, a discussion amongst peers that circulates in specialised journals and congresses without the calculated strategies required in public debate, or the awareness that what is said may be subject to negotiations. One of the most interesting places where we can chart its development is in the performance of obstetric schools, particularly in their growing efforts to differentiate their practices, and in the language, metaphors and analogies they used to build representations of their own.

It was within the field of obstetric surgery, whose expansion can be traced back to the end of the eighteenth century, that the development of two different obstetric schools took place, and have ever since disputed obstetric practice until at least the first half of the twentieth century. One school obtained its prestige by trusting more in the surgical skills of its members than in the natural forces intervening in the process of delivery. The other school promoted a 'contemplative' and 'expectant' attitude with respect to nature instead of an 'interventionist' or artificial one. As conditions in the theatre room considerably improved early in the twentieth century (antisepsis, blood transfusion, and anaesthetics, amongst others), both schools expanded their principles in Western countries by developing techniques that represented their particular points of view in relation to delivery. Thus, the 'interventionist' school perfected the surgical techniques of caesarean section, hysterectomies, and a series of techniques devised to enlarge the pelvis during delivery or to treat myriad of gynaecological diseases. The 'expectant', on the other hand, advocated the use of manual skills that made a limited use of surgical methods, resorting to minor rather than major surgery, like the performance of symphisothomy instead of caesarean section, while preferred the use of instruments combined with proficient obstetric manoeuvres.

In Argentina, each school had its supporters whose location had a rather clear geographical distribution: whilst the 'interventionist' attitude dominated the obstetric clinics of Buenos Aires, the 'expectant' was welcomed among obstetricians in the provinces. Identification with one or another school led to passionate discussions amongst their respective members which sometimes were prolonged in the medical press, a process that reinforced, in turn, the rise of obstetrics as a medical specialty. One illustrative example we find is in the reasons given by the obstetric school from Córdoba, headed by Lascano, in support of their expectant attitude towards childbirth:

> The major comfort of a regulated and quick surgical operation [might appear better] than the hours of waiting, using annoying obstetrical interventions, which are more difficult and prolong the emotions. But the physician owes more to the safety of lives entrusted to him than to his own personal comfort.[82]

For the highly common cases of narrow pelvis, for example, Lascano preferred symphysiothomy, an intervention that, although surgical, implied a simpler and, comparatively, less spectacular operation than the caesarean section at the time. Between the first and second decade, both operations moderated their risks, at the time that marked a new precedent in surgical attitude: those who were more determined to intervene with the scalpel, were more prone to change the primary-vaginal direction of childbirth, placing the obstetric schools in a renewed dispute that was known as, 'abdominal *versus* vaginal methods'. In any case, the methods utilised by both schools were not exempt from contradictions. Especially for the 'conservatives' with their 'classical', 'obstetrical' or 'vaginal' methods, as they used a series of manual manoeuvres combined with mechanical instruments: whether those used for the stimulation of contractions (hot vaginal washes, cervix-vaginal plugging, probes, balloons); those used for the dilatation of the cervix (metallic or manual dilatation, which increased the risks of infection); or those utilised in cases of narrow pelvis (internal version i.e. the shift of foetus presentation, or the use of a variety of forceps).[83]

As commented earlier, Argentinian obstetric schools closely followed developments in Europe, particularly France and Germany during 1890-1930, where many medical students trained in the speciality, contributing on their return a first-hand experience with the clinical tendencies that provided European schools with a recognisable identity. Medical exchanges were also facilitated and promoted by cultural associations and institutions, grants and fellowships, international congresses, and medical journals, notably those especially dedicated to the dissemination of French and German medical culture in Ibero-America that took the form of bilateral undertakings, such as, (France) *Union Médicale Franco-Ibéro-Américaine (1925-1940);* and (Germany) *La Medicina Germano-Hispano-Americana (1923- later Revista Médica Germano-Ibe-ro-Americana until 1938).* Within this framework of well-established, regular academic exchanges, one obstetric school that had a remarkable impact in Argentina around the 1920s and 1930s was the Obstetric School of Strasburg, in the Franco-German border, whose perspective was introduced as a 'conciliating' orientation between the above-mentioned conservative and surgical tendencies. The Strasburg School was led by obstetricians G. Schickelé and his disciple J. Kreis, whose work concentrated on the clinical observation of uterine physiopathology. Kreis proposed around the mid-1920s a method named 'medical delivery' (*L'accouchement medical,* or *parto médico* in Spanish) which consisted of shortening the duration of labour through the artificial and early rupture of the amniotic sac, and to assist or 'guide', by means of new available sedative and antispasmodic drugs the progress of uterine contractions. But if Kreis considered that an 'absolutely physiologic' childbirth (without complications) was a 'rare' event, it is easy to speculate about the interventionist criteria that preceded his actions.

In Buenos Aires, the receptiveness to these ideas was significant, especially in the case of Peralta Ramos, who became one of Kreis' most enthusiastic supporters. As he proudly remarked when the technique became known in Argentina, 'this therapeutic is currently used at the Institute of

Maternity'.[84] The title of the paper where he explained the therapeutic conveyed Peralta Ramos' view without euphemism: 'Government and direction of childbirth'. In his description, it is worth noting the language utilised in Spanish (probably a translation from Kreis' French and German texts) to draw attention to the meaning of childbirth as a process whereby the uterus has become completely dissociated from the female body. Accordingly, the leading role of the action of delivery was moved from woman to doctor, the latter becoming identified with a language that echoed the spirit of the military forces that, in the 1930s, ruled the nation: surveillance and dominance. 'To govern childbirth we need, firstly, to perfectly invigilate the active or functional phenomenon as well as the passive or mechanic ones that are subordinated to it'.[85] This 'taking of government', Peralta Ramos went on to explain, allowed obstetricians to 'accelerate' delivery by means of sedatives and antispasmodics; avoid the 'proof of forces' in order to decide, if necessary, the 'taking over' at the best opportunity, 'neither too early nor too late'. Given the fact that this method was used in cases that did not present grave complications, its aim was 'to shorten its duration and make it less painful'.[86] In this article, Peralta Ramos recalled, evidently still upset, that when he introduced Kreis' ideas at the First Argentinian Congress of Obstetrics and Gynaecology (1931), 'these ideas were challenged with theoretical arguments and objections strongly attached to obstetric classicism, and the old mentality'[87] in reference to 'conservative' obstetric principles that defended a prudent expectation toward women in labour.

Supporters of this method in Buenos Aires had yet another controversial argument to adopt a medical intervention in all delivery cases, when they propose to classify the amniotic sac in 'good sacs' and 'bad sacs'. As one of them asserted: 'our experience demonstrates for that "bad" sacs are in the majority and, therefore, we can justify Kreis' orientation of systematising its rupture in all cases, although "a priori" this might seem excessive'.[88] Finally, studies on the physiology of the uterine dynamic would bring another method, the one proposed by French obstetrician Paul Delmas (1929) named 'childbirth at fixed hour', which consisted of the '*evacuation* of the uterine content at the hour deliberately chosen by the obstetrician'.[89] Basically, it consisted of the manual dilatation of the cervix once it had been previously relaxed by the administration of epidural anaesthetic. In a telling account, an obstetrician from Córdoba detailed the method resorting to mechanical analogies, when he commented: 'the forefinger penetrates like a *screw* in the cervix'; 'clenching one's fist, it should act like a *key* in a *lock* until the dilatation of the cervix *chan-*

49

nel is completed'.[90] The mechanical analogies utilised to express the obstetrician's movements are meaningful but not entirely surprising if we consider that the word 'engine' has long been used as a metonym for 'uterus', hence its associated terms to refer to its capacity to be 'accelerated' at a 'fixed hour'. Obsession with the 'mechanics of the uterus' or the 'physiopathology of the uterine engine', increased the obstetric vocabulary in multiple ways. Another striking example is offered in the next description of the uterine body and the cervix: 'to the normal irritation of the motor elements of the uterine body, corresponds to the inhibition of the cervix's engines'.[91] Accordingly, pathologies such as eclampsia (toxaemias) or the premature detachment of the sac (haemorrhages) stop being named as diseases and became referred to as 'accidents'.

As observed by Emily Martin for the US context, 'medically, birth is seen as the control of labourers (women) and their machines (their uteruses) by managers (doctors), often using other machines to help'.[92] In the Argentinian case, the terminology too resembled a mechanical process, including the one that, in the mid-1930s, reminds us of the industrial fervour of the period and its obsession with time. Revealingly, the Delmas' method was also known as the 'extemporaneous evacuation of the uterus', whose phases were described following a strict control of time, in three steps; 1st) injection of novocaine: 5'; 2nd) manual dilatation: 3'; and 3rd) extraction of the foetus: 3 ½'.[93] It is striking that this chronometric measurement of delivery was, just twenty years earlier, not only absent, but delivery itself was much more controlled by the labouring woman. By 1916, an obstetrician who reported 92.5 per cent of spontaneous deliveries without other medical intervention than observation, claimed from his colleges – who were already concerned with shortening the time of the placenta's expulsion – 'why not systematically invite the parturient to push at the opportune moment, even when she is not spontaneously stimulated to do so?[94] This article was the last one I could find in the medical literature of an obstetrician acknowledging the mother's involvement, as a subject, in the process of childbirth. Her telling absence, in what followed, provides insight into the tacit agreements underlying the opposite attitudes between the 'expectant' and the 'interventionist' schools, showing that disagreements were not about what women's bodies were, or what role they were to play, but about which strategy of intervention would prevail in the profession.

Key ideas underpinning what we now call the medicalisation of childbirth (hospital intervention, safety, risk control) took place in a relatively short period of time, where a new vocabulary of medical concepts, descriptions and representations were crucial in instilling a new meaning for childbirth and women in labour. In this sense, pregnancy was considered as a pathological state, 'our starting point is that a pregnant woman is already an ill-being of a greater or lesser grade', 'The pregnant woman, usually, is not in a fit condition for fulfilling normally the task of being a mother. Why? Because her condition is not absolutely *normal*'.[95] At the same time, there was the pathologisation of delivery itself, 'It is necessary to recognise that the deliveries that are to be considered physiological [normal] are scarce, the majority of them, even those that end spontaneously, suffer numerous anomalies in the course of their different stages'.[96] To this end, obstetricians were not sparing in coining new terms. Dr Josué Beruti, for instance, preferred to say that a delivery was 'approximately physiological' in the best case, making clear that it could never be 'absolutely' normal. Such expressions re-signified the idea of childbirth as an event of high risk in which a wide range of 'accidents' could suddenly endanger the life of the mother or the child. At least two consequences can be articulated in relation to this elaboration of risk: in the first place, obstetricians had no doubts about blaming women for putting themselves under unnecessary risks that only doctors would know how to solve. In the second place, and as Paula Treichler has argued, pregnancy and delivery could only be diagnosed retrospectively as 'normal', when it was evident that mother and child enjoyed a good health.[97]

As far as the underlying ideas used to describe the pregnant body is concerned, it is highly instructive to follow the medical aphorism utilised at different times, for it encapsulates the main medical perception of female bodies more broadly. Thus, the one generally used until the 1930s, as we have seen, was '*muller tota in uterus*' (woman is all uterus), while the one that followed, informed by the rise of endocrine studies, was '*muller tota in ovaries*' (woman is all ovaries).[98] The next chapter is largely devoted to disentangling what the latter meant. Yet beyond the consolidating position that obstetrics as a distinctive specialty was acquiring in these years, specialists' capacity to influence society at large with their elaborated representations of the maternal body would resonate differently as we shall see throughout the book.

Notes

1   E. Coni, *Asistencia y Previsión Social. Buenos Aires Caritativo y Previsor* (Buenos Aires: Ed. Spinelli, 1918).

2   J. M. Álvarez, *La Lucha por la Salud. Su Estado Actual en la Ciudad de Córdoba* (Buenos Aires: Biedma, 1896), 164-82. Unless otherwise stated, all translations are the author's.

3   Álvarez, *La Lucha por la Salud*, 247-48.

4   Y. Eraso (ed.), *Mujeres y Asistencia Social en Latinoamérica, siglos XIX y XX. Argentina, Colombia, México, Perú y Uruguay* (Córdoba: Alción Editora, 2009).

5   D. Guy, 'The Politics of Pan-American Cooperation: Maternalist Feminism and the Child Rights Movement, 1913-1960', *Gender and History*, 10 (1998), 449-69.

6   A. E. Birn, "No More Surprising than a Broken Pitcher?": Maternal and Child Health in the Early Years of the Pan-American Sanitary Bureau', *Canadian Bulletin of Medical History*, 19, 1 (2002), 17-46.

7   E. Cantón, 'Protección a la Madre y al Hijo. Puericultura intra y extra-uterina. Profilaxis del Aborto. Parto prematuro, Abandono e Infanticidio. Maternidad Refugio', *La Semana Médica*, 31, 1 (1914), 39-44: 43

8   A. Peralta Ramos and J. Garrahan, 'Acción Médica y Social de las Maternidades en la Puericultura Postnatal', in A. Peralta Ramos, *Obstetricia, Ginecología y Puericultura, III* (Buenos Aires: Imprenta Mercatali, 1939), 263-77: 263.

9   Peralta Ramos and Garrahan, 'Acción Médica y Social', 264.

10 In 1914, obstetrician Dr J. Beruti lamented that out of 20 illegal midwives identified, only 4 were fined. J. Beruti, 'Nuestro Gremio de Parteras. Reformas Necesarias para su Mejoramiento y Dignificación', *La Semana Médica*, 23, 1 (1916).

11 *Mensaje del Gobernador de la Provincia de Córdoba Dr. Eufrasio S. Loza. 1° de Mayo de 1917* (Córdoba: Imprenta de la Penitenciaría, 1917), 38. As the Governor reported, only 65 women passed the exam, a number that was deemed scarce for a (provincial) population of 850,000 inhabitants, and therefore as a threat for the dissemination of unprofessional ones.

12 B. Galíndez, 'El Aborto Criminal en Córdoba', *RCMC*, 9 (1921), 245-68: 261.

13 For the period 1913-27, puerperal infection accounted for 50 per

cent of maternal deaths due to obstetric cause, and 41 per cent of all maternal deaths. In J. Lascano, 'La Distocia en Córdoba', *RCMC* (1928), 173-93.

14   A. Peralta Ramos, 'La Obstetricia del Médico Práctico', in *Actas y Trabajos del IICNM,* III (Buenos Aires: Casa Editora de A. Guidi Buffarini, 1925), 645-63: 646. In this paper, he also specified the medical interventions that a GP should be allowed to perform, to clearly differentiate them from the ones that an obstetrician was entitled to do.

15   Peralta Ramos, 'La Obstetricia del Médico Práctico', 647.

16   The Association provided support to the university graduates including advice on career prospects.

17   Dr Benito Soria was Professor of Paediatrics at the University of Córdoba; Director of the Service for Infants (1920-23) at the Orphan House; founder of the 'School for Weak Children' (1918) and the Society of Paediatrics. In 1934 he opened a children hospital under his organisation 'Committee for the Defence of Infancy'.

18   B. Soria, 'Obras realizadas en Córdoba en Pro de la Infancia y Escuela de Madres', *Revista de la Universidad Nacional de Córdoba,* 2 (1919), 84-98: 94.

19   Guy, 'The Politics of Pan-American Cooperation', 450.

20   Ibid., 455.

21   For a detailed analysis about the initiatives for the protection of infancy in Latin America and its impact in international health policy see E. Scarzanella, 'Los Pibes en el Palacio de Ginebra: Las Investigaciones de la Sociedad de las Naciones sobre la Infancia Latinoamericana (1925-1939)', *Estudios Interdisciplinarios de América Latina y el Caribe,* 14, 2 (2003) Online at: http://www1.tau.ac.il/eial/index.php (consulted 25.07.2009); and A.E. Birn, 'The National-International Nexus in Public Health: Uruguay and the Circulation of Child Health and Welfare Policies, 1890-1940', *História, Ciências, Saúde – Manguinhos,* 13, 3 (2006), 33-64.

22   D. Barrancos, *Inclusión/Exclusión. Historia con Mujeres* (Buenos Aires: Fondo de Cultura Económica, 2002), 84.

23   B. Soria, 'Educate mothers to assist carefully their children, to inculcate in them the notion of their highest responsibility'. . . 'to arouse in them the triumphal pride of maternity', in newspaper *La Voz del Interior* (7 July 1927), 9.

24 Ibid.

25 Peralta Ramos and Garrahan, 'Acción Médica y Social', 268.

26 Political change also brought about structural transformations within the welfare system, whereby the Society of Beneficence was intervened and deprived of the administration of its institutes in 1946, which became controlled by new national public entities: the Secretary of Public Health and the National Direction of Social Assistance.

27 K. Mead, 'Gender, Welfare and the Catholic Church in Argentina', 91; and Guy, *Women Build the Welfare State*, 48.

28 A. Peralta Ramos, 'Discurso Homenaje. Informaciones Latino-Americanas', *Obstetricia y Ginecología Latino-Americanas,* 3 (1944), 649-59: 657.

29 A. Peralta Ramos, 'Protección de la Madre Desamparada' (Conference paper, 1927), in *Obstetricia, Ginecología y Puericultura*, 307-31: 309.

30 A. Couvelaire, *La Nouvelle Maternité Baudelocque. Clinique Obstétricale de la Faculté de Médecine de l'Université de Paris* (Paris: Masson, 1930). In 1931, the Pan-American Sanitary Office published in its Spanish bulletin a summary of the new features of the Baudelocque maternity entitled '*Maternidad modelo*' ('model maternity'), in *Boletín de la Oficina Sanitaria Panamericana,* Agosto (1931), 986-1022: 992-3.

31 F. Thébaud, 'A Medicalização do Parto e suas Conseqüências: O Exemplo da França no Período entre as duas Guerras', *Estudos Feministas,* 2 (2002), 415-27.

32 These were the Hospital Cochin, the Maternity of Port Royale, the Clinique Tarnier (childbirth) and the children hospital of San Vincent de Paul.

33 The Institute of Maternity was made up of the following sections/ services: 1) pregnant women ('sheltered maternity' and 'common maternity'); 2) childbirth, post-partum and newborns for those in assistance at the maternity; 3) childbirth, post-partum and newborns for those hospitalised in an emergency; 4) separated sector (for septic pregnancies); 5) shelter for mothers (material and moral aid for childrearing, job education); 6) private (pay) assistance; 7) gynaecology; 8) Institute of Puericulture; 9) domiciliary assistance; 10) outpatients consulting rooms (ante-natal care, postpartum, milk station, etc); 11) wet nurses; 12) social assistance (economic and social conditions of mothers). The Institute was partially inaugurated in 1928. By 1930 the second wing of the building was completed. Peralta Ramos,

'Concepto y Organización del Instituto de Maternidad de la Sociedad de Beneficencia de Buenos Aires', *Obstetricia, Ginecología y Puericultura,* 279-99.

34 A. Peralta Ramos, 'Habilitación Definitiva del Instituto de Maternidad', *Archivos de los Hospitales de la Sociedad de Beneficencia de la Capital. Años 1929-1932,* 9-23: 11.

35 Peralta Ramos, 'Protección de la Madre Desamparada', 323.

36 J. Bello, 'Mortinatalidad y Organización Sanitaria', *IVCAOyG* (Buenos Aires: Guidi Buffarini, 1940), 813-17: 814.

37 'Infancia', *Boletín de la Oficina Sanitaria Panamericana* Enero (1936), 27-36: 31.

38 Bello, 'Mortinatalidad y Organización Sanitaria', 814.

39 Scarzanella, 'Los Pibes en el Palacio de Ginebra'.

40 I. Loudon, 'Maternal Mortality: 1880-1950. Some Regional and International Comparisons', *Social History of Medicine*, 1, 2 (1998), 183-228.

41 Other causes were gestosis (toxaemia of pregnancy) 28.3%; infections (24,5%); haemorrhage (24,5%) in M. Torre, 'Mortalidad Materna', *Obstetricia y Ginecología Latino-Americanas*, 16, 7-8 (1958), 233-39: 235.

42 In 1894, the service was re-located to a similarly unsuitable space, but with an increased capacity (11 beds), and it was divided into two rooms: one for pregnant women, and the other for puerperal women, plus one room for surgery, which also served as a teaching room for students.

43 Other outstanding obstetricians from Córdoba who obtained their specialisation in France were: Dr Alfredo Bustos Moyano, who studied in 1911 at both the Tarnier and Baudelocque Hospitals, led by Bar and Pinard respectively. In Córdoba, he was appointed as obstetrician at the Public Assistance, and Associated Professor to the Obstetric Clinic Department. In 1921 he worked in the maternal service at the Hospital San Roque. Dr Benjamín Galíndez was Head of Obstetric Clinic Department (1906-1908) and later, Head of Gynaecology (1918). He also pursued his studies in France at the Tarnier and Baudelocque Hospitals. He became Director of the Maternity Service at the Hospital San Roque. Cfr. Félix Garzón Maceda, *Historia de la Facultad de Ciencias Médicas*, I. (Córdoba: Imprenta de la Universidad, 1927).

44 By 1916 it was estimated that Córdoba, given its population size, should have had six hospitals but in fact it only had three: San Roque

Hospital (160 beds), Children's Hospital (80 beds), and Hospital de Clínicas (300 beds). At that time physicians calculated that 200 beds were necessary for a population of 20,000 inhabitants. Using this standard, Córdoba should have had 1,400 beds instead of the existing 540. *Cfr.* 'Exposición del Senador Arturo Pitt Referida al Proyecto de Ley Sobre Dotación de Obras de Salubridad al Hospital San Roque', in B. Moreyra, F. Remedi and P. Roggio (eds.), *El Hombre y sus Circunstancias. Discursos, Representaciones y Prácticas Sociales en Córdoba, 1900-1935* (Córdoba: Centro de Estudios Históricos, 1998), 270.

45   For the development of eugenic ideas in France, see William Schneider, *Quality and Quantity: The Quest for Biological Regeneration in Twentieth-Century France* (Cambridge: Cambridge University Press, 1990).

46   Stepan, *'The Hour of Eugenics'*, Ch. 3.

47   A. Peralta Ramos, 'La Obstetricia en sus Relaciones con la Eugenesia', in *Obstetricia, Ginecología y Puericultura,* 385-89: 386.

48   'Informe elevado por el Dr. Ernesto del Campillo, director del Consultorio Protector de la Infancia, al Dr. Alejandro Centeno, director de la Asistencia Pública y Administración Sanitaria, referido a la actividad de aquella institución en el período 1904-1905', in Moreyra, Remedi and Roggio, *El Hombre y sus Circunstancias,* 119-26.

49   Lanza Castelli, *Mortalidad Infantil* (Córdoba: Imprenta el Comercio, 1911).

50   These measures were established in order to control wet nurses' practices, as wet nurses were usually blamed for provoking the death of their own offspring by reserving their breast for other children for a salary. 'Proyecto y Fundamentación de Rafael Nuñez sobre la Creación de Cantinas Maternales y Gotas de Leche in 1919', in *La Voz del Interior,* 30 December 1919, 5.

51   'Informe del Dr. Elías Halac elevado al Dr Alberto Stuchi Director de esta Repartición Municipal, Referido a la Instalación de la Gota de Leche en Abril 1930', in Moreyra, Remedi and Roggio, *El Hombre y sus Circunstancias,* 482-85.

52   The classification of infant mortality internationally used was the one elaborated by the French paediatrician Robert Debré and included: 'low': less than 40; 'moderate': from 40 to 69; 'high': from 70 to 99: 'very high': from 100 onwards. P. Dezeo, 'Demografía Internacional', in *Actas y Trabajos del VICNM,* III (Rosario: Est. Gráfico Pomponio, 1939), 612-32: 619.

53 C. Piantoni and P. Luque, 'Protección Médico-social de la Primera
Infancia en Córdoba', in *Actas y Trabajos del V ICNM,* III (Rosario: Est.
Gráfico Pomponio, 1939), 574-78: 575.

54 For the assistance of ill newborns, there were between 15 and 20 cots
at the Children's Hospital, and between 10 and 15 at the Institute of
Maternity.

55 Piantoni and Luque, 'Protección Médico-social de la Primera Infancia',
578.

56 D. Guy, 'Public Health, Gender, and Private Morality: Paid Labour and
the Formation of the Body Politic in Buenos Aires', *Gender and History,*
3 (1990), 297-317: 297.

57 E. Del Campillo, *'La Gota de Leche': Cuatro Años de Funcionamiento del
Consultorio Protector de la Infancia* (Córdoba: Imp. Mitre, 1908), 8.

58 Barrancos, 'Contracepcionalidad y Aborto en la década de 1920'.

59 According to Susana Torrado, the shift from a pattern of natural
fecundity to a planned one took place between 1885 and the beginning
of the 1930s, when birth rates declined below 30 per cent. S. Torrado,
'Transición de la Familia en Argentina, 1870-1995', *Desarrollo Económico,*
39, 154 (1999), 235-60: 237.

60 The condemnation of abortion was a topic highly agitated by Catholic
doctors. In Córdoba, one of them, Dr Bas, calculated that in the 1930s
for each baby born there were 10 abortions. B. Bas, *Aborto y Denatalidad*
(Córdoba: Pereyra, 1942).

61 Nari, 'Las Prácticas Anticonceptivas', 176.

62 D. Iraeta and J. Beruti, 'Protección a la Maternidad Ilegítima', in *Actas y
Trabajos del IICNM,* III, 303-16: 308.

63 M. Acuña, 'Protección a la Mujer Embarazada, a las Madres Solteras y
Madres Abandonadas', in *Actas y Trabajos del IICNM,* III, 269-75: 273.

64 A punishment with a minimum of 6 months to a maximum of 3 years
was applied, '[t]o the mother that, for hiding her dishonour, would kill
her child during birth or during the influence of the puerperal state,
and to the parents, brothers/sisters, husband and children that with the
aim of hiding the dishonour of the daughter, sister, spouse or mother
would commit the same crime'. *Código Penal de la República Argentina*
(Buenos Aires: Zavalía, 1989), 30.

65 Thus by 1934, the statistics for the first twentieth years of the asylum
show for a population of 7,977 in-women, that the main diseases were
as follows: dementia praecox 22,8% followed by a series that Kraepelin

would include as 'maniac-depressive' disorders: 'dysthymias' 19,4%; 'various deliriums'; 13,8% 'mental confusion' 10,2%. In: *Asilo Colonia Regional Mixto de Alienados en Oliva, Memoria Médico-Administrativa de 1934*, 20.

66 H. Marland, *Dangerous Motherhood: Insanity and Childbirth in Victorian Britain* (Basingstoke: Palgrave McMillan, 2004), 203-4.

67 *La Voz del Interior*, 9 October 1922, 6.

68 Acuña, 'Protección a la Mujer Embarazada', 272.

69 S. Torrado, 'Transición de la Familia en Argentina'. For the discussion of illegitimacy in Latin America and at the League of Nations in the 1920s and 1930s, see Scarzanella, 'Los Pibes en el Palacio de Ginebra'.

70 Torrado, 240.

71 A. Peralta Ramos, 'Protección de la Madre Desamparada', 322.

72 Ibid.

73 In Córdoba only one charitable institution (*Patronato de Presos y Liberados*) ran a 'Home for Minor Mothers' from 1918, which provided rooms for 30 young mothers. It also offered them medical assistance, primary education, lessons in 'Domestic Economy', and jobs (i.e. laundry and ironing services) that they performed at the institution for outside clients.

74 There were seven Sisters placed in strategic institutional areas where a rational spending was required: pharmacy, store and kitchen, laundry and wardrobe, and the sterilisation room. In a historical account about the Congregation, it was asserted, 'the director was convinced that the Sisters represented an economy for the institute, for he checked the spending before and after, resulting in a superior economy than when sisters were not there.' In H.F.Lueza, *Breve Reseña Histórica. Congregación de las Hermanas Carmelitas Descalzas de la Tercera Orden: Sus Fundaciones y Obras en las Repúblicas de Argentina y Uruguay (1896-1936)* (Buenos Aires: J. Belsolá y Cia., 1936), 111.

75 A. Peralta Ramos, 'La Asistencia Social en el Instituto de Maternidad de la Sociedad de Beneficencia de la Capital', in *Obstetricia, Ginecología y Puericultura*, 338-56: 355; and J. Lascano, *El Instituto de Maternidad de la Facultad de Ciencias Médicas de la Universidad Nacional de Córdoba* (Córdoba: Imprenta Pereyra, 1937), 70.

76 G. Martínez, 'Introducción al Estudio de la Puericultura', *RCMC*, 3 (1913), 404-16: 408. In that year, the National Council of Education started a campaign at High School level to promote infant care. In

Córdoba the course was titled 'Introduction to puericulture study' and was held at the Normal School (i.e. the educational institutes that were created in Argentina to train teachers for primary school education.

77 Martínez, 'Introducción al Estudio de la Puericultura', 404.

78 Ibid., 416.

79 Soria, 'Obras realizadas en Córdoba', 96.

80 M. Nari, 'La Educación de la Mujer (O Acerca de Cómo Cocinar y Cambiar los Pañales a su Bebé de Manera Científica)', *Mora*, 1 (1995), 31-45: 36-7.

81 In addition to teaching, the discipline allowed women to develop a series of related skills such as the organisation of conferences, the editing of reviews and specialised manuals.

82 J. Lascano and M. O'Farrel, 'La Cirugía Obstétrica en la Placenta Previa', in *Actas y Trabajos del IICNM,* III, 417-51: 444.

83 J. Beruti, J. León, and J. Diradourian, 'La Inducción del Parto por Medios Puramente Médicos en Embarazadas con Rotura Prematura Espontánea de las Membranas Ovulares', in *Actas y Trabajos del VCNM*, V, (Rosario: Talleres Gráficos Pomponio, 1935), 587-91: 587.

84 A. Peralta Ramos and A. Guiroy, 'Gobierno y Dirección del Parto', in *Actas y Trabajos del VCNM*, V, 389-94: 392.

85 Ibid., 390.

86 Ibid., 391.

87 Ibid., 387.

88 A. Guiroy and A. González Collazo, 'La Ruptura Artificial Precoz de la Bolsa de las Aguas', in *Actas y Trabajos del VCNM*, V, 761-67: 767.

89 Delmas quoted in C. Marramá, 'Evacuación Extemporánea del Útero: Método de Paul Delmas', *RCMC* (1939), 1563-90: 1579. My emphasis.

90 C. Marramá, 'Evacuación Extemporánea del Útero', 1579-80.

91 Guiroy, and González Collazo, 'La Ruptura Artificial Precoz', 764.

92 E. Martin, *The Woman in the Body: A Cultural Analysis of Reproduction* (Milton Keynes: Open University Press, 1989), 146.

93 Marramá, 'Evacuación Extemporánea del Útero', 1578.

94 U. Fernández, 'La Asistencia del Parto', *La Semana Médica*, 23 (1916), 312-17: 316.

95 V. Carro, 'El Régimen Alimenticio de la Embarazada Obesa', *RCMC* (1935), 327-47: 335. Italics in the original.

96 Beruti, J. León, and J. Diradourian, 'La Abreviación del Parto Aproximadamente Fisiológico', in *Actas y Trabajos del VCNM*, V, 395-

403: 395.

97 P. Treichler, 'Feminism, Medicine and the Meaning of Childbirth', in M. Jacobus, E. Fox Keller and S. Shuttleworthet (eds.), *Body/Politic: Women and the Discourses of Science* (New York: Routledge, 1990), 113-38:117.

98 J. Lascano, 'La Obstetricia en los Últimos 25 años', *Annaes Brasileiros de Gynecología*, 6, 5 (1938), 1-19: 3.

2

Towards a Taxonomy of Maternal Bodies: Biotypology, Eugenics and Argentine Nationalism (1930-1946)

During the 1930s, the prolonged decline of birth rates in Argentina, along with other factors such as high infant mortality rates and the existence of 'weakening' diseases such as tuberculosis, alcoholism, and syphilis, meant that the 'demographic question' became a matter not only of the quantity, but also of the quality of the population. 'One Argentinian in three grows up to be an inferior man,' a Socialist deputy noted with alarm, later concluding: 'The energies of the nation are in danger'.[1] The immediate effect of such opinions was the creation of the National Direction of Maternity and Infancy (NDMI) in 1936, which reflected the perceived relationship between woman and nation, together with the political possibility of intervention to transform bodies based on a belief in eugenics. This intellectual framework had many points of reference in other countries such as France, Italy, and Germany, where the state intervened in the private sphere to regulate the family, sexuality, reproduction, and particularly maternity, in order to promote biological and social change.

In Argentina, following the French model of *puériculture*, the mother and, by extension, child care became the principal object of eugenics, and maternity and infancy institutes its main centre of action. Explaining this relationship, a prominent obstetrician, Dr Josué Beruti, stated in the Second Pan-American Conference of Eugenics held in Buenos Aires in 1934 that,

> maternity, considered in its broadest sense, encompasses most of the eugenic problems requiring urgent solution, both in our country and in the majority of American nations. Women are overwhelmingly those primarily responsible for the bodily and spiritual health of the people … We must understand, then, the enormous significance that maternity has in relation to eugenics.[2]

Some results of this thinking were expressed on a socio-political level in legislation for the protection of working mothers. Notably, eugenic ideas formed an inextricable part of the creation of the Argentinian welfare state through the establishment of maternity leave (1934), maternity insurance (1936), and the National Direction of Maternity and Infancy as the main institution devoted to the provision of welfare for mother and children.

In medical terms, eugenics in the 1930s became linked with a new tendency in medicine: constitutional medicine, which was developed by focusing on the individual as a morphological, physiological, and psychological unit, within a relational and holistic interpretation. Constitutional medicine was born in and around the 1920s as a reaction to the medical mainstream, as represented by Pastorian analytical medicine and its focus on germs, which had led to specialisation, loss of clinical direction, and a rather dehumanised approach. In attempting to focus on the 'individual behind the disease,' constitutionalists sought to understand individual responses to illness by analysing body-mind relationships along with environmental conditions. To demonstrate the individual's unique reaction to disease, they used complex body-typing schemes, encompassing all the variables they considered to be determinative. In this context, biotypology became a discipline devoted to providing instruments with which to gauge this integral approach to patients, with the aim of enabling physicians to diagnose and treat more effectively.

In the early twentieth century, different schools of biotypology were created in Italy, France, and Germany, which were informed by distinctive strands of scientific thought and shaped by particular national, political, and cultural circumstances. In Argentina, the most influential school was the one first developed by Nicola Pende in Italy in the 1920s and 1930s. Pende had established a typology of the individual based on the study of heredity as well as on the combination of physical constitution (weight, height, muscular mass, cranial and hand proportions, etc.), temperament (neuroendocrine system), and character (psychology). He called this combination 'biotype,' which he considered to include 'all the individual differences of vital manifestation'.[3] Types thus became the result of the combination of continuing variables, for which the English Biometric School, cofounded by Francis Galton and his disciple Karl Pearson, largely contributed the statistical methods.[4] A plethora of taxonomies resulted from the combination of metabolic, endocrinological, psychological, and physical studies, whereby, it was thought, predisposition to disease could be anticipated and, above all, the possibility of individual intervention could be achieved.

Central to the growth of constitutional medicine was endocrinology and its interrelated approach to the body's internal systems, which fostered the perception of the individual as an integrated psychological and physical entity. The study of endocrinology would become essential to dealing with the problems raised by fertility in this decade. Endocrinology's identification of the 'hormonal body,' sexual hormones, and their influence on women's genital and reproductive development proved to be paradigmatic. Unprecedented procedures of intervention on the female body were tested: for example, the manipulating of secondary characteristics to render women fertile when 'constitutionally' they were not. In the combination of constitutional and endocrine studies it is possible to see, first, an unusual taxonomic will that aimed to establish a prototype of the fertile woman – a task undertaken by biotypology – and second, a tendency to correct detected physical anomalies in order to meet ideal types. I shall argue that both procedures were informed by, and contributed to shaping, a distinctive medical practice of eugenics in Argentina. Thus, the desire for ideal fertile bodies reveals in the 1930s a particular concern for the quantity but especially for the *quality* of the population. In addition, the developments in endocrine studies also led to eugenic practices such as 'temporary' or 'biological' sterilisation. By drawing attention to sterilisation practices, I will argue that negative measures of eugenics, although legally banned, still found a subtle application.

As Dr Beruti rightly stated, it was in maternity wards that the obstetrician, the gynaecologist, and the puericultor could develop 'the most correct and prudent application of eugenic principles'.[5] However, it seems that in maternal assistance centres a wide range of practices were performed, many of which would fall outside the classification of 'positive eugenics,' the term that eugenists and historians have usually assigned to Argentina's relatively moderate eugenic measures. Positive eugenics refers to welfare legislation and health measures that aimed to improve social and environmental conditions in order to encourage the reproduction of the fit – as opposed to 'negative eugenics,' which attempted to proscribe the reproduction of the unfit through the use of radical surgical methods. The 1930s, however, witnessed a change, as Nancy Stepan has noted, when a more negative and racist eugenics began to circulate.[6] Indeed, in Argentina it was at a time of conservatism and intensified nationalism that concern about racial consolidation and the 'fitness of the nation' became a prominent theme. But in spite of the negative legislation then in force in some European countries and in the United States, which sanctioned involuntary sterilisation or legalised abortion, Argentina stood within the Latin American mainstream, which had the goal of 'preventing' rather than 'proscribing' hereditary risks of reproduction. To illustrate this turn to the right, Stepan describes a distinctive form of negative reproductive eugenics that took place in Latin America: 'matrimonial eugenics,' which was enforced in the majority of countries through premarital medical examination (in Argentina this became law in 1936).[7]

Stepan's ground-breaking and pioneering study of eugenics in Argentina, Brazil and Mexico offered an account, in her words, 'primarily through the prism of the movement itself'.[8] Such an approach, however, has prevented her from demonstrating the influence of eugenics on medical practices, a topic that constitutes the primary focus of this chapter. In addition, many historians have contributed to our understanding of the influence of eugenic ideas among intellectuals and social reformers (Eduardo Zimmerman, Marisa Miranda and Gustavo Vallejo), in immigration legislation (Susana Ramella), medical-legal discourse (Miranda and Vallejo), welfare policies (Marcela Nari), or ideological groups such as anarchists and socialists (Dora Barrancos).[9] However, it is possible to argue that these studies concentrate on only one side of the picture, in that they raise the question of how eugenics encouraged reproduction of the fit, and proscribed reproduction of the unfit. To evaluate how eugenics actually operated during this period, beyond the legislation and the ideological debates it generated, it is necessary to examine medical knowledge and practices.[10]

In this chapter, I will first explore the political and eugenic assumptions that informed the establishment of constitutional medicine and biotypology with its foundational science, endocrinology, within the scientific-medical scenario. I will then highlight the construction of the biotype of the fertile woman, which promoted a new corporal representation of motherhood conforming to desirable social values (sacrifice, physical strength, and prolificacy), and the obstetric and gynaecological treatments that this prompted. Special attention will be drawn to sterilisation practices and debates in a time when concern over the quality of the population, as I shall argue, occupied a primary position. Finally, I will focus on the social representations of motherhood that this eugenically orientated medical perspective proposed.

A scientific discipline for Argentinian anxieties

The reception of biotypology in the Argentina of the 1930s stemmed from a long tradition of Latin American scientific thought marked by an early scientific adherence to Lamarckian principles. Lamarckism was based on the inheritance of acquired characteristics, and its adherents argued that many of the diseases acquired in the social milieu – such as tuberculosis, syphilis, or alcoholism – could be transmitted to the offspring, causing irremediable traits or racial degeneration. The belief that it was possible to intervene in the milieu where these diseases were produced resulted in political support for social-medical action, which was expected to benefit the racial patrimony of the nation. This neo-Lamarckism, as Nancy Stepan has stated, was the outcome of an early identification with French medicine, the influence of Catholicism, and an initial pessimism toward the heredity theories of Gregor Mendel and August Weismann.[11] The latter had a strong presence in Anglo-Saxon countries, and upheld the idea that the germinal plasma was transmitted from generation to generation independently of human and environmental action.

As the decade progressed, it became less possible in genetic terms to support the neo-Lamarckian doctrine, yet Latin American science continued to be reluctant to reorient itself toward biological determinism. In its place, loyal to the Latin tradition of France and Italy, the theory of constitution or biotypology was embraced, offering a compromise between the two doctrines by recognising both the inheritance of constant characteristics and the influence of the environment in the individual's final adaptation. Indeed, constitutionalists attributed a central role to the environment in shaping the biotype, which ultimately determined individual reaction to disease. One of the greatest influences in Argentina was the American endocrinologist Charles Stockard, who believed that basic characteristics were inherited and remained constant as Mendel had suggested, although he considered that the 'type could only be expressed to the degree allowed by the individual's environment'.[12]

Biotypology's wide uptake was also linked with the need to channel the interpretive and classificatory anxieties of many Latin American states whose populations' racial mix constituted a risk to national cohesion and identity. In Argentina, the census of 1914 found that nearly one third of the population was foreign (mainly Italians and Spaniards) – and in Buenos Aires, the home of intellectuals and social reformers, this percentage astonishingly rose to one half.[13] Although the majority of this migration came from Europe, the immigrants were far from the ideal cultured and civilised Europeans whom Argentinian statesmen had longed to attract to populate the nation: most were poor, illiterate workers fleeing from distressed economic conditions in their homeland. Moreover, their reluctance to integrate into the mores and values of the new society threatened a national unit that soon was interpreted in biological terms. National identity was further challenged by the arrival of new migratory waves from the East (Russians, Syrians, Chinese) in the 1930s, prompting discussions about the advisability of a racial mix in the population: the debates tended toward its condemnation, particularly because many in the 1930s thought that the eastern immigration would enrich very little the national biotype.

However, biotypology was also welcomed because its distinctive perspective on human beings was not based on racial types.[14] Medical constitutionalists insisted that simple observation should indicate the body's anomalies, which then were structured by the doctor's vision. As one of the Argentinian constitutionalists put it,

> these anomalies of mass and form are imposed by all the evidence of geometric facts, because to weigh, to measure, and to appreciate the balance of lines and the external characteristics of an individual requires nothing but the knowledge of the normal geometrical fact, that is, the knowledge of the 'constitutional types in their normal variation.[15]

These ideas facilitated the acceptance of the new medical postulates, although the language on which the types were based internalised hierarchies and segregation among groups of individuals. In a context of political and economic crisis, of social unrest and shifting gender relations, the idea of an 'integral' or 'holistic' interpretation of individuals represented a functional perspective for a state wishing to redress the impulses of modernity. Thus Argentinian supporters of eugenics found in biotypology an instrument not only for the identification and definition of a national type, but also, as I shall argue here, for its improvement. Knowing, recording, and treating the different biotypes that populated the nation would contribute to a better reproduction of the fittest, which would result in a stronger, more powerful nation. In this framework, studies of the morphological profile of the population may be seen as responding to the need to calibrate the existing human potential in order to make it predictable in terms of fertility, health, labour forces, economy, education, and identity.

Biotypological studies, institutions and maternity centres

Within this context of national redesign, it is not surprising that physicians exhibited a nationalistic fervour to justify their intention to classify the population. One of them stated:

> It is necessary to devote all our efforts and sacrifices to achieving the formation of the ideal type that has to perpetuate the species throughout the centuries. When we achieve the formation of superior types, giving aims to nations, orientation to people, and ideals to races, only then will we have accomplished our duties.[16]

We know that this desire was not only rhetorical. The utility of the biotypes had conspicuous social and political implications. The League of Mental Hygiene and the Board of School Physicians undertook several studies and collected a myriad of demographic records. In the case of mental health, Argentinian psychiatrists promoted evaluative tests of individuals in the labour force with the aim of specifying workers' biological and physiological suitability for particular jobs. Some of these tests were carried out by the Institute of Psycho-technical and Professional Orientation and by the Department of Scientific Organization of Work and Psycho-technique within the League of Mental Hygiene.[17]

The studies of childhood also revealed many biotypological concerns and endeavours. The Board of School Physicians was the institution in charge of all the tests on schoolchildren, whose implications for the educational system have not yet been analysed. When the Board was organised in 1920 in Córdoba, paediatrician Dr Benito Soria, proposed that 'it is the school physician who should meticulously evaluate each child, taking all sorts of measurements and weights, with the aim of promoting a selection and distribution of students according to their constitution, predisposition, hereditary antecedents, diseases, etc.'.[18] The aim of these periodic checks was to determine the organic disability of each schoolchild and to pursue an early treatment. Children found to be in need of assistance were admitted to special schools such as the School for 'Weak' Children or psychiatric or judicial institutions. A so-called health card (*ficha sanitaria*) for each child was later implemented by the provincial Education Councils in Buenos Aires (1933) and Córdoba (1934).

More importantly, in the 1930s these studies and procedures had their

focal point in the Argentine Association of Biotypology, Eugenics, and Social Medicine created in Buenos Aires in 1932, probably the most active eugenic institution in South America. The Association created the Institute of
Biotypology, inspired by a similar institution in Genoa led by Nicola Pende,
who personally participated in and directed many of the projects in Buenos
Aires. Pende, who by the 1930s was providing the scientific rationale for
the doctrines of Mussolini, came to Buenos Aires at a time of cultural and
ideological expansion of Fascist ideas, as academic interchanges became part
of the attempt to unify 'Latin science' all over the world.[19] The Association
also created a Polytechnic School of Biotypology and Allied Matters where
students were trained in 'biological eugenics and puericulture' and in 'legal
and social eugenics'.[20]

One of the Association's projects was the study and specification of
the Argentinian biotype. We know nothing about its results, but we do know
that the Institute supported this project through an individual biotypological
record (*ficha biotipológica*), consisting of fifteen pages of meticulously collected
data, showing the use of three different classifications of the cephalic index,
which was scathingly criticised by a Mexican biotypologist for its exaggerated
complexity.[21] More importantly, women's potential fertility became central
to biotypologists because it was through sexual reproduction that the improvement of future generations occurred. Within the Association, the Department of Eugenics, Maternity, and Infancy, headed by Dr Beruti, set up
a centre devoted to medical research, maternal treatments, and educational
campaigns. This centre, along with the Buenos Aires Institute of Maternity
directed by Dr Alberto Peralta Ramos, provided the social and scientific rationale for maternal welfare across the country. It is instructive to consider
that Peralta Ramos regarded the Institute of Maternity as 'constitutes[ing]
the most valuable technical instrument in favour of the ends promoted by
the Argentine Association of Biotypology, Eugenics, and Social Medicine in
relation to health and the social protection of maternity'.[22]

In 1933 Peralta Ramos and Beruti, along with other members of the
Association of Biotypology, presented a 'Plan for the organization of the
welfare of mothers and newborns in Argentina' inspired by the *Opera Nazionale Maternità e Infanzia* founded in Italy in 1925. The plan, with some modifi-
cations, was approved by the National Congress in 1936 (law 12,341), which
created the National Direction of Maternity and Infancy (NDMI) under the
Ministry of the Interior. Its aim was 'to pursue the perfection of future generations,' 'combating infant mortality and morbidity' and 'protecting woman

in her condition as mother or future mother'.[23] The welfare policy of the NDMI – a highly centralised institution with oversight across the country – was both designed and supervised from Buenos Aires mostly by prominent members of the Association, such as Peralta Ramos, who also served at the NDMI's Advisory Committee.[24] The eugenic goals of the NDMI were reflected in the creation of a specific department, 'Eugenics and Maternity', which was responsible for (a) prenuptial, preconception, and prenatal eugenic treatment; (b) measures that assured the medical, obstetric, economic, moral, and social conditions of pregnancy, delivery, and postpartum care; (c) the shaping of social awareness or eugenic sympathies; and (d) the creation and technical direction of the following services: prenuptial and preconception consulting rooms; gynaecological and obstetric prenatal assistance; and Centres of Maternal and Infant Hygiene.[25] In the prenuptial and preconception consulting rooms of the centres, and in the country's main maternity hospitals, it is interesting to observe where eugenic endeavours were concentrated: a voluntary prenuptial certificate (for women); the diagnosis of sexual and maternal capacity; and the treatment of sterility, syphilis, and diseases that might affect the maternal-foetal compatibility (mental, urinary, venereal, and tubercular diseases). The centres were assisted by the departments of endocrinology and biotypology, and were connected to the dispensaries for syphilis and tubercular patients.[26]

By 1938, the distribution of maternal centres across the country was still uneven. While the capital, Buenos Aires, had nineteen centres, the rest of the country had only twenty-three – all located in provincial capitals, and many of them only partially equipped. By 1940 the NDMI had attempted to improve the provision of services by creating twenty-eight Centres of Maternal and Infant Hygiene and four maternity hospitals in the provinces; yet the doctors gathered at the Fourth National Congress of Obstetrics and Gynaecology deemed the improvements insufficient, demanding from the state 'funding to ensure the efficient accomplishment of the work of the NDMI'.[27] Despite the disparities between services in the capital and the provinces, the eugenically-oriented prenuptial and preconception consulting rooms were successfully established in the country's main maternity hospitals and centres after the creation of the NDMI. As we have seen in Chapter 1, some hospitals, such as the one in Córdoba designed by Dr José Lascano in 1932, were already organised along the lines of the Buenos Aires Institute of Maternity. Córdoba's maternity institute represented, in Lascano's words, 'the greatest conception of Peralta Ramos, constituting a model institution for

69

maternal and foetal assistance before, during, and after pregnancy'.[28]

Female types

> All that paediatrics and social welfare could do for the girl in her many
> stages of life in order to obtain a perfect woman, supervising her
> nutrition, games, gym, education, etc., would be the first step in the
> defence of the future mother and her offspring.[29]

In spite of these idealistic intentions, only failures were counted: girls who
died before becoming mothers, and others who accumulated diseases and
misfortunes that, it was feared, one day would not only be theirs. By 1935,
Argentina had a high infant mortality rate of 102 deaths per 1,000 births.
Around 60 per cent of these deaths were attributed to congenital and obstetrical causes. Syphilis and other diseases were considered to be the main
cause for dead foetuses, premature babies, and congenitally weak children
who were considered a 'human waste with permanent traits'.[30]

To make matters worse, the reproductive pattern of the population had
changed drastically during the period of demographic transition: from an average of seven children per woman in 1895 to around three at the end of the
1930s, indicating a clear tendency toward family planning,[31] which vexed doctors engaged in population studies. At the same time, between 1930 and 1940
a perceived change in the sexual composition of the urban population took
place, indicating an increase in the number of women, so that Buenos Aires
was no longer considered 'a city of lonely men'.[32] In this context, women
were thought to be primarily responsible for declining birth-rates – whether
due to their lack of maternal spirit, or their biological weakness. And remarkably, the majority of medical studies were directed toward women, and were
informed by a strong gender bias as we will see at the end of this chapter.

Along with the problem of 'degenerative diseases' such as alcoholism,
syphilis, and tuberculosis, one topic that increasingly worried physicians in
the 1930s was the anomalies of the female body, and in particular, the emaci-
ated woman: both the 'provoked thinness' in the case of working women,
due to poverty and labour exploitation, and the 'voluntary thinness' observable in affluent women, as a consequence of fashion and the imitation of the
silhouettes represented in magazines. This figure of the slim woman gave
rise, in the medical view, to a series of drastic problems that included compromised fertility, low birth-rate, total or partial dysfunction of the repro-

ductive organs, miscarriages, difficult childbirths, lack of lactation, and an array of physical deficiencies that, it was feared, could be transmitted to the offspring.[33] In this sense, constitutional medicine simply added new representations to a female body already designated by the medical literature as an inferior and sickly subject. Considering the constitutional anomalies of the genital apparatus, Pende asserted in his most influential book, *Constitutional Inadequacies*,

> we may say that variants of a slight degree are rather frequent, especially partial variants in the field of function; they are considerably more frequent in the female than in the male, since the former is, as Mathes says, almost physiologically predisposed to conditions of general infantilism, of which sexual hypoevolutionism [retarded development] is the most characteristic side.[34]

It was believed that women's constitution played an overriding role in their fertility and sterility, which explains why constitutional studies were widened to include the diagnosis and treatment of almost all gynaecological ailments. Following the classification of Achille De Giovanni, who had described three constitutional human types according to the structure of the torso – brevilineal (short and fat), normotype, and longuilineal (tall and slim) – Pende defined ten different somatic morphological groups, informed by an analysis of the endocrine system, which he believed conferred an 'individual endocrine formula' that had to be decoded for diagnosis and treatment purposes. The three basic body types marked different fertility types: brevilineal was cast as the most fertile woman at the top of the scale, longuilineal at the bottom, with the normal types in the middle. These three types were also linked to different psychological characteristics, which doctors considered necessary to identify for a more effective treatment: 'The influence of the woman's constitutional type on gynaecological pathologies is so significant that it could be said that in the majority of cases there is a constitutional predisposition for such disorders'.[35]

The classification of female types with their intricate relationships of variables, as utilised by biotypologists in Buenos Aires, provides one perspective on the socio-political aims that the female biotype came to fulfil. To be sure, the biological taxonomy was combined with a classification of behaviour that sought to make women into identifiable and codifiable beings beyond the medical context. Thus, within a classification system sensitive to

71

harmonies and proportions, deficiencies and excesses were easily pathologised. Two groups were identified: the deficient, or 'hypotonic,' and the excessive, or 'hypertonic'.[36]

A. The *hypotonic type* was subdivided into three categories:

(1) The *asthenic* present with flaccidity in the tissues, a lack of vital energy, and pronounced slowness in growth. Within this group, the most frequent type in Argentinian women was the *microsplanchnic*, which Pende described as having a long thorax, a narrow pelvis, small breasts, uterine and sexual hypoplasia (underdevelopment of the organs), a masculine distribution of hair, and limited fertility. Subjective phenomena: general weakness, melancholy, nervousness, frigidity, and vaginismus. 'It corresponds to the type of modern girl who wants to be slim at all costs', doctors Peralta Ramos and Schteingart asserted.

(2) The *infantile* present with physical and psychological characteristics of childhood, severe genital hypoplasia, and secondary sexual characteristics incomplete. Emotionally apathetic and unstable, they also present frigidity and vaginismus. Hereditary cause: syphilis or alcoholism in the parents or, more likely, hypophysis exhaustion of the mother during pregnancy. In general they are sterile, undergo many miscarriages, and produce an insufficient lactation.

(3) The *intersexual* present with the characteristics of the infantile type but, in addition, masculine features observable in the distribution of hair, frigidity, and voice. The ovarian function is diminished, causing sterility, genital hypoplasia, and general asthenia. 'Her life is full of moral and material conflicts'. They have also been classified as schizophrenics.

B. The *hypertonic type* refers to 'physiological gigantism', in which the 'feminine features are exaggeratedly developed' as in the case of obese women, but skinny women also form part of this group. Both types present with several glandular disorders (caused by the hypophysis or suprarenal glands).

In an endocrine-constitutional study of sterile women carried out by the Department of Biotypology of the Institute of Maternity (Buenos Aires), 87 per cent were classified as microsplanchnic.[37] Furthermore, half of these women showed a certain degree of hypoplasia, the other half infantilism, and a quarter presented with intersexualism.

Argentinian biotypologists, however, did not seek simply to offer statistical biotype analysis of female sterility conditions: once women's biotypes were determined, the analysis was continued in the Department of Endocrinology, with both departments (Biotypology and Endocrinology) working together in the prenuptial and preconception consulting rooms of the country's main maternity hospitals. The endocrine study involved a laboratory analysis of the different glands with the aim of providing correlations between body types and specific glandular disorders. Only then was the diagnosis completed and treatment proposed. This provides us insight into the way in which biotypologists combined their interpretation of eugenic ideas. For example, when the biotype indicated a predisposition to sterility, which was sometimes attributed to inherited conditions, endocrine studies provided the possibility of intervention, and thus of improvement of the biotype.

As these studies progressed, some doctors proposed that a semiological analysis of the features of the face was sufficient for detecting ill women. For Dr Antonio Navarro of Córdoba, the most numerous group was represented by the visceral-endocrine-vegetative disorders that corresponded to a number of facial types. The diseases were classified as: hypophyseal (with facial types including acromegalic, infantile, ephebic, and facies characteristic of Frölich syndrome), thyroid (with Basedowian, myxedemic, and cretinised facial types); or gonadic (with ovarian, virile, gerodermic, eunuchised, and matronly facial types).[38] The unreadable classification of female facial types that Dr Navarro embraced meaningfully illustrates a quest for external signs that could be used to convert female diversity into a universal and understandable code. It is revealing that when medical language abandoned such undecipherable technical terms in order to make its meaning clearer, the biotype became reduced to only two terms: maternal and non-maternal. Not surprisingly, an ideal type of fertile woman was soon described, and characterised as a strong, muscular woman with a vigorous and active personality, a long reproductive life, abundant menstruations, and a late menopause.[39] However, such extreme classification in the search for human types must be seen as ultimately political. Not least because despite the number of taxonomies, constitutionalists themselves asserted that the ideal type did not exist. This impossibility demonstrates the fictional function of the biotype in the medical thought and, by extension, in the national politics, ideology, and culture of the time. It was of no importance whether existing women could effectively fulfil the imaginary type. Rather, it was enough to know, as a principle, that a universal female subject was possible and always desirable. Moreover, this classification continued to be used in medical language to describe female bodies, and it was

73

also considered to be a distinctive mark to stereotype women's behaviour, as we will see in the last section of this chapter. We shall now explore the questions of how Argentinians dealt with women's biological flaws and constitutional inadequacies, to what extent the field of intervention was restricted, what therapeutic methods were involved, and whether these were informed by positive or negative eugenics.

Endocrine research and treatments: The improvement of types

Medical responses to female sexual reproduction seem to have oscillated between discouraging advice and therapeutic optimism. To start with, the director of the Association of Biotypology, Eugenics, and Social Medicine, Dr Arturo Rossi, proposed an addition to the existing causes of 'matrimonial impediment' in the Civil Code (leprosy and venereal disease): namely, 'defects in stature, in corporal mass, in weight, and some severe problems of endocrine characteristics'.[40] Although his request was ignored by legislators, it is very likely that in the prenuptial and preconception consulting rooms these and other types of dysgenic women were discouraged from marrying or becoming mothers. Explaining the eugenic importance of those consulting rooms, Dr Peralta Ramos spoke of the resultant advantage: 'we not only avoid the worsening [due to pregnancy] of mothers' pre-existing diseases, but principally we avoid the birth of idiot, deformed, or ill creatures, destined for an early death or to endure a life full of torture and misfortune'.[41]

Second, biotypology was also 'orthogenesis,' the then-current term used to indicate the possibility of correcting individuals who deviated from the type. Gynaecologists believed that with the development of endocrine studies and with the administration of hormones, they could affect and regulate many of those women who did not meet the ideal normal type: 'From our results we deduce that in 80 per cent of cases constitutional sterility is accompanied by alterations in fat metabolism, the hypophysis being the main factor determining obesity or slimness'.[42] This central role attributed to the hypophysis led to a wide range of therapeutic interventions, and gynaecologists enthusiastically credited the 'hormonotherapy of the hypophysis with the successful genital correction of such syndromes as infantilism'.[43]

From the end of the nineteenth century to the 1940s, endocrinology was one of the most dynamic areas of biomedical research and, with bacteriology, was among the first to re-establish its direct utilisation in the medical clinic, after thyroid gland extract proved its efficiency in the treatment of myxedema.[44] Since the discovery of the glands of internal secretion in 1905 (later called hormones), and especially with the study and synthesis of sexual hormones in the 1930s, a strong optimism accompanied endocrine research, which as Nelly Oudshoorn has noted, broadened the possibilities for medical intervention in an unprecedented way.[45] In relation to my wider enquiry, I would argue that not only did endocrinology assure sexual difference through the hormonal body, but hormonal therapy also opened up a field of medical intervention hitherto unattainable. It provided the female reproductive body with a mean of correcting any constitutional deviation or insufficiency, from menstrual dysfunction to infantilism, from which Argentinian women allegedly suffered greatly.

Significantly, it was during the 1930s that Argentina witnessed the rapid development and growing worldwide reputation of its physiological institutes. These institutes formed a network including the cities of Córdoba, Rosario, and Buenos Aires, and were headed by the first Argentinian Nobel Prize winner, Bernardo Houssay. Crucial to this development was the substantial economic support from the Rockefeller Foundation, by then interested in financing studies on endocrine hormones 'that could illuminate issues of growth, body activities, behaviour, old age and sexuality'.[46] Under the patronage of the Rockefeller Foundation, and in close connection with American endocrine constitutionalists, Argentinian physiology expanded studies on the female sexual cycle, hormones, and hormonotherapy. Houssay received worldwide recognition for his findings, notably for his research on the influence of the pituitary gland (hypophysis) in the regulation of carbohydrate metabolism and diabetes, placing the hypophysis, in his words, at 'the centre of the endocrine constellation'.[47] Although he embraced a holistic interpretation in physiology, there is no evidence that his physiological approach was connected with the biotypological perspective. On the one hand, the Rockefeller Foundation funded eugenically oriented programs on the genetics of mental traits in the 1930s; as Diane Paul has stated, 'in the Anglo-American world, eugenists had always emphasised the importance of mental, rather than physical, characteristics.'[48] On the other hand, gynaecologists working with biotypes and endocrine studies were undoubtedly influenced by Houssay's discoveries, clearly in the central role attributed to the hypophysis, for its secretion of both reproductive and non-reproductive hormones. However, Houssay's name never appears in the gynaecologists' articles that I have consulted. Whilst personal sensitivities may have played a part in this lack of recognition, Houssay and constitutionalists were tied to different scientific

75

influences: the American, in the case of the physiological institutes, and the Italian and German, in the case of the Institute of Biotypology.

In any case, gynaecologists' optimism was such that tests did not stop even in the absence of evidence. Commenting on results obtained from the use of follicular hormone in the treatment of infantilism and other ovarian deficiencies, a gynaecologist wrote that 'hormonal therapy can modify abnormal conditions of this organic function, even though the inner mechanism of this action still escapes our knowledge'.[49] It is also revealing that the increase observed in studies of experimental endocrinology and its rapid translation into clinical practice soon came in for criticism from gynaecologists themselves. Seeking to explain the growing number of extra uterine pregnancies in 1940, a gynaecologist from Córdoba asserted that, 'we believe that the hasty use of follicular hormone constitutes an etiologic factor in endometriosis and, therefore, in extra uterine pregnancy'.[50] The National Congress of Medicine in 1934 was another place to observe this 'hasty' enthusiasm, as witnessed by not only the significant number of papers presented there but, more particularly, by the scale that hormonal manipulation and experiments had attained. A good example is the claim, by Dr Pedro Pla of Rosario, that an injection of a pregnant woman's urine – which he tested in both sexes – exercised a 'specific influence on the development of the genital organs',[51] and in the cure of other gynaecological disorders. Reading these clinical experiments against the backdrop of the general desire for population growth, any sort of test seems to have been validated as an effort to convert infertile bodies into fertile ones.

Hormonotherapy was also used to correct abnormal weight in pregnant women because this was thought to cause toxaemia of pregnancy (hypertensive states, superimposed on chronic hypertensive vascular or renal disease), which caused a significant number of infant deaths as well as premature and weak babies. It was estimated that pregnancy should add no more than 20 per cent to a woman's normal weight. Concerned by those who exceeded that norm, and acting according to the classification of female body types, Dr Víctor Caro of Córdoba treated his patients with a nutritional plan combined with the administration of thyroid extract, which he considered of 'great utility . . . to obtain the ideal weight of the woman which is the goal of the treatment'.[52]

Another platform where the significance of hormonotherepay could be observed is in the Fifth Argentine Congress of Obstetrics and Gynaecology (1940), where two of the four main topics were devoted to endocrine matters. One of these focused on the constitutional problem of 'genital hypoplasia'. In a paper entitled 'Social Factors of Genital Hypoplasia', a well-known female gynaecologist, Dr Mercedes Rodríguez, signalled the influence of heredity and poor working conditions on the malformation of bodies, bone lesions, abortions, premature foetuses, and congenital weaknesses. She advised that a eugenically oriented endocrine treatment, by 'tending to the harmony and perfection of bodies through the milieu in which they were developed,' was the best way to deal with those tenuous female bodies.[53]

Endocrinology was instrumental for biotypologists in more than one way: as well as providing much of the scientific rationale for knowledge of the fertile potential of the population (female biotypes), and contributing therapy for the 'correction' of that potential, it also provided a biological means of sterilising women temporarily. Further examination of sterilisation methods will allow us to assess whether these methods were also used for eugenic purposes.

Temporary and definitive sterilisation

The conservation of the species is due to endocrine-glandular balance; for this reason deliberate biological sterilisation results from the disruption of that physiological harmony.[54]

As may be expected, biological methods of temporary sterilisation disrupted more than a 'physiological harmony.' Not least because the availability of new means and methods of sterilisation was closely intertwined with the controversial topic of the artificial prevention of pregnancy. Indeed, before the advent of hormonal temporary sterilisation, many procedures were performed to find ways of ensuring sterility for a variable period, avoiding the more complicated temporary surgical methods. Grafts of ovaries or placenta, injections of corpus luteum and of the anterior lobe of the hypophysis, were widely tested in laboratories and in women's bodies. By the mid-1930s, one of the most prevalent procedure was the injection of sheep spermatozoids, both because of the method's accessibility and because it was considered less apt to spread tuberculosis, syphilis, and gonococci.[55] The resultant immunization lasted about one year, a period that could be extended by reinoculation.

The legal context in which sterilisation took place in Argentina was anything but straightforward. On the one hand, definitive sterilisation was banned by the Penal Code, which in its article 91 sanctioned 'imprisonment

77

for three to ten years, if the lesion produces . . . the loss . . . of the capacity to conceive'.[56] However, in practice, jurisprudence authorised doctors to practice sterilisation on the same grounds that legally authorised them to perform a 'therapeutic abortion' (article 86, sect. 2), 'to avoid a danger to the mother's life or health'.[57] In the case of sterilisation, jurisprudence trusted to the knowledge, discretion, and prudence of the specialist, and only in 1967 would 'a clear therapeutic indication' be demanded by law.[58] The medical literature that I have reviewed for the period indicates that this legal framework seems to have neither restrained nor worried doctors in their practice; they were acting in a fairly permissive field, which aimed to safeguard the mother's life or health in cases where pregnancy was thought to complicate a pre-existing disease. Chronic or temporary tuberculosis, cardiovascular illnesses, diabetes, haemophilia, and a wide range of urinary, renal, endocrine, obstetric, and mental diseases fell into this category.

For a Catholic country with a powerful, influential Church, however, there was a moral restraint that resolutely opposed the practice of sterilisation and abortions, regardless of the medical circumstances. The dogmatic principles of *Casti Connubii* – the encyclical of Pius XI (1930) that, among other things, condemned both temporary and definitive sterilisation[59] – were to be fiercely defended by the international and national Consortium of Catholic Doctors (*Consorcio de Médicos Católicos*, CCD), which the Pope himself urged be set up across the Catholic world. Undoubtedly, the moral condemnation raised by the encyclical and by the doctors gathered at the CCD was reflected in the caution with which obstetricians expressed in public their opinions and experiences of sterilisation. In practice, however, medical or therapeutic indications proved to be more important than religious ones, as we shall see later.

In a decade of eugenic debate, proposals, and institutions, and in light of the enactment of involuntary sterilisation laws in the United States and Germany,[60] sterilisation in Argentina became entwined with other, more questionable, aims: those destined to prevent the birth of undesirable beings. The absence of a sterilisation law, which has contributed to the notion of 'positive eugenics,' should not dissuade us from analysing this topic and its potential eugenic uses in subtle 'negative' practices. It is instructive to note that, for the Latin American eugenists gathered at the Pan-American Conference of 1934, the main objection to a sterilisation law was a lack of certainty regarding the laws of heredity. Yet not all doctors agreed: in Argentina there were many voices that recommended and sympathised with a eugenic sterilisation law (lawyers, legal physicians, hygienists, and psychiatrists), proposals

78

on which I am not going to dwell on this chapter. I will instead discuss obstetricians' and gynaecologists' opinions and clinical experiences.

The most influential obstetrician of the period, Dr Peralta Ramos, defined eugenics as the 'science of healthy generation', with the aim of 'combining generators in order to obtain the physical and intellectual improvement of the human species, and in particular, with the aim of combating the effects of the fatal inheritance arising from toxic and infectious diseases, such as alcoholism, syphilis, tuberculosis, and so forth'.[61] Such statements raise the question of whether sterilisation methods formed part of the therapeutics used for that aim, particularly for those who thought that the laws of heredity did apply in certain cases.

Biological methods for obtaining temporary sterilisation were generally well accepted – particularly by those obstetricians who considered temporary sterilisation by surgical methods to be a façade, since women later transformed it into a definitive procedure: 'it is very rare that someone comes to the clinic to ask for the reinstatement of the suppressed function', as one of them complained.[62] This positive perception can also be detected in medical records. Unlike the care evidenced in the protocols for 'definitive sterilisation', temporary biological procedures had far fewer data and specifications. This suggests that biological sterilisation was a field in which experiments and practices developed more freely – or, in other words, a space where the problem of moral conscience may have been less restrictive, or control over reproduction more effectively achieved. In one protocol presented by Drs Peralta Ramos (father and son) and Dr Mario Schteingart, involving more than 141 women at the Institute of Maternity, they described satisfactory results with the use of sheep spermatozoids. They omitted to specify, however, which women they had decided to sterilise, referring to them only vaguely as 'ill women.' Not a single reference is made to the kind of pathologies in which sterilisation was practiced: that is, whether it was to save the mother's life or to avoid the birth of weak children – an omission not found in recorded cases of definitive sterilisation.[63] A group of doctors from the city of La Plata (province of Buenos Aires) used this same biological method in 1937, with the difference that they explicitly commented on the indications that had preceded the sterilisation. First were cases of disease that put the mother's life in 'imminent danger', and second, a different category that they called 'a series of sociological indications' – namely, alcoholism, syphilis, and mental alienation.[64] The latter were clearly eugenic justifications.

This social, eugenic perspective was also to be found in cases of definitive sterilisation. In 1928, Peralta Ramos performed a therapeutic abortion followed by sterilisation on a woman with leprosy, which he justified by alluding to 'medical, eugenic, and social reasons'; and regarding the eugenic reason, he explained: 'The possibility of a hereditary transmission, the risk of contagion during delivery, the birth of a weak and sick child'.[65] This case also illustrates that 'therapeutic abortion,' like sterilisation, was performed to preserve the mother's health and life, and like sterilisation, too, its widely extended practice probably formed part of the same shadowy, ambiguous zone of eugenic use.

The relevance that the practice of sterilisation was acquiring during the 1930s can be traced through the increasing number of articles published in both non-Catholic and Catholic medical journals.[66] A good 'state of the question' is found in the Fourth Argentine Congress of Obstetrics and Gynaecology (1940), at which sterilisation was one of the two main themes. The main commentator of the Congress, Dr Manuel Pérez, director of the maternity centre at the Hospital Alvear in Buenos Aires, presented a detailed analysis of the history, methods, and indications of sterilisation. He devoted extensive commentaries to the eugenic indications, and reviewed each of the diseases covered by the German law (1933).[67] He concluded that sterilisation due to eugenic causes should be 'performed exceptionally,' and only in cases of indisputably hereditary disorders. He explicitly commented: 'we adhere to the practice of sterilisation in women with congenital feeblemindedness [idiocy, imbecility], manic-depressive psychosis, and alcoholism with psychopathic crises'.[68] He also added epilepsy, blindness, and deafness – as long as these were also confirmed in other family members. This shows that, despite frequent allegations about the shortcomings of theories of heredity, when heredity was thought to be proven, then sterilisation was accepted.

The second commentator in the Congress, Dr Arturo J. Risolía, presented a paper on the techniques involved in different sterilisation methods, which provide an insight into the growing development of these procedures. Some doctors successfully practiced temporary sterilisation through vaccinations of human and animal sperm (biological methods); others used X rays to obtain both temporary and definitive results – a technique practiced in the Institute of Radiology and Physiotherapy in Buenos Aires; and finally, some doctors considered surgical methods (tubal ligation) the most effective means of achieving either temporary or definitive sterilisation.[69] Dr Risolía also presented the results of a survey that he had sent to fifty obstetric and gynaecological services throughout the country, asking for details of the methods of temporary and definitive sterilisation used in the service; opinions on the surgical, radiological, and biological methods; numbers of cases treated; and their success and failure rate. Only eleven heads of service responded – a number that raises some speculation. The responses give us some idea of the practice of sterilisation, but not of specific cases in which it was performed. Overwhelmingly, doctors provided limited information. For example, Dr José Lascano from Córdoba reported only nine cases of 'definitive sterilisation' for the period 1918–39.[70] However, Lascano did not refer to 'temporary sterilisation,' which he had supported in an early study of tuberculosis and pregnancy. In that study, he recommended temporary sterilisation for young and working-class women (in the latter case, because he considered their access to other contraceptive methods to be nearly impossible), and the 'definitive method' for multiparous women.[71] Although he referred to the practice of sterilisation to avoid the deterioration of a tubercular patient, he preferred not to discuss whether moral, social, religious, or economic reasons should also be considered, leaving the decision to physicians' consciences. It is quite likely that obstetricians encountered this situation more than once, since tuberculosis was the main cause of death between 1900 and 1946, and its hereditary transmission, in both bacilliform and 'ultra virus' cases, was considered possible.

Overall, physicians made scant reference to their moral conscience in medical congresses. Obstetricians always tried to avoid confrontation with other colleagues, from the dogmatic Catholics to the more controversial scientific objections of those for whom the existence of recessive characteristics could 'annul, deviate, or modify hereditary determinism'.[72] It is revealing that Peralta Ramos celebrated the special treatment of sterilisation as a main topic in this Congress, given 'its medical importance, as much as its vast social and eugenics implications' – but in his paper he deliberately decided to 'remain in the medical domain . . . therefore, we will avoid all eugenic, social, professional, moral, and even religious considerations of this issue'.[73] He detailed eighty-six cases of definitive sterilisation (1928–39), sixteen of them performed jointly with abortion. Revealingly, the omission of the above mentioned case of the woman with leprosy confirms that he was referring *only* to cases that were medically, not eugenically, indicated. Of these, 43 per cent were driven by an apparent concern with the biotype – that is, with women suffering from narrow pelvis and intersexualism. It is striking that, in Peralta Ramos's data, narrow pelvis constituted the majority of cases (twenty-nine women with one previous caesarean, and seven with two previous ones),[74] for this condition was rarely a cause of sterilisation. Analysing the international tendency, Dr Pérez concluded: 'today [sterilisation] is abandoned thanks to the caesarean operation'.[75] He also stated that unless there were other concomitant factors, he performed sterilisation on patients with narrow pelvis only after the third caesarean section. Commenting on the sterilisations carried out by a psychiatrist in Brazil who had justified them on the basis of the 'perversity syndrome' of his patients, Stepan wrote a footnote with a legitimate suspicion, which I would extend to the obstetric field, she commented: 'This makes one think that eugenic sterilisations, perhaps disguised as purely medical procedures, were more common in mental and correctional institutions than is realised'.[76]

At the Congress of 1940 other speakers' contributions were sympathetic toward sterilisation, such as that of Dr Benjamín Galíndez, who considered temporary sterilisation 'a completely acceptable intervention', although he had never performed it.[77] In Dr Roberto Herrera's opinion, 'sterilisation, whether for medical or social-eugenic indications, is largely a way of helping nature in the selection of the fittest'.[78] The only negative response came from Dr Carlos A. Castaño, president of the Argentinian Consortium of Catholic Doctors, whose condemnatory speech was likely to have moderated the enthusiasm of some of his colleagues.

The rather restrained commentaries of some Argentinian obstetricians contrasted with those of the delegates from Uruguay, who related their cases and opinions with a great deal of determination and confidence. 'I have always performed it without any scruples of conscience',[79] stated one – an attitude probably reflecting the permissive legal framework provided by the Uruguayan Commission of Hygiene, something that did not exist in Argentina at that time. But contrary to what an initial view might suggest, the frugal, unrecorded, implicit, and therefore suspicious framework in which all sterilisation was performed in Argentina seems to have created a permeable space for its practice. Following the comments of the American eugenist Paul Popenoe, who stated that many U.S. official institutions carried out an increasing number of sterilisations with the agreement of the patient but without the authorisation of the law, Dr Ariosto Licurzi, a Cordoban supporter of the eugenic sterilisation of degenerates and criminals, concluded: 'This also happens in other countries, even in ours, although less frequently, without making them public, so the statistics do not appear to increase'.[80] It seems that by the end of the decade, obstetricians and gynaecologists, although acting without the framework of a sterilisation law, had managed to place this practice in a secular, more flexible, and more permissive domain. Those from a militant Catholic position – a minority – who would have liked to question the doctors who performed sterilisations during this period, would have had to be satisfied with the following assertion:

> When a competent and worthy physician recommends sterilisation for medical reasons, we believe him liberated of all immorality. These are problems of professional conscience ruled by deontology and medical ethics.[81]

Within this framework, the practice of sterilisation for eugenic purposes had the capacity to generate further practice, favourable opinions, and few clear condemnations. In any case, its presence deserves scholarly reinterpretation. While Stepan has concluded that, 'on the whole, the eugenists operated in a political, cultural, and religious climate in which birth control, abortion for any but the most strictly defined medical reasons, and sterilisation, whether for eugenic or feminist purposes, were unacceptable',[82] I have argued that the legal framework was insufficient to define the medical practice. The medical literature I have discussed for the decade of the 1930s and 1940s shows that some doctors carried out sterilisations to prevent the transmission of certain traits, although we do not know exactly how widespread this practice was. Others preferred not to comment publicly or to discuss whether eugenic justifications should be considered, leading to the suspicion that their viewpoint was nearer agreement than rejection – after all, if the legal, cultural, and religious climate opposed sterilisation, it would have been much the easier course for doctors to openly declare themselves against it rather than to go against the grain. In the last section, I would return to the rather distinctive way biotypologists shaped representations of motherhood by merging women's biological type with social behaviours.

Mother's new social representations

In an article suggestively titled 'Voluntary undernourishment in modern woman. A study of medicine, gynaecology and social obstetrics', Dr Beruti described with alarm what he thought was a 'collective illness': The voluntary loss of weight in women. Such a tendency distressed obstetricians, not only for the supposed harms inflicted on women's health, but more importantly, for its potential challenge to gender roles. According to Beruti, the 'prototype

83

woman of the epoch' was the one that, in the search of stylised lines, imitated the 'Anglo-Saxon model of the slim woman with unattractive rectilinear lines',[83] voluntarily putting herself on ridiculous diets to lose weight, obsessively and unnecessarily. The outcome was aesthetically devastating: 'haggard and angular faces, narrow thorax, fallen shoulders, skinny legs, . . . tiny and atrophied breast, reduced hips, rectilinear sizes'.[84] In addition, this prototype woman showed, Beruti went on to say, 'a suggestive tendency to make herself masculine'.[85] In other words, the image of the 'new woman' much contrasted with the traditional Argentinian matron, very prolific, rather fat and thick, with clear curves, big breasts, and in line with the canon, 'feminine'. Not surprisingly, this new 'masculinised' woman, ultimately, compromised something worse: 'her maternal capacity'.[86]

Medical metaphors of saving-spending were formulated by doctors to refer to a supposedly female energy, which according to the industrial times, were expressed in economic terms. If femininity, by means of sex hormones, became something that women could dispose of (not that they definitely had), then it became something quantifiable that could be increased as much as it could be wasted. Thus, for many doctors, the habits of the 'new woman' were producing an 'inestimable waste of female energies' that should be kept as a supreme good to carry out the primary and fundamental mission to which every woman was destined for: her maternal function.[87]

> To this ultra-refined type of masculine woman, to whom 'pregnancy and rearing' are little less than swearwords, the mention of procreative functions and the conservation of the species would result for her more and more disgraceful, harder, and sicker. [88]

Behind this perception of the 'ultra-refined type' of woman, can be found a parallel with fascist Italy, which as discussed earlier, is hardly surprising given the constant exchange of medical ideas that Argentinian doctors had with their Italian peers. As Lesley Caldwell has noted, the Italian campaign set up to increase the population as much as the defence of the 'stirpe' during fascism, and included the spread of a particular maternal image that was intended for woman to imitate. Thus, the robustness and curved forms were the most extended images in literature and visual representations of the period. 'The fascists demanded that mothers should not be elegant since elegance was a bar to fecundity, and 'slovenly' women were far more prolific'.[89] On the other hand, the Italian *Opera Nazionale Maternità e Infanzia* insisted on the dangers that fashion images were instilling through advertisements that promoted a thin, fragile female figure. These and other advice directly reached Buenos Aires's women through the Italian documentaries broadcasted by the *Argentine Association of Biotypology*, in the framework of its 'maternology campaigns' initiated in 1936.

The stigmatisation of slim women under their masculine aspects, undoubtedly responded to the activism of feminists and the liberation of social female practices, which, in its diversity, showed women's rejection of being identified as merely reproducers of the nation. It is also interesting to note how these perceptions were class linked. The commonly or occasionally fasting woman, the one who had a rather quiet social life (school teacher, student, secretary and store assistant) was thought 'to follow' the method in order to adapt herself to the exigencies of fashion, practising diet because of 'ingenuity and frivolity'. Yet the most voluntarily undernourished women were thought to belong to the well-to-do classes. 'They have a lot of external activities, a life in perpetual movement, where there predominate sporting activities, massage, walking, and even dancing'.[90] Not surprisingly, upper-class women were the ones who concerned gynaecologists and obstetricians the most for their exemplary potential as models who could create habits and behaviours later disseminated to the rest, especially to the middle classes, of whom doctors feared their latent tendency for imitation. Middle-class women, on the other hand, could endanger maternity for other reasons. Explaining their rejection to seek medical assistance during pregnancy, Dr Lascano thus described them,

> Resources are insufficient to afford a doctor's appointment because the style of modern life demands them to pretend to belonging to upper classes, with frequent changes of car models, radios, fur coats, dresses, travel, parties, cigarettes, food and diners that, for sure, are not the most hygienic for their condition; so for such a normal function [pregnancy], there are no savings left, except for the indispensable such as the need to dress the baby as well as they can, and pay, when they do, a modest midwife.[91]

Given the possibility of social mobilisation for Argentinian middle-classes, it was common place for the positivist medical discourse to regard the behaviour of the ascending middle classes, the 'nouveaux riches', with suspicion, and to stigmatise their conduct as moved by greed and social ambition. This is why middle-class women were considered as trivial subjects absorbed by the idea of money, and above all, by the idea of appearance and simulation. For the most poor and prolific segments of society, however, the corporal reading of the slim women was less condemnatory given the evidence of a deficient diet and malnutrition of vast sectors of the population alongside deplorable working conditions. Thinness was here interpreted with more compassion, although under certain limits, since working mothers continued to be seen as the chiefly responsible for the health of their own bodies and their children.

Beyond these stigmatisations of female bodies, by the 1930s it was clear that Argentina had shifted its fertility pattern from natural to voluntary fertility. If we disaggregate this process by social class, we find that the upper classes were the sector that started earliest, followed by the urban middle classes and, far later, by the unskilled urban and rural workers. By 1936, women from the most affluent neighbourhoods in Buenos Aires had an average of 1.9 children, while the average in marginal social areas was 3.9 children.[92] In this sense, female typology became inextricably linked with the search for a solution to the perceived decline in birth-rates, especially among those deemed as the biologically fittest. To confront the threat presented by the changing composition of the family and, in particular, by an increasingly elusive female identity, a catalogue of biotypes was established, and attempts were made to codify fixed identities. But aspiring to universal typification, makes taxonomy fail. The ideal type of the fertile woman, physiologically specified and sociologically described in her gender role, seems to have been as far from reality as the search for an 'Argentinian biotype' within a racially and ethnically mixed population.

Throughout this chapter we have seen how a focus on medical practices in maternal centres, rather than on maternal welfare legislation or debates on matrimonial law, can shed new light on the techniques and methods used by eugenists to improve the reproduction of the fittest and to prevent the reproduction of the unfit. Argentinian eugenists' subscription to constitutional medicine, with its elaborate body-typing schemes influenced by the Italian school of Pende, provided them with a new scientific language to describe the biological composition of the population. Endocrine methods seemed promising for the treatment and improvement of the constitutional inadequacies of female bodies, the treatment of infertility, and the corrections of genital and hormonal dysfunctions. More importantly, the broad area of gynaecological problems and their potential hormonal treatments allowed eugenists to achieve a direct intervention in the improvement of types, beyond the more indirect measures aimed at improving environmental conditions. The combination of biotypology and endocrinology services in the preconception and prenuptial consulting rooms organised by the NDMI in 1936 gave this approach, already practiced in Buenos Aires, a larger scope.

In addition, I would suggest that the eugenic purpose of the consulting rooms may have contributed increasingly to dissuading dysgenic women from marrying or becoming pregnant: no law would have prevented them from doing so, since the prenuptial certificate introduced in 1936 was compulsory only for men and restricted only those infected with venereal disease.[93] It was not that the advice offered to women in the consulting rooms was illegal, since the consultations took place, and the advice was formulated, within the organisation of the NDMI. Rather, I argue that to concentrate on the prenuptial certificate law as the only eugenic impediment to marriage is to ignore an important part of eugenic practice. The work of the consulting rooms in preventing the reproduction of dysgenic women was not the only negative practice observable in Argentinian eugenics: sterilisation was another. This, too, took place outside, or in spite of, the legal framework. Although sterilisation was completely banned under the Penal Code, this legal impediment did not preclude doctors from practicing sterilisations to save a mother's life – as demonstrated by the development of surgical techniques (for definitive and temporary sterilisation), about which Dr Eduardo Baldi eloquently commented: 'few are the gynaecologists who have not created a personal variant, seeking with each to obtain the most secure way of preventing the possibility of a future pregnancy'.[94] With the exception of the doctors gathered in the Consortium of Catholic Doctors, who bluntly rejected sterilisation and abortion even when the mother's life was seriously at risk, the rest of the medical profession, with greater or lesser emphasis, supported both practices. Furthermore, and as the next chapter will suggest, even some Catholic doctors sought to accommodate eugenic ideas within the dogma, thus giving the broader idea of the reproduction of the fittest new ground for its dissemination. The biotype had a lasting presence in Argentinian medical discourses and, as we have seen, it affected a great deal of medical treatment especially during the 1930s and 1940s. The following chapters will focus on the extent to which the biotype, along with other medical ideas previously analysed, pervaded the social representations of motherhood in other fundamental areas of the cultural field and the social imaginary.

Notes

1   'Creación del Departamento Nacional de Maternidad e Higiene Infantil', in *Congreso Nacional: Cámara de Senadores* (Buenos Aires: Imprenta del Congreso, 1937), 10-16: 12 and 284-95.

2   *Actas de la II Conferencia Pan-Americana de Eugenesia y Homicultura de las Repúblicas Americanas* (Buenos Aires: Fascoli y Bindi, 1934), 164.

3   N. Pende, *Constitutional Inadequacies. An Introduction to the Study of Abnormal Constitutions* (Philadelphia: Lea and Febiger, 1928), 244.

4   The 'Biometric School' was set up in 1892 at University College London. In its origins conflated, on the one hand, biologists' interest for quantifying their discipline (morphological studies), and on the other, Galton's eugenic studies, which were oriented to measure inheritance. In 1901, both tendencies merged in the laboratories of 'Biometric and Eugenics'. Cfr. D. MacKenzie, *Statistics in Britain 1865-1930. The Social Construction of Scientific Knowledge* (Edinburgh: Edinburgh University Press, 1981).

5   *Actas de la II Conferencia Pan-Americana*, 166.

6   Stepan, *'The Hour of Eugenics'*, 102-103.

7   Ibid., 103.

8   Ibid., 14.

9   Cfr. Zimmermann, *Los Liberales Reformistas*; M. Miranda and G. Vallejo (eds), *Darwinismo Social y Eugenesia en el Mundo Latino* (Buenos Aires: Siglo XXI Editores, 2005); and 'Formas de Aislamiento Físico y Simbólico: La Lepra, sus Espacios de Reclusión y el Discurso Médico-legal en Argentina', *Asclepio*, 60, 2 (2008), 19-42; M. Nari, 'La Eugenesia en Argentina, 1890-1940', *Quipu*, 12 (1999), 343-69; D. Barrancos, 'Anarquismo y Sexualidad', in D. Armus (ed.), *Mundo Urbano y Cultura Popular* (Buenos Aires: Sudamericana, 1989), 15-37, and *La Escena Iluminada. Ciencia para Trabajadores 1890-1930* (Buenos Aires: Plus Ultra, 1996); M. Miranda, 'La Antorcha de Cupido'; S. Ramella, 'Ideas Demográficas Argentinas (1930-1950): Una Propuesta Poblacionista, Elitista, Europeizante y Racista', *Revista Persona*. Online at: http:// www.revistapersona.com.ar/Persona11/11Ramellatesis.htm (consulted 4.03.2009).

10 For an analysis of the influence of eugenic ideas and its practice in a psychiatric institution see Y. Eraso, 'A Burden to the State'. The

Reception of the German 'Active Therapy' in an Argentinian Colony-asylum', in W. Ernst and T. Mueller (eds.), *Transnational Psychiatries. Social and Cultural Histories of Psychiatry in Comparative Perspective, c. 1800-2000* (Newcastle upon Tyne: Cambridge Scholars Publishing, 2010), 51-79.

11 Stepan, Ch. 3.

12 S. Tracy, 'An Evolving Science of Man: The Transformation and Demise of American Constitutional Medicine, 1920-1950', in Ch. Lawrence and G. Weisz (eds.), *Greater Than the Parts: Holism and Biomedicine, 1920-1950* (New York: Oxford University Press, 1998), 161-88: 170.

13 In 1914 Argentina had a population of 7,885,237, of which a 29,9% (2,357,952) were foreigners. Foreign population was composed of 40,6% of Italians and 36,3% Spaniards, followed by those from other European and neighbouring countries. For the period 1930-1940 the arrival of immigrants was the lowest since 1880. The percentage of foreigners over the total population of that period was reduced from 23,5% to 18,4%. In M. Lobato and J. Suriano, *Atlas Histórico, Nueva Historia Argentina* (Buenos Aires: Editorial Sudamericana, 2000), 308 and 370.

14 For the analysis of constitutional medicine in Europe and USA *cfr.* Lawrence and Weisz (eds.), *Greater Than the Parts*. For the case of Mexico, see A. Stern, 'Mestizofilia, Biotipología y Eugenesia en el México Pos-revolucionario: Hacia una historia de la Ciencia y el Estado, 1920-60', *Relaciones*, 81 (2000), 57-91.

15 A. Navarro, 'Anomalías del Desarrollo Somático y Morfológico, *RCMC* (1939), 1811-55: 1811.

16 B. Soria, 'Protección a la Infancia', *Revista de la Universidad Nacional de Córdoba*, 2 (1924), 32-48: 30.

17 E. Vidal Abal, 'Consideraciones sobre Profilaxis Mental a Propósito del Tema Praxiterapia', *Boletín del Asilo de Alienados en Oliva*, 16 (1937), 119-26: 126.

18 Soria, 'Protección a la Infancia', 36.

19 E. Scarzanella, 'Criminología, Eugenesia y Medicina Social en el Debate entre Científicos Argentinos e Italianos, 1912-1941', in H. Troncoso and C. Sierra (eds.), *Ideas, Cultura e Historia en la Creación Intelectual Latinoamericana: Siglos XIX y XX* (Quito: Ediciones Abya-Yala, 1997), 217-34.

20 E. Díaz de Guijarro, *El Impedimento Matrimonial de Enfermedad.*

Matrimonio y Eugenesia (Buenos Aires: Kraft, 1944), 330. The degrees awarded by the Association were: Biotypologists, Teachers for Disable People, Nutritionists, Techniques in Social Hygiene, and Counsellors on Professional Orientation.

21 J. Comas, 'La Biotipología de Arturo Rossi', *Boletín Bibliográfico de Antropología Americana,* 7 (1943), 99-113: 106-107.

22 Peralta Ramos, 'La Obstetricia en sus Relaciones con la Eugenesia', 389.

23 'Creación del Departamento Nacional de Maternidad e Higiene Infantil', 287.

24 Along with Peralta Ramos the Advisory Committee was made up of the following members: the President of the National Hygiene Department, the President of Public Assistance of Buenos Aires, a representative of the Board of Infancy, and a professor of obstetrics appointed by the Faculty of Medicine of Buenos Aires. 'Creación del Departamento Nacional de Maternidad e Higiene Infantil', 287.

25 J. Lascano, 'Aspecto social de la Asistencia Obstétrica. Reseña Histórica y Legislación Argentina', *Revista de la Universidad Nacional de Córdoba,* 28 (1941), 1449-75: 1468.

26 A. Peralta Ramos, 'Plan de Organización de la Asistencia Social de la Madre y del Recién Nacido en la Argentina', in *Obstetricia, Ginecología y Puericultura,* 364. See also E. Boero, 'Institutos de Eugenesia y Maternidad', *La Nación,* 9 January 1931, 13.

27 J. Bello, 'Mortinatalidad y Organización Sanitaria', 817.

28 J. Lascano, 'Asistencia Pre-natal', in *Actas y Trabajos del V ICNM,* III (Rosario: Est. Gráfico Pomponio, 1939), 528-52: 547.

29 Lascano, 'Asistencia Pre-natal', 533.

30 Ibid., 534. For data on infant mortality, Cfr. Dezeo, 'Demografía Internacional', 613.

31 S. Torrado, 'Transición de la Familia en la Argentina', 238.

32 Between 1930 and 1940 the male:female ratio in Argentina declined from 1.12 to 1.075, in Lobato and Suriano, *Atlas Histórico,* 369.

33 J. Beruti, 'La Desnutrición Voluntaria en la Mujer Moderna', in *Actas y Trabajos del IV CNM,* VI (Buenos Aires: Spinelli, 1932), 339-61: 340-58.

34 Pende, *Constitutional Inadequacies,* 199.

35 A. Peralta Ramos and M. Schteingart, 'Los Factores Endocrino-Constitucionales en la Obstetricia y Ginecología', in *Actas y Trabajos del V CNM,* V (Rosario: Talleres Gráficos Pomponio, 1935), 686-94: 687.

36   The following characterizations are extracted from ibid., 686–94.
37   G. Peralta Ramos, M. Schteingart and I. Chasín, 'Constitución y Esterilidad', in *Actas y Trabajos del VCNM*, V (Rosario: Talleres Gráficos Pomponio, 1935), 432-40: 433.
38   A. Navarro, 'Semiología de las Facies', *RCMC* (1941), 273-81: 281.
39   Peralta Ramos and Schteingart, 'Los Factores Endocrino-constitucionales', 686.
40   A. Rossi, *Tratado Teórico Práctico de Biotipología y Ortogénesis*, I (Buenos Aires: Ideas, 1944), 157.
41   Peralta Ramos, 'La Obstetricia en sus Relaciones con la Eugenesia', 386.
42   Peralta Ramos, Schteingart, and Chasín, 'Constitución y Esterilidad', 438.
43   Ibid., 439.
44   Ch. Lawrence, 'A Tale of Two Sciences: Bedside and Bench in Twentieth-century Britain', *Medical History*, 43 (1999), 421-50: 443.
45   Oudshoorn, *Beyond the Natural Body*.
46   M. Cueto, 'Laboratory Styles in Argentine Physiology', *Isis*, 85 (1994), 228-46: 234.
47   B. Houssay, 'The Role of the Hypophysis in Carbohydrate Metabolism and in Diabetes', Nobel Lecture, 12 December 1947, in *Nobelprize.org*. Online at: http://nobelprize.org/medicine/laureates/1947/houssay-lecture.html (consulted 25.02.2011).
48   D. Paul, 'The Rockefeller Foundation and the Origins of Behaviour Genetics,' in K. Benson, J. Maienschein, and R. Rainger (eds) *The Expansion of American Biology* (London: Rutgers University Press, 1991), 262–83: 270.
49   I. Chasín and M. Schteingart, 'Las Inyecciones Endovenosas de Foliculina en las Menorragias', in *Actas y Trabajos del VCNM*, V (Rosario: Talleres Gráficos Pomponio, 1935), 441-44: 441.
50   H. Dionisi, 'Embarazo Ectópico', *RCMC* (1940), 2313-29: 2316.
51   P. Pla, 'El Tratamiento de la Insuficiencia Genital en Ambos Sexos con Inyecciones de Orina de Embarazada', in *Actas y Trabajos del VCNM*, V (Rosario: Talleres Gráficos Pomponio, 1935), 445-50: 447.
52   Carro, 'El Régimen Alimenticio de la Embarazada Obesa', 346. It is also important to signal that the professorship of nutrition was among the titles awarded by the School of Biotypology since 1932.
53   M. Rodríguez, 'Los Factores Sociales en la Hipoplasia Genital,' in *VC*

AOyG (Buenos Aires: s.n., 1943), 806–11: 806.

54 A. Risolía, 'Esterilización en la Mujer', in *IVCAOyG* (Buenos Aires: Guidi Buffarini, 1940), 122-299: 126.

55 Norman Haire is reputed to have been the first to apply biological sterilisation to women, in 1928.

56 *Código Penal de la República Argentina*, 31.

57 Ibid., 30.

58 In 1967, the National Law on Medical Practice, Dentistry and Auxiliary Practices 17.132, in its article 20, (18) forbade doctors 'to practice interventions that result in sterilisation without any clear therapeutic indication and without having depleted all the conservative resources of the reproductive organs', in 'Ley Nacional N° 17132. Ejercicio de la Medicina, Odontología y Actividades Auxiliares', *Notivida*. Online at: http://www.notivida.com.ar (consulted 6.02.2010). Previously, the Medical Ethical Code (1955) approved by the Medical Confederation of Argentina, in its article 19 stated, 'the doctor could not sterilise a man or a woman without a perfectly determined therapeutic indication', in *Confederación Médica de la República Argentina*. Online at: http://www.comra.org.ar/ (consulted 6.02.2010).

59 *Casti Connubii*. Encyclical of Pope Pius XI (31 December 1930) Online at: http://www.vatican.va/holy_father/pius_xi/encyclicals/documents/hf_p-xi_enc_31121930_casti-connubii_en.html (consulted 23.09.2010).

60 By 1930 a total of thirty three states had enacted such laws.

61 Peralta Ramos, 'La Obstetricia en sus Relaciones con la Eugenesia', 386.

62 Risolía, 'Esterilización en la Mujer', 281.

63 G. Peralta Ramos and Schteingart, 'Esterilización Temporaria por Método Biológico', in *Actas y Trabajos del VCNM*, V (Rosario: Talleres Gráficos Pomponio, 1935), 656-58.

64 A. Gordillo et al., 'Esterilización Biológica Temporaria de la Mujer', *Revista de la Asociación Médica Argentina*, 50 (1937), 291-96: 292.

65 M. Pérez, 'Esterilización, Definición, Historia, Indicaciones', in *IVCAOyG* (Buenos Aires: Guidi Buffarini, 1940), 47-121: 86.

66 Between 1930 and 1940, I could find 24 articles and 7 monographs only devoted to tests of methods of sterilisation. In the case of the Catholic literature, there were 7 such articles in the medical journal *Iatría*, and 3 in *Criterio*.

67   The German law included the following diseases: congenital
     feeblemindedness, manic-depressive psychosis, schizophrenia, epilepsy,
     Huntington's Chorea, blindness, deafness, severe alcoholism and severe
     physical deformities.

68   Pérez, 'Esterilización, Definición, Historia, Indicaciones', 109 and 121.

69   Taking into account the Congress of 1940, as well as other literature
     consulted, the following list of physicians, although incomplete, is
     representative of the use of sterilisation methods during the period:
     Biological methods: Alberto and Guillermo Peralta Ramos, Mario
     Schteingart, Nicanor Palacios Costa, Ricardo Pastorini, Pedro A.
     Tapella, Carlos A. De Pierris, and Rafael Araya (Buenos Aires);
     Alberto Gordillo, Rodolfo Romero, Aderbal Bisso, and Juan Pinto
     (La Plata); Manuel Vázquez Amenábar, Pablo Arata, and Rodolfo
     Calaberry (Córdoba); Hugo Magistris (Rosario). Surgical methods:
     Juan M. Sánchez, Arturo Risolía, Alberto Peralta Ramos, Daniel Rojas,
     Eduardo Baldi, Roberto Herrera, Manuel Pérez, Juan Gabastou, Juan
     C. Ahumada, Juan C. Llanes Massini, Tomás A. Chamorro, Josué
     Beruti, Orestes Palazzo, Antonio Molfino, Raúl Boero, Juan Viacava,
     and Enrique S. Garré (Buenos Aires); José Lascano (Córdoba); Ricardo
     Schwarcz (Santa Fe). X-ray methods: Eduardo Lanari, José Molinari,
     and Federico Vierheller (Buenos Aires).

70   Risolía, 'Esterilización en la Mujer', 286.

71   J. Lascano and G. Sayago, 'Tuberculosis y Embarazo', in *IICAOyG*
     (Buenos Aires: Caporaletti Hnos., 1934), 38-75: 57.

72   J. Belbey, 'La Esterilización Humana por el Estado', in *Actas y Trabajos
     del VCNM*, VIII (Rosario: Talleres Gráficos Pomponio, 1935), 325-29:
     327.

73   A. Peralta Ramos and G. Peralta Ramos, 'Indicaciones y Técnica de la
     Esterilización Artificial Definitiva de la Mujer', in *IVCAOyG* (Buenos
     Aires: Guidi Buffarini, 1940), 309-25: 309.

74   Peralta Ramos and Peralta Ramos, 'Indicaciones y Técnica de la
     Esterilización Artificial Definitiva de la Mujer', 323.

75   Pérez, 'Esterilización, Definición, Historia, Indicaciones', 100-101.

76   Stepan, *The Hour of Eugenics'*, 113.

77   Risolía, 'Esterilización en la Mujer', 288.

78   R. Herrera, 'Consideraciones Acerca de la Esterilización', in *IVCAOyG*
     (Buenos Aires: Guidi Buffarini, 1940), 304-5: 304.

79   C. Escuder, 'Discusión' in *IVCAOyG* (Buenos Aires: Guidi Buffarini,

1940), 325-31: 328.

80 A. Licurzi, 'La Esterilización Eugénica de Degenerados y Criminales,' *Revista Médica de Córdoba* (1937), 207–25: 209.

81 Peralta Ramos and Peralta Ramos, 'Indicaciones y Técnica de la Esterilización Artificial', 326.

82 Stepan, *'The Hour of Eugenics'*, 201.

83 Beruti, 'La Desnutrición Voluntaria', 340.

84 Ibid.

85 Ibid., 346.

86 Ibid.

87 Ibid., 354.

88 Ibid., 354. Among the organic consequences enumerated, there were: ovary dysfunction, dystocic pregnancy, abortions, long and painful deliveries, impossible or insufficient natural lactation, etc.

89 L. Caldwell, 'Reproducers of the Nation: Women and the Family in Fascist Policy', in D. Forgacs (ed.), *Rethinking Italian Fascism. Capitalism, Populism and Culture* (London: Lawrence and Wishart, 1986), 110-41: 113.

90 Beruti, 'La Desnutrición Voluntaria', 348.

91 Lascano, 'Asistencia pre-natal', 541.

92 Torrado, 'Transición de la Familia en la Argentina', 255.

93 Law 12.331: Prophylaxis of Venereal Diseases, article 13, in Díaz de Guijarro, *El Impedimento Matrimonial*, 147–50. The prenuptial certificate became mandatory for women in 1965.

94 E. Baldi, 'Sobre algunas Observaciones de Fracasos de la Esterilización Quirúrgica,' in *IVCAOyG* (Buenos Aires: Guidi Buffarini, 1940), 305–9: 307.

PART II: THE TEXTUAL RECORD

3

The Catholic Press and the Strategic Uses of the Marian Cult

The great crusade of modern times is the press, and we all should be involved with it

    Priest Angel Clavero[1]

In 1899 Pope Leo XIII gathered, for the first time, a Plenary Council with Latin American Bishops with the aim of reinforcing the role of the Church in a liberal and secular world. Gathered in Rome, the Council sought to initiate an overarching process of reform of the Latin American Church under Roman supremacy, a direction that the Vatican had already secured in Europe during the Catholic resurgence of the end of the nineteenth century. As the guardian of authority and moral order, the Church, the pontiff insisted, should promote welfare and pacify social conflicts, while combating the dangers that threatened the Latin American faith: 'superstition, ignorance, Socialism, masonry and the bad press'.[2] Practical rules to prevent the advance of such evils soon followed suit, set up by the bishops attending the meeting for whom the expansion of religious education, a wide and strategic mobilisation of the laity, and the promotion of the Catholic press became a priority. Indeed, the latter was one of the themes in the agenda to be discussed at the Episcopal Conference in Argentina in 1902, where bishops especially called upon lay Catholics to publish and disseminate Catholic newspapers, at the time that they alerted the flock about the pernicious involvement (whether in writing or consuming) with the 'bad press', that is, publications contrary to the Church.[3] Similarly, in 1906, the bishop of Córdoba called a Synod to draw out a plan of religious education, involving the clergy and lay organisations, while declaring liberalism the main enemy of the Church. The special condemnation of the 'pornographic novels, magazines, and the liberal newspapers'[4] that the Synod declared reflected the Bishop's main and enduring concern with the secularising forces that permeated society, which he perceived as threatening the Church's legitimate social role. As he expressed with alarm, 'in this hour of such an active propaganda against the religious dogmas'; 'in this hour of religious indifference, of laicism and blasphemy'.[5]

The development of a Catholic press that bishops were urged to promote on their return from Rome is a process that, although weak and limited, had already started in Argentina during the nineteen century, as the existence of a handful of Catholic newspapers testifies.[6] But the creation of new daily publications at the turn of the century, as a phenomenon specifically advanced by the clergy, had an uneven response in Argentina's main cities: thus, in Buenos Aires, the main referent was the paper *El Pueblo* (1900-1960) founded by priest Federico Grote, who was notable for the creation of Catholic Workers' Circles; Santa Fe turned to the confessional press *Boletín Eclesiástico de Santa Fe* (1900) as the main organ of the diocese, alongside the weekly *El Heraldo*, creating only much later, during the period of 'Catholic renascence', the first Catholic newspaper, *La Mañana* (1937-52);[7] while Córdoba, on the other hand, had *Los Principios* (1894-1982), the longest running newspaper of the period that became a referent of the Argentinian Catholic press. The significance of *Los Principios*, in many respects, exceeds that of *El Pueblo* (The People), not only for its longevity, but particularly for the alliance that the clergy accomplished with Cordoban lay Catholics, the support it enjoyed by larger segments of society and the ruling class, and the wealth of its economic resources, which allowed *Los Principios* unproblematically to adopt the technological advances of the modern press. In addition, while *El Pueblo* was less doctrinaire and dogmatic and had the ambition of becoming a popular paper,[8] as its title suggested, *Los Principios* (The Principles) on the contrary, was 'the standard-bearer of religion and champion of the Church's rights'[9] having since its foundation both laymen and priests as members of its editorial board and directorate. Furthermore, it was not driven by a popular interest or aimed to reach out to the masses it was, on the contrary, concerned about the 'vulgarisation of religious themes' for which it drew attention to the quality of Catholic writers, stating that, 'the dignity of Christian doctrine suffers ... when inept pens, without theological and literary studies throw themselves to doctrinarian discussion without noticing that they discredit religion' forcing the paper's decline, impeding it 'being the honourable means of the Catholic cause'.[10] It can be argued that in the absence of a strong, national, Catholic paper (an unaccomplished desire of the Argentinian ecclesiastic authorities) *Los Principios* managed to disseminate, particularly in the decades post 1900, the hierarchical, clerical and doctrinal character that was thought as necessary to instil in a liberal, secular state. Founded by a group of influential Catholics and clergymen, the paper sought the protection of the 'Society of Catholic Youth', in an attempt to 'liberate it from personal, political influences'.[11] Its public was clearly the Catholic elite and the ascending middle-classes, to whom it aimed to shape in Catholic, moral values, and to offer a prescribed response to the problems of individuals' everyday life. A Catholic vision on political, economic and cultural issues also characterised the paper as it developed a strong profile as an opinion-maker. In the 1930s, the Catholic press in Argentina acquired a greater visibility and circulation, as we will see later in the case of *Los Principios*, while it increasingly became engaged in the political debates of the time. The importance of the press in moulding the opinion of the people was, however, acknowledged from an early stage by Córdoba's Catholics, as observed by one of *Los Principios's* main collaborators on the occasion of the paper's thirtieth anniversary:

> It is fascinating the influence that the newspaper exerts on its readers ... it is a true educator of the people. ... The masses, incapable of having ideas of their own about the multiple current problems that the world poses to humankind, think like the newspaper that they read.[12]

Nevertheless, and despite its significant role, as arguably papers and the press became central to people's engagement with their society, such a prominent position has been underexplored as historians have tended to see newspapers as sources of historical information rather than as cultural objects in their own right. Form and character, style, layout and design, will be touched on in my analysis but more attention will be given to content and its changing nature in the context of broader socio-cultural developments. More specifically, I am interested in the representations that the paper elaborated concerning the mother figure and on motherhood more generally, to gain insight into how the Catholic press offered a distinctive representation, but also how it became affected and implicated with the medical one, giving rise to new forms of representation that emerged from the very dynamic of relational configurations.

As in other newspapers of the period, there was a gender divide in the pages of *Los Principios* where women found 'their' pages in the so-called 'Social Section', although articles appealing to women were also to be found quite often, scattered in editorials and in the central pages dedicated to men. The 'Social Section' was the one that conveyed messages addressed directly to women and mothers, and it was composed of different types of articles:

from all those issues that concerned housework (food recipes, medicines, gardening, etc.) to advice to mothers, and young ladies about themes that directly involved their role within the family: engagement, matrimony, familial affairs, mother-child relationships and, especially, mother-daughter relationships. These articles reflected a growing concern with the 'female question', whose seriousness merited long spaces within the principal sections too, as anxieties grew over the changing patterns introduced by modernity, especially in respect to gender relationships, the family and motherhood. Drawing on Catholic literature the paper's writers, mostly priests and lay intellectuals and professionals, aimed at instilling and reinforcing what was considered to be acceptable behaviour for female readers. Articles in the 'Social Section', sought to instil notions of women's appropriate behaviour including that of the 'mother's mission', and they were characterised by a prescriptive and instructive language, with headings easily distinguishable, such as 'mothers' or 'women', to prompt women's reading. Many of these articles stemmed from what was perceived as a secularisation in mothers' behaviour, as their Christian role was thought to be challenged by both the rising presence of Buenos Aires's feminists, and by the consumption patterns and ostentatious behaviour of elite women, who were regarded as being absorbed into a stream of vanity, frivolity and wealth. To keep these women under the spiritual sphere of Catholicism, and its supernatural, transcendental reign, implied a constant reminder that access to this sacred sphere was to be accomplished not only inwardly, but through clear external gestures. The importance of the spiritual over the material was a recurrent exhortation that was devised along gender lines, since women, unlike men, were expected to secure the moral values of the home. To this end various female attributes and demeanours were presented as normative, natural qualities, as showed by the following passage, 'A woman without heart is a monster of nature. How many times the instinct of a mother's heart equals and overtakes the perspective of great men?'[13]

Women's heart, however, was being tempted by other types of recognition. The fashion industry was instrumental in the emergence of women as new consuming subjects, and newspapers and magazines were the places where this fast-growing market was publicised. Style and fashion became notes of distinction for an increasingly consumerist society, whereby, 'good taste' became a social regulator that brought forth new forms of femininity, and with them too, the possibility to display alternative identities. Not surprisingly, the dangers of following a luxurious fashion were soon pointed out as improper behaviour in an attempt at controlling abuses and excesses.

The perceived threat that the feminine dress represented, heavily concerned Catholic writers from the Pope, who devoted encyclicals and official documents with precise instructions on feminine clothing,[14] to the local clergy responsible for spreading his message among the flock.[15] In the numerous articles that appeared in *Los Principios* it is possible to observe that women's clothing preoccupied pious men in at least two different ways. The insistence on observing 'decorum and decency' indicated an attempt to control the female sexual body; whilst the exhortation on 'modesty and simplicity' was directed to those in whom extravagant dressing indicated a predilection for materialistic values. In both cases it was clear that the new codes of female visibility were in need of regulation to preserve a Catholic, feminine image. In this sense, mothers were made responsible for controlling these worldly temptations in their daughters. As one article written in a personal way recommended, 'Please understand my dearest readers that the most terrible enemy for woman is the luxury with which mothers accustom their little daughters to dress'.[16] It also warned that, 'modesty and simplicity is the principal ornament that a man looks for in the woman that he will choose as his companion, the angel of home and the mother of his sons', thus contending women's possibility of forging a female subjectivity independent of masculine desire.[17]

As women were gradually establishing their presence in different areas of the public sphere, newspapers became instrumental in accompanying that process by disseminating women's activities, but also by imposing new forms of female visibility and new forms of representation. This widely-observed phenomenon that took place in most Western societies, which scholars have termed the 'feminisation of the press', was developed under gendered premises and implied a wide range of characteristics that varied according to the newspaper's style (broadsheet or tabloid) and profile.[18] The notorious increase of the 'Social Sections' devoted to women, the participation of women's journalists, the raise of advertisements and the shift in news' presentation towards a more visual style, indicated the definitive incorporation of the female public as established readers. Following this tendency, and to counteract women's representation in the liberal press, *Los Principios* too increased the number of editorials devoted to women, as well as the length of its 'Social Section' with the view of delineating the Catholic woman's profile. The material support of the paper largely facilitated this process as the incorporation of new technology notably expanded the number of pages and increased the number copies. Initially, *Los Principios* appeared in a print run of 500 copies, financed by the subscription of the members of the Catholic Youth. By 1901, it printed four pages in a broad-sheet design of approximately 150 cm. The incorporation of new, modern rotary presses in 1909, 1914 and 1924, increased the number of pages to eight, twelve then thirty-two respectively, while its print run rose to 22,000.[19] A timely modernization of the paper was evidently carefully considered by the editorial board, which rapidly embraced technological changes as a way of securing the continuity of the paper among its readers.

This extended format allowed for a deeper analysis of the many facets of modern woman's behaviour as well as for a detailed description of the active role Catholic women were called to perform as the counter-figure to the liberal, defiant, destabilising one of the 'new woman'. Considerable efforts went, for example, into restricting the pernicious influence of the cinema, clothing, literature and children's entertainment for which mothers were called to exert their sphere of authority. These demands attempted to enhance the mother's mission in society as an irreplaceable subject. The more women in public were portrayed in the circulating press, the more insistent *Los Principios* became on their private role, and their spiritual duties at home.

Above all, the figure that concerned the paper the most was the one of the feminist. During the first three decades of the twentieth century, the fear of feminism largely structured the newspaper's discourse about women and mothers. For clergymen, feminism epitomised the liberalisation of women's behaviour in a way that exceeded the discussion on specific feminist ideas and demands of the time, such as, the vote, divorce, or female work. To a great extent, feminism became a concept that Catholics recognised as a reference to what was wrong in woman's role. However, in an effort that tells us more about their fears than the real expansion of feminism across the country, clerics re-signified its message with Catholic values and presented it to women as a 'true feminism'. To this aim, the newspaper resorted to both text and the persuasive power of visual images (photojournalism), as we will see in more detail in Chapter 6.

From Feminism to Mary

Early in the century, the development of a feminist movement in Buenos Aires was perceived by the Church as part of the secularising process initiated by the state whose laws in civil matrimony and lay education directly attacked the Church's influence and its undisputable ascendance on the family, overshadowing religion as a force in national life. The gradual transformation of the family in liberal Argentina was variously noticed through other unsettling factors such as the rapidly growing immigrant population, and by the entry of women into spaces, until then, preserved for men. Women's slow entry into the labour market, for example, was negatively perceived by *Los Principios*, in writings that combined doses of irony to emphasise a disapproving tone. Under the title 'Female invasion', an article criticised the decision of the national government to equalise, for both sexes, the teaching programmes of telegraphy, an area of services (communication) where women became swiftly integrated. The article argued,

> We already have telephonists and women employed in the post. Soon we will have the telegraphers and then, why not? the deputies.
> What we will obtain is simply this: the struggle for life will be more and more difficult, and men will not have any other option than to become babysitters. . . .
> Nature has put limits to both sexes that cannot be violated. Let's respect those limits and not withdraw woman from the family, where she is the queen, to make her an employee, poor and under remunerated.[20]

The argument attempts to raise awareness of the dangers of women's work, both in terms of household roles, and in economic terms, and it does so in a way that chimed with the initial view of the liberal press and even that of Anarchist and Socialist papers in their perception of women's salaried work outside the home as a disarray that required rectification.[21] Motives differed, however, in that for the Church, women's work was viewed primarily as against the natural order. Nature provided the paramount reason to justify an order of things, for each sex, that should not be subverted by the cultural domain.

In 1902 a piece in the central space of the front page made it impossible to miss. Big headlines in bold read, 'Feminism'. The article describes the participation of feminists in the Pedagogic Congress that took place that year in the capital of the Republic. It states that feminism, 'is blowing things up for many women, especially for distinguished ladies and young ladies from Buenos Aires'.[22] Undoubtedly, the fact that 'distinguished ladies' were the ones being won for 'the cause' in Buenos Aires constituted the main fear among Córdoba's Catholics, because of its potential dissemination in the province.

103

The fear was well grounded. With a large number of elite women already mobilised in the provision of welfare, as members of charitable organisations, the perceived threat seemed all the more plausible. Not surprisingly, feminism continued stimulating articles to be read in the 'serious' pages of the paper, as they were intended for the male readership. In another editorial, feminism is associated with women's education and professionalisation,

> If her predominance in the field of art, science, trade and industry
> is to be accomplished at the cost of the decline of home, the ruin
> of society, the abandonment of orphans and the poor, the cruelty
> of pain in the heart of the masses, it is imperative to refuse such
> predominance and to keep woman in the condition and sphere that
> nature itself has taught to her, by choosing her to hold the sublime
> responsibility of maternity.[23]

As it is made clear here, once again, nature (maternity) operates as contrary to culture (science and education). However, the need of Catholics to set maternity in a clearly differentiated domain, and one that was opposite to feminist ideas, may have presented difficulties given the characteristics of Argentinian feminism, which was precisely built on maternalist premises. This may explain the fact that, from 1910 onwards, Catholic discourses started to re-signify the term 'feminism' to indicate a positive notion under Catholic principles. Revealingly, this started to take shape when the paper translated and article written by the French Abbé, Henry Bolo, which were probably extracts of his book *Feminism and the Church* (1902) where he analysed the situation of the movement in France, the same country that Buenos Aires's feminists identified with in their defence of maternity as a 'social function'. Drawing on the French society, Bolo argues about the existence of different types of feminisms, proposing a classification that would later become appropriated by writers of the local Catholic paper. 'There are half a dozen feminisms', says the Abbé, which should not be confused amongst them: the 'revolutionary' that 'preaches anarchy'; the 'socio-economic' that strives for improvements in this area; the 'Christian', which 'claims these reforms and asserts that the fate of women in society depends on the fate of the Gospel';[24] the 'literary', the one that 'dreams and makes novels'; and finally, the 'religious feminism', which 'puts all the resources of Catholicism to be at the service of women's dignity and weakness, and is doing so since the foundation of the Church'.[25] Undoubtedly, the proposed classification aims to elide the meaning of feminism as a movement striving for women's rights. Yet its upmost intention is to set up an improbable notion, which is the so-called 'religious feminism'. Bolo laments that the only feminism that drew women's attention is the first one, the 'revolutionary' or 'insurgent' kind, which he considers, is not the 'first in date', nor 'wiser' in its claims, or 'sincere' in its declarations. With a 'religious feminism' at hand, whose existence could be traced back to the appearance of Catholicism, the real problem seems to be a semantic one, 'the worst misfortune for women who want to improve their social condition is that the pure and simple name of feminism seems to designate *only* that one [the revolutionary one]'.[26]

In tandem with this religious appropriation of the term, Córdoba's bishop said to the charitable ladies of the Society of Ladies of Saint Vincent de Paul, speaking at the Society's annual meeting, that 'feminism', when 'well understood, should not take mothers away from the household and make them neglect their affections'.[27] But this was not merely a semantic reaction. Catholic clergy and laymen endowed the content of this acceptable 'feminism' with new meanings and imagery, claiming for Catholicism the credit for women's 'liberation'. Coinciding with national debates on female suffrage and discussions on women's civic rights – the latter finally sanctioned in 1926 – a new ideal of womanhood became essential for Catholics to oppose to the one claimed elsewhere.

It was within this context that the figure of the Virgin Mary started to be used as a foundation to fulfil this 'accepted feminism'. The Marian cult in Córdoba was developed early in the 1920s, and its connection with the fear of feminism seems, as I will argue here, all the more evident. This Marian cult was mainly developed discursively, through the printed press, for which *Los Principios* became instrumental in its dissemination. Although masses and liturgy (performance) played a significant part in the extolling of Mary's figure, the ritualised culture of Mary reached its apogee in the next decade, when it conveyed a slightly different meaning, as we shall see later. In this sense, I would argue that it is possible to identify in Córdoba two different moments in the development of the Marian Cult, which conveyed or corresponded to different meanings and representations of motherhood.

Let's concentrate on the first of these moments, the one developed in the 1920s that stemmed from the fear of feminism and the need to consolidate a positive role for Catholic women. In *Los Principios*, the main rationale to link Mary with women's earthly destiny was provided by the Virgin's main commemorations: the Assumption and the Immaculate Conception. The

105

Virgin's Assumption contributed the most powerful one, since the ascension to the reign of God was easily metaphorised with the ascension of women in society. This association was clearly proposed in the title of a long essay written in 1924 by a priest, member of the editorial staff, entitled, 'The Assumption of the Virgin and the social elevation of woman'. All antique civilizations, explains the author, with the exception of the Jews have despised, degraded and humiliated women, until a Mary appeared, embodying 'all divine and humane graces'. In the elevation of Mary to heaven (the Assumption), he continues, many have seen 'extolled woman's prestige', since it was 'in the bosom of the Church itself where women started to be elevated.' Mary, 'whose marvellous *elevation* has *descended* over the beautiful half of humankind [women], for their greater glory and influence that they enjoy in society'.[28] In another compelling article, under the heading 'The Social Mission of Woman', it is also emphasised that Catholicism was the only force that brought about women's liberation. In this case, however, the author establishes less symbolic associations to directly address feminists' demands. Convinced that 'none can speak of oppression in a century of liberties', he acknowledges that women have not been granted political rights, although he believes there were fundamental reasons for that,

> Women have distorted the path of their mission, and then we see them claiming and demanding rights that they believe theirs, among others, the suffrage. . . .
> Woman's influence is not in the committee but at home . . . from there she rules society, because in her hands is the destiny of tomorrow's men, and if she educates her sons with austerity, love and justice, she will be the real queen of the world! [29]

It is also interesting to note that the article considers that an 'idealised, moderated feminism, logical and adequate to the environment, is a fair and legitimate aspiration for modern woman, but she has to resort to the means to attain it.' And these means were, as above-mentioned, naturally stated, 'before anything she is a woman and her primordial destiny is motherhood'.[30] Thus, Mary's Assumption was emphasised not only to illustrate to women where the 'real' social elevation resided, but also as a meaningful image of motherhood, women's primordial role. Whilst Mary represents the two most valuable female qualities, virginity (Immaculate Conception) and maternity (Assumption), it is not a fortuitous fact that the Marian cult started by praising the second one, especially if we take into account that the Assumption of the Virgin was not yet a dogma of faith as the Immaculate Conception was. For the doctrine, the Assumption celebrates the motherhood of Mary, not her virginity. It indicates the recognition of the Son to his mother's earthly motherhood, for which Mary was prized with the quality of redemption. It only became a dogma of faith in 1950. The reappraisal of the Immaculate Conception in sociological terms soon followed suit, as the paper sought to reinforce the role of Catholicism in liberating women's condition. In priest Clavero's view, the great respect that Christian woman deserved in the contemporary world was due to Mary's pureness: it 'elevated Mary to the dignity of mother of God, thus, all women were rehabilitated and liberated from slavery to become queens of home, angels of charity, blazons of peace, and nuncios of fortune'.[31] It is instructive to remember that in this case the dogma of the Immaculate Conception was declared in 1858 on the pope's sole authority – it 'was revealed by God' as Pius IX declared – setting up a controversial precedent of papal infallibility. The dogma stated that 'the Virgin Mary was, in the first instant of her conception, preserved untouched by any taint of original guilt'.[32] According to contemporary writers Nicholas Perry and Loreto Echeverría the opportunistic character of the dogma 'was of the essence of counter-revolution'. It was a response to the European upheavals and social protests of the nineteenth century and the accompanying wave of irreligiosity, while 'the [dogma] definition is acknowledged by its supporters in more recent times as a master-stroke in the struggle against secular thought'.[33] In this sense, it seems that the precedents that surrounded the declaration of the dogma opened up other opportunistic uses of its content in other scenarios and contexts where secular thought threatened to erode Catholic values.

As we have seen for the case of Córdoba, the emergence of maternalist feminism, its public demands in Buenos Aires and internationally through the child congresses, was perceived as threatening women's role in society for which Catholic men evoked and re-signified the content of the Marian veneration to present it as the 'real feminism'. Along with this strategic use, the exalted figure of Mary in the press left women with exemplary attributes to follow during the 1920s. On the one hand, Mary represented women's elevation, dignity and purity because of Her earthly motherhood. On the other, the mother and child bond stressed through Mary, placed mothers in a strategic position which was superior to any familial relationship, endowing them with a greater influence over their children's secular and spiritual values. In this way, maternity was surrounded by positive attributes too, as it empowered women in society, making them unique, sublime, pure and honourable. In the 1930s, however, Mary's figure was emphasised differently, both in its ritual repertoire and in its content. It has been suggested by a number of scholars that the Catholic elaboration of motherhood was that of the virginal, kind, loving, and abnegated mother. I would argue that a more authentic perspective may be gained from a distinction among the different concepts used and their timing of appearance as they reveal how Catholicism brokered, rather than rigidly stated, its representations of motherhood in response to specific challenges posed by the period.

The 'Catholic Mother' and the 'New' Mary in the 1930s

When Pius XI wrote the encyclical *Lux Veritatis* in Christmas of 1931 to celebrate fifteenth hundred years since the Ephesus' Council that declared the Divine Maternity of Mary (the first of the Marian dogmas), he recalled the Nazareth family in the words of Leo XIII as an example proposed for the imitation of all: Fathers should be inspired by the 'vigilance and paternal prudence' of Joseph, mothers should find in Mary an example of love, 'modesty and submission', and children should have in Jesus a model to imitate. [34]
He later made the following claim:

> But in a more special manner it is fitting that those mothers of this
> our age, who being weary, whether of offspring or of the marriage
> bond, have the office they have undertaken degraded and neglected,
> may look up to Mary and meditate intently on her who has raised this
> grave duty of motherhood to such high nobility. For in this way there
> is hope that they may be led, by the help of grace of the heavenly
> Queen, to feel shame for the dishonour done to the great sacrament
> of matrimony, and may happily be stirred up to follow after the won-
> drous praise of her virtues, by every effort in their power.[35]

The 'special' call to 'weary mothers' to make 'every effort in their power' to sustain the example of the Nazareth family, had, however, a different tone regarding that emphasised by Leo XIII at the end of the nineteenth century. In Pius XI the idea of motherhood as *sacrifice* and *abnegation* was particularly emphasised. As he had previously demonstrated with the encyclical *Casti Connubii*, his ideas responded to a different type of concern: women's birth-control practices and women's liberal behaviour towards family and home. To counteract this tendency, the Divine Maternity was emphasised with his 1931 encyclical, alongside 'a liturgical monument of this commemoration, which may help to nourish the piety of clergy and people towards the great Mother of God'.[36] With it, a reminder to mothers in the 1930s, that Mary and her sublime maternity was not only love, elevation and purity, as established by previous encyclicals, but also the most magnificent example of *maternal sacrifice*. Female 'martyrdom' was now vigorously claimed.

To interpret the impact and scope of this new maternal attribute in Argentina I would trace its inscription to the broader changes operated in the nation during the 1930s, when Catholicism witnessed an unprecedented resurgence with a remarkable militant spirit. The Church's main initiatives were channelled through the creation of the Argentinian branch of the *Catholic Action* (1931), the worldwide movement fostered by Pious XI to promote and strengthen lay activities 'in the apostolate of the hierarchy'. The participation of the laity was directed towards the provision of a moral and spiritual foundation for the re-Christianisation of society, through an active involvement in different spheres, political, economic, educational, professional as well as public culture.[37] The increasing visibility of Catholic ideas in the cultural realm, was reflected through the circulation of a wide range of literature (newspapers, bulletins, magazines, and books), the presence of new publishing houses, and most notably, the intellectual debates organised by the 'Courses of Catholic Culture' (from 1922) and the prestige and influence acquired by the weekly magazine *Criterio* (1928-present). Arguably one of the most recognisable features of this period was that the spirit of religious *reconquista* (reconquest) was unreservedly staged on the streets. Catholic acts, parties, ceremonies and demonstrations were organised by the multiple branches of the Catholic Action, which alongside the peregrinations and magnificent parades staged by the clergy, generated an unprecedented climax of Catholic public fervour.

In this sense, it is exemplary to observe the remarkable changes that took place in the ritual and the cult of Mary in Córdoba, through the practices of veneration of the Virgin of the Rosary and Miracle, who was made Patroness of Córdoba by Leo XIII in 1892. This Virgin, the oldest image of Mary that the city sacredly kept since its arrival from Peru in 1592, had ever since become the central focus of the city's devotion. The image represents a maternal Mary with a child in her left hand, a sceptre in the other, and a large Rosary hanging from her hands. As the most venerated image of Córdoba, the Virgin had been paraded on the city's streets only on specific occasions, exclusively linked to important historical events (wars) and public claims of miracles in times of calamities (cholera epidemics, or droughts). The austerity of her public presence on the streets and the special moments in which her physical attendance was formally requested (only seven times between 1592- 1934), reveals, for the early twentieth century a Marian cult adjusted to a time of growing secularisation. It is very telling that when Bishop Zenón Bustos y Ferreira dedicated a pastoral letter in 1917 to commemorate the twenty-fifth anniversary of the Virgin's coronation, he asked his flock to imagine and follow 'with their thoughts, the imposing procession that led the Virgin out of her sanctuary to the throne [in the street] where she was to be crowned'.[38] Although he did organise a peregrination to the sanctuary, he decided not to parade the Virgin. This situation changed dramatically when, in 1934, Fermín Lafitte, Archbishop of Córdoba between 1934 and 1958, decided to parade the Virgin in ostentatiously and carefully-staged ceremonies with a multitudinous congregation of the faithful.

Unlike the few occasions that until then had justified her presence on the streets, Archbishop Lafitte organised a massive parade of the Virgin without feeling compelled to provide explanations in support of an otherwise extraordinary event. He did, however, have things to celebrate, which remind us the inroads that the Argentinian Church was making not only at national level. For example, Lafitte enumerated the Vatican's choice of the city of Buenos Aires to host in 1934 the International Eucharistic Congress; he also celebrated the 'first anniversary' of the First Diocesan Eucharistic Congress in Rosario (Santa Fe), and more importantly, the promotion to the status of Archdioceses of the diocese of Córdoba (1934). All these momentous events deserved, according to Lafitte, a celebration for which he prepared the festivity of Christ Rex on the 28th October in the city's Cathedral. An occasion, the latter, as he went on to say 'to associate his divine Mother', for which he ordered a parade of the Virgin, just a week in advance, as a 'homage of Marian piety, and a worthy preparatory for the following feast consecrated to Christ Rex'.[39]

Lafitte's statement symbolically reinforced the long tradition of the Marian cult as it was organised after the Counter-Reformation, whereby control over the mother, represented in Mary, passed from noble men to the 'sons' (celibate priest). As Luisa Accati has perceptively observed, the worship of Mary as well as her representation and imagery became strictly controlled by the clergy.[40] In this sense, I would argue that the unusual decision of parading the Virgin – simply to gather momentum for a major festivity devoted to Christ – made by the Archbishop of Córdoba should be read both in the frame of the reinvigorated Marian cult of the 1930s, encouraged by Pius XI, and as a renewed exercise of the power of the 'sons' over the mother. As Pius XI recommended, Mary's motherhood deserved this kind of liturgical boost to stimulate her imitation among unruly mothers. Consequently, a highly theatrical ritual characterised the Marian machinery in the 1930s, particularly in corporative, nationalistic states such as Italian Fascism and Spanish Falangism where a renewed and closed collaboration between church and state was forged.[41] In Argentina, Mary has been the protector figure in the main battle fields, exercising an enduring maternal patronage over Argentinian military forces since the country's Independence in 1810. This liaison was accentuated after the military *coup d'état* of September 1930, when the prominence of integralism positioned Catholicism as the 'true' cultural matrix of the Argentinian nation. Whilst 'homeland and Catholicism' became synonyms, the Marian devotion recovered its traditional maternal protection over the armed forces, now enhanced with staged military-like religious ceremonies.[42]

In this pious climax, the festivities for the Divine Mother took place in Córdoba, the city that Lafitte renamed 'the Argentinian Rome'. The organisation of the procession was widely covered by *Los Principios*, with large pictures, commemorative articles, and detailed information on the activities programmed for the event. From there, we learn that the main street where the Virgin's parade took place was occupied by the 'Catholic family', whose performance dominated the central stage. The different places assigned to each of its members can be seen as projecting a notion of family in its relationship to the private and public spheres. The parade started with separated columns of boys and girls of Catholic schools, who were followed by the members of the Catholic Action, with its branches divided by sex and age. As in all Catholic ritual in the 1930s, gender was all-pervasive. Thus, children were besides the columns of ladies and, on the other side of the road, they were followed by young ladies. Female branches, in turn, were followed by male ones (men and young men) in a disposition where sex was conveniently separated by age. The masculine columns in both sides of the road were the ones that escorted the Virgin. In front of Her, the 'hierarchy' with the representative authorities of the three orders of society, first the ecclesiastical ones, and at a 'considerable distance', the military and civil ones. Beyond the Virgin, the police music band was followed by the cavalry troop. Finally, the people, as the newspaper specified, 'will march behind the troop and in the streets but without entering in the columns of the [Catholic] associations'[43] In this way, the people were separated from the main parade, guarded by the representatives of the 'Catholic family', while at the same time, they were patrolled and contained by the troop.[44]

Following a request of Archbishop Lafitte, this Virgin was also named by Pius XI patroness of the Archdioceses of Córdoba in 1936, an event that was magnificently celebrated in the following year in October, the Virgin's month. Ever since 1934 the most venerated image of Córdoba left its sanctuary in the Dominican church to parade through the city's streets escorted by its retinue of favourite 'sons'. Bringing up the rear, the 'Daughters of Mary' and other female associations accompanied in safe proximity. In addition to these parades, Mary's public presence was ubiquitous, multiplied through the processions of near nine different images during their respective festivities.

As part of the perceived revitalisation of the Marian cult another important Catholic festivity was organised since 1933 by the League of Catholic Ladies, the 'Day of the Catholic Mother', celebrated on the 11th of October in all the parishes of the province.[45] Moreover, the Catholic Action requested from the Córdoba's government that this day were celebrated in all public schools with commemorative lessons, something that the minister of Public Education conceded. By 1935 the festivities of the Catholic mother occupied long passages in the pages of *Los Principios*, with announcements of the celebrations in each parish, Eucharistic workshops, schedule of masses and commemorative activities. Also significant were the celebrations held on the two main maternity centres of the city, the maternity ward of the San Roque Hospital and the Institute of Maternity, where masses were celebrated in the hospitals' chapels, and charitable ladies distributed clothes and stamps of *Our Lady* to the poor mothers there hospitalised.[46] The day of the Catholic mother celebrated on the 11th of October was preceded by another maternal celebration, the one of the Virgin of the Rosary, celebrated on the 7th of the month, with both festivities mutually reinforcing the other. During October the pages of *Los Principios* were saturated with commemorative articles, becoming instrumental in the dissemination of the contents of the Marian cult, especially in its remarks to Catholic mothers. Accompanying photographs also played a significant role in conveying this message, for they made explicit issues that were often implied in the articles, as we shall see in Chapter 6.

Long, dull and repetitive editorials and opinion pieces were devoted to the meanings of the 'Catholic mother', whose editorial efforts illustrates the tensions over the interpretative work to fit in and to make Catholic doctrine compatible with a convincing image of a Catholic mother in touch with the realities of the 'true woman'. The figure of the 'sacrificial mother' pervaded both the exhortatory and commemorative writings of the press, as an antidote for the perceived dissolution of the family, raised at the time by the debates on a divorce bill in 1932. In one article, priest Vera Vallejo revived the tone of the encyclical *Lux Veritatis* whereby the idea of 'maternal sacrifice' was overly stressed. The example of 'divine maternity' came to remind earthly mothers that pain should be borne heroically,

> The mother of God started by calling herself the slave of the Lord; the Christian mother should be so, subjecting herself too, to the abnegation of the most sublime mission and accepting its sacrifices, if needed, heroically.[47]

In another commemorative article, another local cleric commented on the importance of celebrating the day of the Catholic mother with a scolding tone, as he addressed another pressuring social problem of the 1930s, the limitation of maternity:

> We celebrate not the 'mother' but the 'Christian mother'. Not the woman driven by passion, flightiness or by other non-confessional ends, who assumes the enormous responsibility of being 'mother' without having the condition for being so. We refer to the Christian mother, the one that knows what is to be a mother, the one that understands her sublime mission; the one that took her nuptials to the altar to receive the benediction of God and borne that sweet weight that Jesus made sacrament [matrimony], to become the relief of her husband and a good and saintly mother of the sons that God may send to her. Not the sons that she would like in limited number, by means of the excesses condemned by *Casti Connubbi*, but the Christian mother that would accept all the sons that God would send to her, convinced that her best ornament are her sons, and they . . . are her rewards.[48]

The content and emphasis of the writings in the 1930s thus reveals a discontinuity in the representation of the Catholic mother, as motherhood seems to be constituted by a conglomerate of duties more than prerogatives, as they were stressed in the 1920s. Arguably, the Marian cult was strategically

113

used across the Catholic world with different political meanings, although with similar aims within the backdrop of nationalist and conservative governments of the 1930s. In Argentina and Córdoba specifically, as we have seen, Mary's ritual was fostered to symbolically sustain a military order whose spiritual strength relied on the Church's proposed mission of 're-Christianisation of the nation'. But the most powerful meaning of the Marian devotion during this time was her 'divine maternity', whose attributes were emphasised to delineate the figure of the Catholic mother. With her, arrived a less promising prospect for Córdoba's mothers if we compare it with the content of the journalistic literature of the 1920s that highlighted 'woman's liberation' through the Assumption and the Immaculate Conception. Certainly, the Mary of the 1930s onwards left the sanctuary to parade another message on the city's main streets, one that was much closer to the *Mater Dolorosa*, in that it recalled the sorrowful mother whose strength overcame the most inconceivable pain for the sake of her son. Throughout the 1940s, both the Marian cult and the message of the Divine Maternity continued being reinforced by the Church, the Catholic Action and the press. In a column entitled 'Message to mothers' that appeared in *Los Principios* during 1945 and 1946, it was written, 'When we see ourselves under physical and moral tests, we should consider that the pain is the path that leads us to heaven . . . didn't (Jesus) fulfil Mary, his beloved mother, with affliction and pain?'[49] In another article of this column it was affirmed that divorce and the artificial control of birth 'destroys woman's dignity and the sanctity of the home'.[50]

By then, neither the clergy nor laymen were alone in shaping the mother's role and its associated representations. As we have seen in Chapter 2, Catholic doctors contributed a vital medical interpretation to support and voice the doctrine too. Yet their perspectives and their influence through the positions many of them held in medical institutions, hospitals and health offices across the country have been little studied by historians of medicine. Here, I will approach their ideas on motherhood and I will do so mainly through the prism of the press.

Los Principios and the spread of medical knowledge

The spread of medical ideas in the Catholic press was inextricably linked to two main but different sorts of sources, one doctrinal, produced by the Pope and theologians, and the other medical, produced by local Catholic physicians. Papal intervention in topics concerning the practice of medicine became more prominent from the 1930s, with the encyclical *Casti Connubii* and Pius XI's call to organise professional associations of Catholic doctors across the world. Faithful Catholic doctors, on the other hand, had an active participation in the Argentinian parliament, academic societies, sanitary structure, and in public and private health services, an influence they had managed to exert by occupying strategic positions since the beginning of the expansion of the healthcare system. Early in the century, and parallel to the formation of a group of liberal, positivist hygienists that filled the first vacancies in the National Department of Hygiene, there was a group of Catholic hygienists who attempted to sway state policy with the stamp of Catholicism. Many of them were appointed in the various hospitals administered by the ladies of the Society of Beneficence in Buenos Aires, and by different female charitable organisations with close connections with the Church. Catholic doctors had also an important presence in the government of Argentina's state-run universities, and its medical faculties, departments and institutes. Their longstanding intervention in the country's oldest University, the University of Córdoba, was vigorously contested by students during the University Reform (1918), generating a left-wing ideological movement of university youth whose ideals soon spread nationally and to other Latin American countries. Catholic doctors were also instrumental in the creation and direction of the Medical Circles, which were created to protect the interests of the profession, like the one founded in 1910 in Córdoba by, amongst others, the ultra-Catholic ex-Chancellor of the university, Dr Antonio Nores, who was its first director. It is worth mentioning that Nores also integrated the directorate of *Los Principios* in the 1920s.

With such an influential position in the academic establishment Catholic physicians largely intervened in the process of state legitimisation of the medical field at both the national and provincial level. Crucial to this process was the political career that many of these doctors developed along with their medical profession, thus strengthening the bonds that linked medicine with state policy. Among them, stands out the parliamentary work of two prominent Cordoban doctors, Dr Félix Garzón Maceda (1867-1940), and, especially, Dr Juan F. Cafferata (1877-1957) who served as deputy in the National Chamber for nearly 30 years. Both hygienists politically represented the most progressive sectors of Catholicism in all matters related to the country's health and welfare system. According to health historian Héctor Recalde, Catholic hygienists, like their Socialists fellows, shifted the centre of preoccupations of the sanitary field, from the nineteen-century focus on 'hygiene-civilisation' to the one centred on the 'hygiene-social question'.[51] This generation of hygienists and 'social reformers' denounced workers' labour and material conditions, and claimed for a greater state intervention in the improvement of welfare provision. Their visions, however, differed considerably, to put it in Cafferata's words:

> The Catholic and the Socialist are happy in defending the legitimate demands of the proletariat; in improving the working class housing; in combating the terrible consequences of alcoholic intoxication; in procuring the lower prices for subsistence. But between the Catholic – who considers material improvement as a means to attain moral progress, and man's ultimate aim which is eternal happiness – and the Socialist – who denies the immortal soul and seeks only an earthly happiness – there is an abyss. The discrepancy in aims is due to the divergence of principles.[52]

Catholic hygienists added a moral component to the parliamentary debates on public health and healthcare provision, which was only sometimes compatible with Church doctrine. From the state, they demanded labour legislation, programmes of assistance for alcoholics and tuberculosis sufferers, and housing projects for the working classes. The latter became a primary concern due to the fear of 'moral promiscuity' generated by overcrowded lodgings, whose urban presence multiplied with the arrival of mass immigration. From individuals, they demanded charitable work and an active involvement in lay Catholic groups as a way of smoothing social conflicts and extending the public influence of Catholic social action. Provided their commitment to the Church's principles was unquestionable, something that not always was apparent, their projects and proposals found support in *Los Principios*. Professionals and legislators found there a tribune for the dissemination of medical and welfare ideas, through the publication of parliamentary projects and speeches given at the annual celebrations of charitable organisations, where many of them served.

Concentrating our attention on the paper's treatment of mother and child issues, it is possible to assert that *Los Principios*'s editorial policy did not differ from the one sustained regarding other health or sanitary problems existing at the time. In this sense, the paper largely endorsed the proposals of the elite of Catholic specialists (paediatricians and obstetricians) acting in the period, and it did so according to particular political circumstances, that is, when Catholic forces needed to publicly demonstrate their commitment for social problems. The same applied in relation to the initiatives of state authorities, mayors and governors, in this area, whenever their candidacy and election to office had been supported by the Church and Catholic political forces.[53]

During the first decades, and reflecting what was the main concern at the time, articles addressing issues of infant well-being outweighed those that revealed an interest for mothers' welfare. Only in 1930, when the lack of maternity services in Córdoba was notoriously absent, a piece emphatically requested from the President of the Republic, Hipólito Yrigoyen, to send the 'promised funds' to inaugurate the Maternity Institute.[54] But here again, politics prevailed as this article, along with others that appeared in *Los Principios* systematically questioning the President, was part of a nation-wide journalistic campaign that ended with Yrigoyen's overthrow by a military *coup d'état*. Equally political was the omission in the piece, to name obstetrician José Lascano, mentor of the Maternity Institute, who had been vigorously demanding for the provision of funds necessary to inaugurate the institute. This might be explained by the fact that Lascano did not form part of the medical Catholic circle.

As far as the medical education for mothers is concerned, in the sampled issues I selected for the period, *Los Principios* offered virtually no advice to mothers on how to look after their children, either in terms of hygiene or in terms of potentially dangerous diseases, nor did it recommend them to seek medical advice during pregnancy and delivery. It is true that this was also the case for the liberal press, as we will see in the next chapter. There is very fragmented evidence as to suggest that this was also observed in other provincial newspapers. If this was indeed the case, then historians should be more precise in their appraisal of a 'medicalised' society during this period even when the advertisement of medical products appeared in newspapers, or medical advice related to childrearing practices were found in specialised magazines. It is however, interesting to reflect on how the Catholic press engaged with the problems of maternity and infant mortality, how it politicised the public discussion (feminism *vs.* the Catholic mother, or by supporting Catholic doctors) and foreclosed the discussion of the physical aspects of maternity at the same time. It is well known that any public description that involved the biological body, like the act of breastfeeding, was interpreted as awakening the instincts and therefore relegated to the private domain. The moral obstruction that prevented discussion on female corporal issues was

117

counterbalanced by the instruction on the spiritual aspects of motherly tasks, mainly in the 'Social Section', which as discussed earlier, encouraged mothers to instil in their children an education and habits grounded in Catholic values. This was, on occasions, supported from a medical point of view, but remarkably, this found expression through the literary narrative. Dr Cafferata, most enthusiastically, believed in the didactic potential of writing social novels and short stories as a way of instilling medical teaching in a Catholic frame.[55] It is difficult to discern if the resort to fiction stemmed from an awareness of growing competition from secular magazines and novels, or because they believed this was a more suited genre for women to understand. In any case, the Catholic doctor articulated a reinterpretation of the biological component of his secular discipline into a version of 'nature', rather than the theological discussion or the Marian verb, to claim that mothers' role was naturally ordered rather than socially constructed or medically regulated:

> Nature guides and illuminates [parents], holds the mother as a custodial angel at home, makes her body light, her hand sweet, provides to her weak organism a new strength, and awakes and inspires such feelings and tenderness that shape the path of love whereby the child's soul is naturally introduced in the bosom of society. [Nature] Establishes between these two hearts a mysterious and unlimited sympathy.[56]

The supremacy of the spiritual over the material implied that scientific knowledge ranked lower on the divinely ordained scale of values. As we have seen, in a time of fervent antagonism between clerical and anticlerical supporters, Catholic hygienists drew attention to the moral question to address a myriad of public health challenges posed by a growing urban population. Differences were not a mere question of diverging perspectives on specific policies, or on attitudes regarding those thorny issues that directly contravened Catholic faith, such as abortion, illegitimacy, or sexual education. Catholic doctors perceived themselves, and their practice, medical research, and role in society, as being informed by a substantially different interpretation of science as they sought to agree its principles with the magisterium of the Church. What divided a 'medical materialism' from a Catholic one was, according to Monsignor Gustavo Franceschi, the main intellectual referent of the Catholic magazine *Criterio*, that,

The scientist declares that nothing exists beyond what his intelligence perceives; he disregards, following Comte, the problems relative to the First Principle and the Last End, and he proclaims himself materialistic. Or, on the contrary, he humbly recognises that his knowledge and his potential have limits, and he prostrates himself towards God.[57]

It is interesting to note, as this reminds us, too, of the scope of Catholic ideas in the capital district during the 1930s, that this article was inspired by a speech given by the Dean of the Faculty of Medicine of Buenos Aires, who lamented that the 'strictly technical doctor of today' had replaced the 'doctors of aforetime' 'confessor of souls, consolation for the sufferer, and the inspiration of hope with his presence'. [58] Franceschi also paraphrased Ambroise Paré to emphasise the utmost principle of the Catholic physician as a mere 'instrument' in a divine plan, 'I looked after him, God cured him'. Underlying these assumptions, there was a conception of bodily pain and suffering not only spiritually, but physically grounded, which pervaded medical practice as well as the very notion of illness. To those sufferers of incurable diseases, an article in *Criterio* recommended, 'See in suffering a supernatural perspective, and therefore, [we should] not attempt to annul it, nor overcome it, but to make the most of it as an instrument of individual purification, since wisdom consists of taking advantage of the holy utility of pain'.[59]

Physical and spiritual suffering pervaded the exhortatory writing produced in *Los Principios*, particularly, in its fictional representation of maternal problems, where suffering and/or poverty appeared as ennobling. Little short stories published during the period, represented in fiction a reality that indicated high infant and maternal mortality rates, lack of assistance and poverty. Yet the paper's sentimentalised portrayals, such as those written by Cafferata, provided no practical considerations on how to improve mothers' conditions or a suggestion that poverty was unfair. Almost invariably, the paper emphasised the need of a strong faith as the best 'medicine' that mothers could have to confront deprivation, a son's death, or any distressing circumstance that affected her motherhood.

Towards the end of the 1920s, the dichotomy of science/spirituality deepened in the Catholic world, having an unprecedented impact within the structures of medical corporations, as proved by the international creation and rapid dissemination of the associations of Catholic Doctors.

Towards a moral medicine: The Consortium of Catholic Doctors

Specific doctrinal guidelines clearly addressing medical practice had a starting point in the 1930 encyclical *Casti Connubii,* which banned abortion, birth control, sterilisation and eugenic measures as contrary to Catholic principles. These principles were later to be guarded worldwide by the associations of Catholic Doctors, the guild heavily promoted by Pious XI whose international presence rose after the first international meetings gathered in Budapest (1930) and Paris (1934).

In Argentina this process was accompanied by the development of a wide range of specialised and popular medical literature, including medical journals, books, and magazines. The role of the Catholic press, as I will analyse through *Los Principios,* was significant in that it spread the activities and goals of the Consortium of Catholic Doctors – as they were called in Argentina – firstly, in conveying the distinctiveness of the Catholic doctor in the frame of a medical profession that was rapidly increasing its number of graduates, and secondly, in raising awareness, amongst its readers, about the ethical component involved in 'the art of healing'.

To understand the reception of the Vatican's ideas and the creation of 'Catholic Consortiums' in Argentina there are at least two convergent phenomenon to be analysed, firstly, the professionalisation and legitimisation of the medical field *in* the state, a process that associated the physician as a 'state employee' rather than a 'liberal professional'; and secondly, the growing biologisation of medicine and eugenically-oriented state policies to the detriment of the Church's moral authority within the sphere of family, reproduction and sexuality. In relation to the professionalization of medicine, we need to consider that the development of a sanitary structure since the end of the nineteenth century, a process undertaken by both the state and female charitable organisations, implied that the hospital became the institution of medical practice *par excellence,* and at the same time, one that endowed doctors with prestige and reputation. This process, however, left medical professionals largely dependent on gaining a hospital appointment, generating a supply of doctors that could not be fully absorbed by the hospital itself. Training hospitals, whether university clinics or charity hospitals, on the other hand, were dominated by a patronage system that largely controlled university appointments or were dependant on the equally restrictive system of appointment established by charitable ladies. As the number of graduates increased

120

in the 1920s, doctors started to question the disadvantages of the hospital system, formulating the first attempts at medical unionisation. This malaise in the profession also shed light on another problematic issue, which was the gradual decline of, and the difficulties in keeping, a private practice. This was denounced with alarm by Dr Cetrángolo in 1935, who stated,

> The tragedy of the physician is that he, who has made the hospital with his efforts and hard work, who has given the hospital its prestige by the progress of medicine, [he] is today threatened by being absorbed by the hospital.[60]

In contrast to the preponderance of services offered by the hospital, the private consulting room was losing prestige, as for many new graduates it was unable to secure an acceptable income, and more importantly, it could not offer the technology or the specialisation of services of modern medical treatments. While this phenomenon affected all the members of the medical profession, only Catholic physicians feared another important one, the ideological problem. With public health expanding its areas of intervention, the delineation of health policy was increasingly under state control. This situation particularly concerned Catholic physicians who questioned, in ideological terms, the right of the state to rule in all orders of society. The deep-rooted dispute about the temporal versus the spiritual order that had historically problematised State-Church relationships in Argentina, in this area too, framed the discussions. For Catholic doctors this often implied a tension between the exigencies of a moral doctrine and those of a secularised science, whose distance was being widened by the state due to the transformation of the medical profession into a state profession. In addition, the biologisation of medical knowledge informed by eugenic theories in the 1930s discussed in Chapter 2, would lead to an unprecedented state intervention into the individual's private sphere, by regulating issues concerning the family, sexuality, reproduction and especially maternity in order to promote biological and social change. The most militant and representative figures amongst Catholic doctors fiercely opposed the lack of morality that informed an eugenically orientated medicine in issues such as therapeutic abortion, sterilisation, prenuptial certificate, and so on, whose practice took place within the state sanitary structure. In this sense, the creation of the countrywide Consortium of Catholic Doctors (*Consorcio de Médicos Católicos* - CCD) provided them with an institutional platform to voice their concerns.

121

The CCD were encouraged by the Vatican as part of the overarching project of re-Christianisation of the social order by means of the laity's participation in corporative associations tightly controlled by the ecclesiastical hierarchy of which the Catholic Action was its most accomplished form. In Argentina, the first CCD was created in Buenos Aires in 1929, with the aim of 'defending the principles of the Catholic moral following the norms and doctrines of the Church in all matters related to medicine'.[61] Organised under the patronage of the Archbishop, who supervised their activities, the CCD also joined the Catholic Action once the chapter was created in 1931.[62] Their ideas were published in the medical journal *Iatria*, which, in its first number, contained a papal message addressed to the international congress of doctors gathered in Budapest (1930) to discuss nothing less than 'sexual ethics'. Pius XI there stated,

> Adulterating the directions and principles of the Church, the impious and immoral teaching of disgraceful procedures are so widespread that they are turning the physician from being the saviour and regenerator of the family and society into its most despicable corruptor.[63]

It may seem strange that in Córdoba, 'the city of bells', the CCD was created only in 1938, almost a decade after the one in Buenos Aires.[64] Three main reasons may explain this delay. Firstly, cultural differences between cosmopolitan, liberal Buenos Aires, and traditionalist, religious Córdoba have played a role in the different reception of eugenic ideas, as we have seen in Chapter 2. Secondly, Catholic physicians exerted in Córdoba a much more important influence than their peers in the capital of the Republic, because of their significant presence in the University and in public and charity hospitals. Thirdly, the timing for the creation of the Consortium should also be linked to the secular health policies initiated by the leftist government of Dr Amadeo Sabattini (1936-40), from the Radical Civic Union party, who amongst other measures, implemented prophylactic campaigns on venereal diseases while promoting sexual education.

Following the articles of *Los Principios*, which became the organ of diffusion of the CCD's activities, we can trace their proposals and aims. The inaugural meeting in 1938 was announced by the paper with big headlines and photographs in a broad coverage that spanned two days. The paper reproduced the speech of the CCD's president, Dr Ramón Brandán, who was Chair of Clinical Medicine at the National University of Córdoba, Con-

122

sulting Physician of the Institute of Maternity, and Director of the charity hospital for tubercular patients, Hospital Tránsito Cáceres de Allende. He started by thanking Archbishop Lafitte for calling for the foundation of the Consortium, a call that according to Brandán, doctors had responded to with 'satisfaction', since 'the religious truth, [is] so noble even more than the scientific one'.[65] After explaining the principles of the Thomistic philosophy, where Catholic doctors turned for guidance and inspiration, he addressed the problems that modern medicine, especially an eugenically-orientated one, was posing at the time,

> The lack of philosophical culture has resulted in deviations and lamentable mistakes in this modern scientific movement, such as the pansensualism of Freud, already happily overtaken by Adler and others, or those for whom the human soul is nothing more than the result of a harmonious constellation of glands of internal secretion. A philosophical argument of the current doctrines of racism – a direct consequence of the Protestant Reform and liberalism – seeks to improve men with the same criteria applied to the improvement of the genetics of horses.[66]

Brandán fervently criticised the sexological tendency of medical knowledge, especially through the intervention of eugenics and endocrinology, since, in his view, they led to the denigration of the medical profession while it conspired against the morality that should rule the constitution of the family. His unsympathetic remarks on Freud are also very telling, as psychoanalysis had an enduring penetration in Argentinian intellectual and scientific circles. Its inception in the medical field was related to the dissemination of constitutional medicine and its focus on a holistic interpretation (physiological and psychological) of disease aetiology. During the 1930s married life and its hidden sexuality started to be scrutinised especially by those specialists engaged in the growing field of endocrine gynaecology, who started to associate uncertain cases of uterine and ovary dysfunctions with women's episodes of psychological *disequilibrium*. Parallel to the circulation of a popular sexual literature, where psychoanalysis found its major source of dissemination in Buenos Aires' culture,[67] the increasing attention to the private order of intimacy, passions and sexual dissatisfaction also spurred the elaboration of a medical interpretation of sexual discontent. At this juncture, Catholic doctors claimed for a moral orientation of medical explanations, grounded

123

in the 'natural principles' of the family, in the divinely appointed sexual roles in society, and in the natural function of maternity. During the 1940s as the question of *dénatalité* reached the status of a national problem, Brandán for example, taught to his students that the cause of several organic gynaecological disorders was in the psychological damage produced by contraceptive practices.[68]

In tune with the highly ritualised Catholic culture of the 1930s, the activities of the CCD were constructed around pious rites.[69] Their mission was not only morally to influence colleagues in their daily practice, but also to sway, as a medical institution, state health policy. The CCD's conferences were dominated by the themes that loomed large in the public agenda of the period, namely the regulation of human reproduction and its associated topics, birth control, induced abortion, temporary sterilisation, inheritance law, prenuptial certificate, venereal disease, tuberculosis and pregnancy, and sexual education, amongst others. As mentioned above, during the 1940s, the decline in birth rates prompted a renewed concern for demographic problems in Argentina, particularly after the military *coup d'état* of 1943, which created a National Commission of Dénatalité with the aim of studying and finding a solution to the problem of depopulation. In Córdoba, a member of the CCD, Dr Bernardo Bas, who was Professor in the Department of Clinical Obstetrics and Director of the Hygiene Department (1943-46), was appointed member to the Commission. Bas spearheaded an anti-abortion campaign, as he wrote in *Los Principios*, 'with moral authority and patriotic spirit, to reach the bosom of households in order to return dignity to mothers and a sense of virile responsibility to the head of the home'.[70] His statistics on population growth made him come to the conclusion that wealthier and bourgeois families were the ones that had fewer children (something that was statistically evident since the 1930s). Yet, what was less evident in previous discourses on population decline was not the assumption of contraceptive practices, which Bas also acknowledged, but the practice of abortion. As part of the new rhetoric that charged well-off families for the moral decay, for their indulgence in an 'easy life' with little space for familial responsibilities, and less so for patriotic duties, the condemnation of criminal abortion resonated in a wide spectrum of perspectives and health policy-makers.[71] For Bas, voluntary or criminal abortion seemed to be the main cause that lay behind Argentinian demographic decline, or at least the cause that disturbed him the most. As director of the Department of Hygiene, Bas' anti-abortion campaign was well covered by the press (*Los Principios* and the daily *Diario*

124

Córdoba), where his articles made explicit aspects that were inspired by the pro-natalist, Catholic position leaded by Alejandro Bunge (1880–1943), one of the most recognised figures on Argentinian demography.

The construct class-race-civilisation present in Bunge was informed by ongoing preoccupations in industrialised countries for the 'decline of the white race', which in Bunge's adaptation was translated into an anxiety for the low fecundity of the affluent classes whom he identified as embodying the 'highest interests of nation and race', while he expressed dismay at the fecundity pattern of the 'inferior people'.[72] Bunge's natalist plans were analogous to those proposed by the Italian eugenist and fascist Corrado Gini,[73] with proposals that ranged from the stimulation of population growth in the interior of the country, to financial and legal measures that attempted to increase the number of legitimate unions. Like other Catholics who embraced eugenic ideas, and followed those who brokered in Italy an acceptable church-eugenics ideological conciliation, Bunge's pro-natalist ideas were supported by *Criterio*'s writers, and other prominent members of the CCD. In this sense, the reduction of a group of Catholics preoccupied with Argentinian demography to their religious militancy, as Hernán Otero has rightly noted for the case of Bunge, does not sufficiently account for the connexions and multiple nuances that have informed their theoretical perspective.[74] Resuming the ideas of one of Bunge's followers in Córdoba, Dr Bas, whose pro-natalist approach was perhaps more restricted that that of Bunge, in that it was exclusively directed to eminent and well-off families. It is interesting to see that, unlike the proposals aiming at reducing infant mortality, the teaching of puericulture, illegitimacy, and all those measures that sought to increase the vigour of the population, in Bas' proposals, working-class mothers and families did not warrant any comment. To be sure, Bas was not worried about the reproductive patterns of the lower segments of society, nor was he interested in those incentive measures proposed by Bunge as a solution for population growth. Bas' class-ridden concern for demographic growth was reduced to a moral/patriotic obligation from the 'right people' to breed, and to the legal, criminal prosecution of their abortive practices. Not surprisingly, on the one hand, he angrily attacked doctors, rather than midwives, as the main agents involved in this illegal trade, thus assuming a clientele of wealthy women able to afford the payment of a professional; and on the other, he targeted middle and upper-class mothers' behaviours with resentful reproaches. In one of his journalistic articles, he commented that,

Society has habituated itself to the new type of woman that has replaced the true mother and spouse. To this modern product, semi-
mother, semi-spouse; to the superficial female, fearful of losing com-
fort or the slenderness of her flesh if she engenders children; who if
she is well-off, will know sports, fashions and social display, will live
with fierce selfishness and for the detailed care of her appearance.[75]

To this social representation of the 'new woman' he added physical features
that, he assured, would unmistakably unveil to society the woman who had
aborted. When biological laws were broken, 'grave and innumerable physiological alterations occur,' whose marks, he warned, were easily visible:

It is commonly observable to both physicians and laypersons how the
physical aspect of women with many children contrasts with those
with many abortions: healthy-looking and youthful the former ones;
faded, prematurely aged and decadent the latter ones.[76]

This attempt to pathologise modern women's behaviour with distinctive
medical features supports the multiple Catholic representations that functioned at the time to control women's sexuality and their decisions about
motherhood. These representations cannot be separated from perceived social indicators, such as, women's birth control, on the one hand, and a secular medical perspective on reproduction that sought to protect the biological composition of the population, on the other. The latter became evident
through statutory health measures and in a wide range of medical practices,
such as temporary and definitive sterilisation, hormone-therapy, therapeutic
abortions, prenuptial certificates and preconception advice. The spiritual figure of the 'Catholic mother' in the 1930s, with its emphasis on self-denial and
child-devotion was thus reinforced by the one offered by Catholic doctors,
who attempted to support its spiritual values with physical signs of social
recognition. This also reveals the emergence of new 'bio-moral' articulations
in the 1940s, where endocrine medicine is made to agree and support an anti-
birth control stance, which as noted before, became more strident according
to the ascension of population groups in the class structure. The dissemination in this particular church-controlled newspaper of these medical ideas
gives us insight into the irremediable public involvement of Catholic culture
in ongoing discussions of demography and reproduction in a way that Mary's
cloak alone could no longer sufficiently secure.

Visual representations of motherhood in the newspaper *Los Principios*, through photojournalism, would take the imprint of Catholic ideas a bit further, as we shall see in Chapter 6. But so will too the Catholic novel (analysed in Chapter 5), a literary genre that grew out of the deep-seated fear of secularism and moral dissolution. Representations of motherhood in Argentinian society, this study argues, appear as disperse statements elaborated by different registers. Somehow the virtue of the ubiquity of the Catholic one, of the little explored vast and I would emphasise varied penetration of a Catholic culture that was becoming more heterogeneous in its formulations and sources of inspiration is that it helps us to see that there were no fixed places for its enunciation, and that the 'sons' that represented the mother were not only the spiritual, celibate ones. There were also the son-doctors and journalists, and as Nora Domínguez has argued for the fictional representation of motherhood, the son-narrators.[77]

Notes

1   A. Clavero (priest), 'Variaciones Sobre el Periodismo Católico', *Los Principios* (9 July 1924), 27.

2   P. Gaudiano, 'El Concilio Plenario Latinoamericano (Roma 1899). Preparación, Celebración y Significación', *Revista Eclesiástica Platense*, 101 (1998), 1063-78.

3   N. Auza, *Aciertos y Fracasos Sociales del Catolicismo Argentino: Grote y la Estrategia Social*, I (Buenos Aires: Docencia y Don Bosco, 1988), 93.

4   *Sínodo Diocesano Celebrado en Córdoba por el Iltmo. y Rmo. Señor Obispo Don Fray Zenón Bustos y Ferreira el Año del Señor de MCMVI: Resoluciones y Apéndices* (Córdoba: Tip. La Industrial, 1907), 4-5. Fray Zenón Bustos y Ferreira was bishop of Córdoba between 1905 and 1925, although from 1919 when he suffered a stroke and until his death in 1925 he was replaced by priest J. Anselmo Luque.

5   Z. Bustos, *Libro de Autos y Visitas Parroquiales, 1885-1916* (29 January 1906), folio 5, Archivo de la Arquidiócesis de Córdoba.

6   In Buenos Aires there were the following Catholic papers, *La América del Sud* (1876-80), *La Unión* (1882-90), *La Voz de la Iglesia* (1883-1911); in Córdoba, *El Eco de Córdoba* (1862-86) and *El Porvenir* (1886-94). In the case of the latter, the majority of its editorial board subsequently

founded *Los Principios* in 1894. For the development of the Catholic press in Córdoba during the nineteenth century, see P. Vagliente, *Indicios de Modernidad. Una Mirada Socio-Cultural desde el Campo Periodístico en Córdoba, 1860-1880* (Córdoba: Alción Editora, 2000).

7   L.A. Quintana, 'La Constitución del Diario Católico *La Mañana*, Santa Fe 1934-1937. Aportes Para un Uso Didáctico de la Cultura Católica', *Clío & Asociados*, 13 (2009), 13-33. Online at: http://www.fuentesmemoria.fahce.unlp.edu.ar/art_revistas/pr.4623/pr.4623.pdf (consulted 20.05.2011)

8   L. Miranda, 'Una Modernización en Clave de Cruzada: El Diario Católico de Buenos Aires en la Década de 1920: El Pueblo', *Revista Escuela de Historia*, 7 (2008). Online at: http://www.redalyc.org/src/inicio/ArtPdfRed.jsp?iCve=63818509004 (consulted 20.05.2011)

9   *Los Principios* (9 July 1924), 27.

10   *Los Principios* (9 July 1924), 18.

11   *Los Principios* (9 July 1924), 2.

12   *Los Principios* (9 July 1924), 27.

13   *Los Principios* (15 July 1908), 2.

14   Pope Benedicto XV in his Encyclical *Sacra Propediem*, 1921, stated, 'From this point of view one cannot sufficiently deplore the blindness of so many women of every age and condition; made foolish by desire to please, they do not see to what a degree the indecency of their clothing shocks every honest man, and offends God. Most of them would formerly have blushed for those toilettes as for a grave fault against Christian modesty; now it does not suffice for them to exhibit them on the public thoroughfares; they do not fear to cross the threshold of the churches, to assist at the Holy sacrifice of the Mass, and even to bear the seducing food of shameful passions to the Eucharistic Table where one receives the heavenly Author of purity.' *Vatican Web Site*. Online at: http://www.vatican.va/holy_father/benedict_xv/encyclicals/documents/hf_ben-xv_enc_06011921_sacra-propediem_en.html (consulted 17. 08.2010). At the end of the 1920s, Pius XI delivered specific instructions to be observed and disseminated into the community by bishops about the modesty in clothing: 'A dress cannot be called decent which is cut deeper than two fingers' breath under the pit of the throat, which does not cover the arms at least to the elbows, and scarcely reaches a bit beyond the knees. Furthermore, dresses of transparent materials are improper. . .'. Quoted in the

Spanish newspaper *La Vanguardia*, (11 July 1929), 10. Online at http://www.lavanguardia.com/hemeroteca/index.html (consulted 30.04.2011).

15 The Bishopric of Córdoba issued Pastoral Letters and extensively commented in its official bulletin on the indecency of female clothing, to which it considered as a 'grave sin'. It also gave precise instructions to parish priests on how to interrogate and admonish women during the confessional act. In *Boletín Eclesiástico de la Diócesis de Córdoba*, 1 (1930), 23-27.

16 *Los Principios* (17 July 1919), 2.

17 Ibid.

18 See Patricia Holland, 'The Politics of the Smile: 'Soft news' and the Sexualisation of the Popular Press', in C. Carter, G. Branston and S. Allan (eds.), *News, Gender and Power* (London and New York: Routledge, 1998), 17-32.

19 *Los Principios* (11 July 1924), 2.

20 *Los Principios* (3 January 1901), 2.

21 On the perceptions of women's work by other social groups see M. Lobato, *Historia de las Trabajadoras en la Argentina (1869-1960)* (Buenos Aires: Edhasa, 2007); and from the perspective of the Catholic Church see C. Wainerman, 'La Mujer y el Trabajo en la Argentina desde la Perspectiva de la Iglesia Católica', *Cuadernos del CENEP*, 16, Centro de Estudios de Población (1980), 1-30.

22 *Los Principios* (1 March 1902), 1.

23 *Los Principios* (9 August 1908), 2.

24 French Catholic women identified themselves as "feministes Chretienes" in 1896.

25 *Los Principios* (29 July 1910), 3.

26 Ibid.

27 *Los Principios* (20 July 1920), 2.

28 D. Velasco, 'La Asunción de la Sma. Vírgen y la Elevación Social de la Mujer', *Los Principios* (15 August 1924), 3. My emphasis.

29 O. Walker, 'La Misión Social de la Mujer', *Los Principios* (27 August 1924), 4.

30 Ibid.

31 *Los Principios* (8 December 1924), 1.

32 N. Perry and L. Echeverría, *Under the Heel of Mary* (London and New York: Routledge, 1988), 118.

33 Ibid.

34 *Encyclical Lux Veritatis* (25/12/1931), *Papal Encyclicals Online*, Online at: http://www.papalencyclicals.net/Pius11/P11VERIT.HTM (consulted 7.02. 2011).

35 Ibid., (para. 50).

36 Ibid., (para. 52).

37 P. Misner, 'Catholic Labor and Catholic Action: The Italian Context of "Quadragesimo Anno"', *The Catholic Historical Review*, 90, 4 (2004), 650-74.

38 *Los Principios* (11 August 1917), 1.

39 *Boletín Eclesiástico de la Diócesis de Córdoba*, 11 (1934), 348-50.

40 Accati, 'Explicit Meanings', 245.

41 For the Spanish case, see M. Vincent, 'Gender and Morals in Spanish Catholic Youth Culture. A Case Study of the Marian Congregations 1930-1936', *Gender & History*, 13, 2 (2001), 273-97.

42 Linda Hall has investigated the Marian devotion of the Virgin of Luján in Buenos Aires by the military state of the 1930s, and also the resonances of the Marian cult in Argentinian political life through the figure of Eva Perón, in L. Hall, *Mary, Mother and Warrior: The Virgin in Spain and the Americas* (Austin: University of Texas Press, 2004), Chs. 7 and 8 respectively.

43 *Los Principios* (20 October 1934), 4.

44 Ibid.

45 The 11th of October was the date chosen by the Argentinian Church to commemorate the Divine Maternity of Mary.

46 *Los Principios* (11 October 1935), 6.

47 *Los Principios* (10 October 1935), 2.

48 *Los Principios* (11 October 1935), 8.

49 *Los Principios* (4 May 1945), 10.

50 The article was entitled, 'Women who do not appreciate themselves', and it reproduced a radio broadcasted conference in Paris delivered by the director of University of Notre Dame, who stated that 'the best thermometer of people's strength, and more importantly of its moral strength, is the appreciation or dismissal of the Christian concept of motherhood, ennobled by the Mother of God. The disdain of Her dignity is the first sign of the moral decay of a nation.' *Los Principios* (4 July 1946), 12.

51 H. Recalde, 'Transformaciones Dentro del Discurso Higienista', in R. Salvatore (ed.), *Reformadores Sociales en Argentina, 1900-1940: Discurso,*

Ciencia y Control Social, DTS 119, (Buenos Aires: Instituto Torcuato Di Tella, 1992), 40-45: 42.

52 J. Cafferata, 'La Eucaristía en la Vida Social', in Moreyra, Remedi and Ruggio, *El Hombre y sus Circunstancias*, 313.

53 In 1926 the paper celebrated the sanction of a municipal bill by the Catholic and conservative Mayor, Emilio Olmos, ordering the creation of *crèches* in industrial work places with 20 or more working mothers to breast-feed their children. 'Infant's health should be a primary preoccupation of the public power.' . . . 'we welcome all the initiatives that pursue social improvement' . . . 'especially of the infants exposed to the risks of poverty or to becoming orphans', in *Los Principios* (8 November 1926), 1.

54 *Los Principios* (6 July 1930), 1.

55 Among Cafferata's literary works are: *Esther*, a novel published in *Los Principios* in 1910, to teach about the evils of tuberculosis through the story of a girl from a wealthy family; and *El Secreto del Bargueño o el Hijo del Anticuario* (1918) a novel featuring the tragedies of an alcoholic man also against the backdrop of a traditional, well-to-do family.

56 *Los Principios* (25 September 1932), 7.

57 G. Franceschi, 'Dios y la Fisiología', *Criterio*, 317 (1934), 295-97: 295.

58 R. Bullrich quoted in G. Franceschi, 'Dios y la Fisiología', 295.

59 C. Lerena, 'Eutanasia y Eugenesia', *Criterio*, 293 (1933), 206-7: 206.

60 A. Cetrángolo, 'La Crisis de la Profesión Médica', *Revista Médica de Córdoba* (1935), 341-52: 547.

61 C. Carranza Casares, 'Consorcio de Médicos Católicos', *Iatría*, 78, 189 (2008), 6-7: 6.

62 On the CCD in Buenos Aires see O. Acha, 'El Catolicismo y la Profesión Médica en la Década Peronista', *Centro Cultural de la Cooperación*. [s.d.] Online at: http://www.centrocultural.coop/descargas/historia/el-catolicismo-y-la-profesion-medica-en-la-decada-peronista.html (consulted 17.08.2010); and *A. M. T. Rodríguez*, 'La Perspectiva Católica Sobre la Salud y la Práctica Médica en la Argentina de los Años Treinta. La Visión de los Médicos Confesionales', *Anuario de Estudios Americanos*, 65, 1 (2008), 257-75.

63 Quoted in Acha, 'El Catolicismo y la Profesión Médica', 4-5.

64 In Córdoba, Catholic medical students organised a Catholic Centre of Medicine in 1932, which held seminars and conferences prior to the creation of the CCD in August 1938.

65 *Los Principios* (7 August 1938), 3.

66 Ibid.

67 See H. Vezzetti, 'Las Promesas del Psicoanálisis en la Cultura de Masas', in *Historia de la Vida Privada en la Argentina. Tomo III. La Argentina entre Multitudes y Soledades: De los Años Treinta a la Actualidad* (Buenos Aires: Taurus, 1999), 173-97.

68 R. Brandán, 'Patología de la Contracepción. Síndrome de Sedillot', *Revista de la Facultad de Ciencias Médicas,* Universidad Nacional de Córdoba, 5, 5 (1947), 537-75.

69 At the inaugural conference in Córdoba, Dr Castaño, obstetrician and President of the CCD of Buenos Aires, delivered a speech on 'physicians and the moral', which ended with a plea to the audience to pray. He was followed by the blessing of the ceremony by Archbishop Lafitte. The conference was attended by fifty-six doctors, who became the first members of the Consortium. Their annual sessions took place in the Seminar of the Archdiocese of Córdoba, where they also celebrated with mass and communion the 'day of the doctor' (18th of October) in commemoration of the festivity of St. Luke, the patron saint of physicians. The Archbishop, on the other hand, supervised and approved the CCD biannual reports, which were published in *Los Principios*.

70 *Los Principios* (18 October 1944), 6.

71 Dr Aráoz Alfaro was one of the main opponents of abortion at the beginning of the 1940s, see Reggiani, 'Depopulation, Fascism, and Eugenics', 314-15.

72 A. Bunge, *Una Nueva Argentina* (Buenos Aires: G. Kraft Ltda., 1940).

73 Bunge established academic links with Corrado Gini with whom he collaborated as member of the advisory board of the journal *Metron* that Gini directed.

74 H. Otero, *Estadística y Nación: Una Historia Conceptual del Pensamiento Censal de la Argentina Moderna, 1869-1914* (Buenos Aires: Prometeo Libros, 2006), 236. For the 1940s debates on demographic proposals see also C. Biernat *¿Buenos o Útiles?: La Política Inmigratoria del Peronismo* (Buenos Aires: Editorial Biblos, 2007); M. Miranda, 'La Biotipología en el Pronatalismo Argentino (1930-1983), *Asclepio*, 57, 1 (2005), 189-218, and A. Reggiani, 'Depopulation, Fascism, and Eugenics'.

75 B. Bas, 'Porque la Denatalidad es un Peligro para la Nación y el Individuo', in B. Bas, *Artículos Sueltos* (Córdoba: Pereyra, 1945), 35-48: 47.

76 Ibid., 45.
77 N. Domínguez, *De Donde Vienen los Niños,* 16.

4

The Liberal Press and the Political Uses of the Maternal

Analysing the transformations of the Latin American press at the turn of the nineteenth century, literary and cultural critic Julio Ramos queried the extent to which Jürgen Habermas' theorization on the changes experienced by the press in Europe and America were echoed in the region. His analysis was specifically related to what Habermas characterised as a perceived change from a politically-partisan and opinion-maker newspaper to an independent, autonomous and news-focussed press.[1] Ramos concluded that, 'The transformation of social communication was quite uneven in Latin America', and taking leading Argentinian newspaper *La Nación* as an example, he asserted that it was 'an extremely hybrid newspaper, which preserved vestiges of traditional journalism, even as it radically modernised its discursive and technologised organization'.[2] Ramos's observations can be extended to other Argentinian newspapers, which were less influential at the national level but were significant in provincial contexts, in particular those that continued circulating or started to do so after 1900. The case of *La Voz del Interior* in Córdoba is an instructive case in point. Founded in 1904 through the initiative of two local tradesmen who were sympathisers of the new political force, the centrist party Radical Civic Union, the paper developed a strong profile as an opinion-maker while rapidly becoming identified with radicalism, the party that mobilised the political participation of the middle-classes and urban masses. Right from its first issue, *La Voz del Interior* became the voice of liberal and anti-clerical thought, giving room to a wide spectrum of professionals and young university leftist writers including Socialists, Radicals, feminists and freethinkers. By using a direct and caustic prose style, *La Voz del Interior* soon developed a combative tone that encapsulated what the paper envisioned as 'the battle of ideas' against Catholics and their press (*Los Principios*), generating a level of antagonism that at its highest resulted in proscription, in violent attacks to its editorial office, and in the imprisonment of journalists.

The modernisation of the paper through print technology, the increase in advertisements, alongside the incorporation of the style that characterised the 'new journalism' throughout the period did not hinder the closeness of the paper to its public nor his struggle to control public political opinion. It rather seems to have stimulated its presence, forgoing a new sense of immediateness with the reader that somehow belies a process of 'transition from a press that took ideological sides to one that was primarily a business'[3] that Habermas and others have observed in industrialised countries during this time.[4] On the one hand, the incorporation of printing technology allowed the paper to increase its daily print run from 300 in 1904 to around 35,000 in 1930.[5] On the other, in those decades, sales and profitability were secondary to the paper's primary goals of political and cultural influence. Indeed, one telling example was the way in which *La Voz del Interior* secured the communication of scoops, where instead of publishing bulletins, which other newspapers used as a source of revenue, the paper found through the use of a blackboard an innovative device to project itself in the public space.[6] Placed outside the building of the editorial office in town, the blackboard communicated breaking news in a creative way: they were announced by means of resonant firecrackers to the thousands of passers-by in the city.

Yet the paper's appeal to a mass readership was not based in scoops and exclusives but in a political and anticlerical crusade as well as in an understanding of the emergence of a new reading public and its desire to be informed, persuaded and entertained. Through its pages it is possible to sense the paper's perception and portrayal of a society that was unmistakably changing in all its main structures. Amongst these perceived changes, the 'female question' and its wide range of associated topics, civic and civil rights, motherhood, welfare, work, sexuality and behaviour, occupied a considerable space. The decades of the 1920s and 1930s saw plenty of articles that tackled different aspects of the 'female question' that, in the case of *Los Principios*, as we have seen, were perceived as threatening the values of a traditional, Catholic society. The treatment of these themes in *La Voz del Interior,* and the opposing perspective it offered to the Catholic paper, renders the analysis of the press not only as a more complex cultural artefact, but it offers to the representations of motherhood a more authentic viewpoint by incorporating the different registers that mapped out the representations on which motherhood could be recognised.

The changing patterns of the 'new woman', especially with respect to her behaviour as a consumer was encouraged by an expanding fashion market opening up other representations of the feminine, most notably the 'flappers', to which the liberal press also helped to expand. And although *La Voz del Interior* offered a more liberal representation of women's clothing and attitudes, it did not escape attempts at the normalisation of a female identity that was under considerable transformation. I would argue that the paper functioned both to spread new images of women's social role, which affected the representations of motherhood, and as a locus of cultural and political exchange. In this sense, the treatment of feminism provides a good example of the former, while the topic of women, welfare and maternalism serve to illustrate the latter.

The development of feminism as a phenomenon and the ideas that it prompted beyond the specificities of the Argentinian movement largely featured in the national and the local printed media where it was unevenly received, but nowhere with such an unwavering opposition as in the religious press, which built upon the fear of its expansion a particular representation of the 'Catholic mother'. In *La Voz del Interior*, on the contrary, feminist ideas and activities at national level received considerable attention, something that was especially important in the absence of a local feminist movement and in the lack of a female press. If feminism seems to provide a meaningful topic from where to trace the paper's own social representation of motherhood, the mother's welfare stands out as another area where the paper articulated discourses of the maternal in a rather unconventional way. As we will see in the following pages, the paper spearheaded a 'maternal campaign' in the 1920s, which convincingly illustrates the political uses of the maternal during the time.

A third area of special focus will be the treatment of medical ideas both in the extent to which *La Voz del Interior* became instrumental in their spread, and in the ways that it contributed to reformulate its postulates. Feminism, welfare and medical ideas constituted the main spaces where discourses of the maternal circulated and were formulated offering us insight into the papers' own representation of motherhood. In so doing, they provide understanding more broadly of the interface of the biological and cultural that cut across the maternal during the period.

The feminist stamp

In the year of its inauguration, *La Voz del Interior* published in its editorial column an article entitled, 'The emancipation of women', a title evidently chosen to honour the famous homonymous essay that Cordoban feminist and writer María Eugenia Echenique (1851-1878), wrote in 1876.[7] The article of 1904 started by reproducing one of the resolutions of the International Women's Congress gathered in Berlin in that year, which stated: 'Men and women are born free and equal as independent members of society. Equally endowed with reason and capacity, they are equally entitled to exercise political rights'.[8] After pointing to the virtues and vices of famous women through history, and affirming female physical capacity to work, the article finished by inviting women 'to take part in the fight' to bring to power rulers that would respond to 'mutual aspirations'.[9] The author used a pseudonym, Raúl de Nanci, composed by two forenames, one masculine and the other feminine, suggesting, in an somewhat satirical way, a reversed 'dominion' to the traditional composition of surnames in Spanish married women, i.e. which adds to the woman's surname the one of her husband with the preposition 'de' ('of'). In this case, it was a man's name followed by or placed under the dominion 'of' a woman's name. However, it is the content of the article more than the chosen pseudonym that suggests that the author was a woman. In fact, *La Voz del Interior* had at least two women journalists in its early years, one of them was the writer and journalist Leonor Allende (1883-1931), who became a member of the editorial staff during the first decade of 1900s.[10] As this piece was probably the first in the local press in defending women's enfranchisement, one might expect, therefore, that it should have provoked a strong reaction among a readership mostly composed of men. This seems even more likely if we consider that the male vote was granted only in 1912 in Argentina, through a bill that declared it 'universal [meaning all classes], secret and compulsory'. There is no doubt that the paper was introducing a debate on a topic that was just starting to be articulated in society, following the participation of women – most of whom later became feminists – in newly formed middle and working-class parties (radicalism and Socialist Party).

Women's enfranchisement continued to be discussed in the following days, in the same editorial column, and most probably by the same author, who under different pseudonyms, fabricated a debate where men exchanged editorial letters arguing in favour and against it. The supposed 'debate' was striking for the exposition of ideas that became key arguments of Argentinian maternal feminism. In the last article that brought the debate to a close, for example, the writer resorted to a core argument of maternal feminism when he/she questioned, 'if the Nation is considered as a great family, why is it denied to her [woman] the entry into political affairs? What is a mother for? What is a spouse for?'[11] In his/her view, the mother's contribution to the

137

state needed to be translated into laws that empowered women. Men, said the journalist, have left to woman 'the most needed work and the worst rewarded one', to later create laws that have made her 'a slave of masculine egoism'.[12] Here it is possible to detect the more radical branch of Argentinian feminism of the early twentieth century, especially in its emphasis on the connection between maternity and political legitimacy. More importantly, this pseudo editorial debate demonstrates the extent to which the new paper was willing to give room to novel ideas emerging in a society that was starting to move along the path to modernity. And feminist ideas, as the paper let its readers know, were part of that process.

The two above mentioned women journalist are likely to have written – sometimes under pseudonyms, others without signature – most of the pro-feminist articles that I will be commenting on along this chapter. The topic of women's political rights in exchange for maternal duties was a recurrent one, but not the only one. Another area where the feminist stamp could be unmistakably traced is in education, and more specifically, in the role of maternal education. In an article entitled 'Mothers', its importance was explained by remarking on maternity's social function. There, it was asserted that,

> The first and the most powerful educator is the mother . . . What a work, what a sublime mission corresponds to woman in human destiny! She is more effective than man, she is more powerful. In her hands is the future of humankind. . . . Do mothers realise this?[13]

More revealingly, the article was built upon the recommendations of Johann Pestalozzi, the Swiss Protestant pedagogue, from whom the writer transcribed many passages to highlight the importance of mother-child education. In doing so, the role of motherhood, as it was delineated by the first wave of Argentinian feminism was voiced. Pestalozzi's ideas were first introduced in the country by the feminist writer and teacher Juana Manso (1819-1875), a campaigner for lay and free education, who embraced the Protestant faith to the hatred of the Catholic Church and conservative circles alike. Nineteenth-century Argentinian feminists, such as Echenique, Manso and Manuela Gorriti, extolled the mother's role in child education, and vigorously campaigned for women's instruction under the conviction that a well-educated mother would better accomplish her domestic duties, which ultimately underwrote a platform of liberal and professional education for women. To

138

fulfil that 'powerful mission', women's education should not only be granted but renewed and advanced by introducing them to the study of science and philosophy.[14] Another piece with the heading, 'It's about time', expressed in a complaining tone that 'woman's education is very poor, although she constitutes the basis of the family and shapes the hearts of future generations who will administer the country'.[15] The article also expanded the educational topic beyond the mother-child sphere to install it in the wider framework of education for work. It condemned the 'vanity' and 'elevated ideas' of some women who considered paid work as 'vile', while in other nations female work, the article argued, was the foundation of its happiness.

The second decade was marked by the First World War, whose events were widely covered by the international pages of *La Voz del Interior*. The wide interest awakened by the war, in a city like Córdoba, is explained by the large number of European immigrants among its population for whom the newspaper constituted the only means of communication. Interest in the war resulted in review articles, editorials and new sections, such as, 'Judgements and episodes of the Great World', devoted to analyse social aspects of the conflict. Some of these articles were exclusively dedicated to praising women's accomplishments during the war, particularly, women's work[16] as well as other female endeavours that emerged as a direct consequence of their contribution during the war. 'The triumph of Feminism', reads one of these headlines, to celebrate the arrival of the first woman into the American Congress. The article further praised the achievements of Miss Jeannette Rankin, a Republican candidate, who won a seat in a Democratic state, to whom it described as a '34 years old, slim, physically good looking and with an unusual intelligence',[17] a description that contradicted the masculine-like image with which feminists were commonly portrayed.

The powerful boost that the experience of the war gave to feminist movements across the Western world was echoed in *La Voz del Interior*, which kept its readers informed about some of the achievements and activities of feminists on both sides of the Atlantic. Such an attention is all the more striking if we consider that Córdoba did not develop a local feminist movement at the time. More importantly, the paper also lent its support to feminism in different ways, by endorsing its main claims, especially women's enfranchisement, by debunking feminists' stereotypes, and significantly, by using feminist ideas to review women's condition in Córdoba society. Women's involvement in local politics, for example, was always informed with encouraging words. Some articles contained or reproduced the ideas of women militants in the

139

radical party, the political force that the newspaper supported, while other pieces praised women's political contribution in sometimes lengthy obituaries.[18] At the same time, women's suffrage bills, like the one put forward by Socialist national deputy Mario Bravo in 1919, were enthusiastically welcomed.[19]

Criticisms of the feminist movement, at the same time, were not absent, although they were formulated in a constructive and thoughtful perspective. An article that appeared in 1921 entitled, 'Practice of ideals', provided insight into the few accomplishments of the movement in Argentina, and explicitly, into the causes that hampered the organisation of feminist group in Córdoba,

> Our feminism has been orientated to religious tendencies; this is why what it can and must do has not had another character than exhibition when it should be inspired by the concept of duty.[20]

Although not explicitly alluded here, the author's sceptical vision may also have stemmed from the increasing enrolment of Cordoban charitable ladies in the Patriotic League, a right-wing, Catholic organisation formed in 1919 to combat communism and socialism.[21] Arguably, the association of feminism with the figure of the charitable Catholic matron as opposed to a progressive, liberal, feminism reflected the divide that since 1910 (as discussed in Chapter 1) had split the women's movement at national level.

As the decade of the 1930s progressed, women's civic rights were supported by the paper through the coverage of the activities of the 'Argentinian Union of Women' (1936), an intellectual female organisation created primarily as a defence of women's civic rights which were under threat by a projected presidential reform to the Civil Code. [22] *La Voz del Interior* welcomed the foundation of the Union, in which women from Córdoba also participated, and, in particular, celebrated two goals of the Union's programme: Firstly, the non-partisan aim of the organisation, and secondly, the 'fight for the dignity of the mother, regardless of her civil status',[23] a topic unwaveringly defended by the paper, as we shall see later.

In addition, the advocacy of women's suffrage continued to feature prominently in the paper, as for example, when in 1934 the female vote was sanctioned in San Juan province – becoming the second place in Argentina after it was granted in Santa Fe city (1927). The article that announced the event conveyed the optimism of a time when women's vote was very close to being sanctioned in the National Parliament. Its language placed enfranchisement as a symbol of progress and culture,

> Woman's civic right, thus recognised, is not anymore the object of
> ironic smiles like before, for even those who most opposed the claims
> of Eve's daughters already accept that we are far from the times in
> which woman was considered a domesticated beast, or a reproductive
> machine and to whom no education or participation in current or
> future affairs should be given.[24]

The anti-Catholic connotations are provocatively pointed here through the
affiliation of women with Eve, in a time when her counter-figure, Mary, was
saturating the streets of Córdoba in an unprecedented exaltation of the Marian cult. Thirteen years later, when the political scenario in the Republic had
considerably changed after the arrival of Perón to power, in 1947 the vote
was finally granted to all Argentinian women. The article that *La Voz del
Interior* published after the bill obtained the approval of one of the chambers
was, like the ones that appeared from 1904 on, written by a woman. The
piece was predictably joyous and celebratory, not only in the recognition of
the right itself, but in what was envisioned as future political consequences
for women's condition, 'the effectiveness of the female vote will reside in
that women will influence legislators in those laws that tend to improve their
situation'.[25]

Mother and child welfare was high in the agenda of Argentinian feminist, and their related ideas, as we have seen in the case of women's education, civic and political rights, had an influence in the liberal press and in the
way papers like *La Voz del Interior* perceived mother's welfare conditions too.
But welfare ideas, particularly before the rise of the welfare state, were not a
solid, coherent set of political or economic proposals that parties or groups
could adhere to. In what follows, I will focus on a 'maternal campaign' initiated by *La Voz del Interior* which will give us an idea of the extent to which
motherhood, when associated with welfare, was subject to different political
uses. It will also illustrate how the liberal press managed to articulate a specific representation of the maternal which passed into circulation.

Mothers and the newspaper's politics of motherhood

In 1922 *La Voz del Interior* started a long, dedicated campaign that took mothers as both subjects and objects of what I understand as a particular form of

'politics of motherhood'.[26] By then an overtly political category, maternity, as we have seen, was being enunciated by different actors while its multiple ideas materialised in diverse scenarios from monumental buildings to the streets' parades, from the Catholic press to international health congresses. In these displacements, the locus where ideas of maternity are articulated offer specific connotations that need to be interpreted according to the inner characteristics of the field in question. The perceived changes in journalism at the time, from the incorporation of a new style, the so-called 'new journalism' (short and snappy stories, with big headings and sub-headings, large photographs, etc.), competition for a reading public, and the redefinition of newspapers' profiles will frame the maternal campaign as a journalistic event with both internal and external ramifications. In any case, the maternal reveals itself as a sufficiently laden concept to be appropriated to serve various interests.

In 1918 with a new editorial director and a renewed editorial staff, *La Voz del Interior* shifted toward a more sharp and critical content. In its new version, it openly attack clericalism and *Los Principios* (to whom it called 'Tartuffe' in reference to the pious fraudster character in Molière's novel) with scathing and sarcastic comments, if sometimes too obsessively, a style that was not restricted to its leading articles. In that same year, Córdoba witnessed the upheavals of the University Reform, which the paper strongly supported against the Catholic forces that ruled the university government, giving rise to an ideological battle that was largely staged through the press and lasted well into the following decade.

The maternal campaign extended until 1930 and it had two main directions. First, it considered single, working-class and indigent mothers as subjects and, in so doing, it recognised them as actors in need of welfare assistance and social recognition in a society that harboured strong prejudices against them. At the same time, the paper took mothers as objects by politically utilising them to criticise the Catholic ideology – especially charities with church connections – and to a lesser extent, the social policy of conservative governments. By hearing the mothers' needs and giving voice to their claims *La Voz del Interior,* and this is most striking, installed itself as an actor of social assistance, seeking to offer solutions that institutions were providing insufficiently. In doing so, it introduced to the circulating discourses of motherhood class considerations, and it did so within the framework of the press and its own agenda and style underpinning its elaboration. By revealing the conditions of working-class, and poor single mothers, the collective 'mothers' and its universally associated values was broken up due to the differentiations that class revealed.

Catholic discourses on motherhood, and to great extent medical ones, were based on a traditional vision of the family, where gender roles were clearly separated into different spheres; the masculine, public sphere of economic provision, and the feminine, private one that stressed mothers' responsibility for children's spiritual education, and for their healthy upbringing. However, this ideal concept of family did not reflect the actual experiences of working-class mothers. A working father who earned enough to allow his spouse and children to withdraw from the labour force constituted a model more fitted to the middle classes. For working-class mothers, work and family did not represent different spheres. Nor did the concept of the nuclear family adjust easily to mothers, since for many of them 'family' meant children, sometimes parents, but not husbands.

As mentioned earlier, an important feature of the paper's 'maternal campaign' was its profound anti-Catholicism, whereby the process of clericalisation of the public life that immediately followed the University Reform was fiercely contested in *La Voz del Interior*. Furthermore, for a welfare system where female charitable organisations were more important than the state, the majority of which were run by lay Catholic ladies, it is not surprising that their work was directly targeted by the paper. There were, however, three charitable organisations whose activities the paper almost always supported and in whose responsibility lay the most important welfare institutions: the Society of Beneficence (*Sociedad de Beneficencia* responsible for the Children's Hospital, Psychiatric Hospital for Women, Tuberculosis Hospital for Women and Children); the *Sociedad Tránsito Cáceres de Allende*, which ran the Tuberculosis Hospital for both sexes; and the Ladies of Providence (*Damas de la Providencia* who administered the Orphan House). The first two were considered, to some extent, state institutions subsidised by the province and administrated by ladies of the elite, although fund raising granted them a more secure source of income. To give an idea of the aggressiveness of the paper's campaign against charitable institutions, a sub-heading of 1925 stated,

Only three big institutions of real action deserve to be helped – the Orphan House, the Society of Beneficence and the Society Tránsito Cáceres de Allende. Beyond them the others are collectors to maintain the lazybones of the churches. The public powers have the duty of controlling the mania of false fund-risers.[27]

143

In this way, a considerable amount of welfare provision delivered by the largest female voluntary organisation of the time, the Society of Ladies of Saint Vincent de Paul (*Sociedad de Señoras de San Vicente de Paul*), was starkly ignored. However, as I have analysed elsewhere, it was the Vincentians who quickly detected the problems that single poor mothers confronted, and they did so in spite of the Church limited support for their organisation.[28]

In what follows I will dwell on further aspects of the paper's campaign taking into account only a handful of the articles that constituted it. The first one appeared in 1922 under the headline, 'A mother is needed. A little woman is given. A call to the feelings of good people'.[29] The event was told to the newspaper by a girl who came to the editorial office to publish a note in the children's section. In her visit, the girl narrated the facts to the journalists, in a dialogue that was reproduced to demonstrate closeness with ordinary people's concerns.

> [girl] - A baby has just been offered to my mum . . . She is very little, red like a strawberry, I liked her very much but . . .
> [journalist] - But what? we asked interested
> [girl] - . . . My mum already has many. . .
> Without *listening* more, we went off *in search* of the big-little woman to find out what it was about. In the journey from *our house* to the address that we've been told . . . we *made the story* by evoking all the *via crucis* of those loves, ordinary loves, those that society do not recognise and that, however, we see in many places and that are the typical plot of novels.[30]

The mother's misfortune remains 'evoked' but her particular reasons for abandoning the child deliberately remain untold. The paper has placed itself directly amongst ordinary people, 'listening' 'dialoguing' and taking immediate action (in 'search of'). It is also worth noticing the 'humanisation' of the newspaper as a 'house' and the journalist as an individual, who listens, acts, thinks and shows compassion with human misfortune. Biblical phrases such as *via crucis* would become token expressions, strategically used to show/ denounce both, where the 'real' *via crucis* was (poor people), and to expose what was perceived as the absence of religious commitment in the clergy and lay Catholic organisations. The paper's displacement to the woman's home, the reproduction of dialogues written in informal language, and the use of photographs as irrefutable proof, were some of the strategies utilised to transmit closeness to the problems of the needy. This marked a difference with other techniques of communication used by the popular press, such as the correspondence columns. Although these columns reproduced people's words, and set up an intimate bond between paper and readership, they still constituted a mediated relationship, as it was kept in the space of the editorial office. The face-to-face relationship with people set up by *La Voz del Interior* and its reporters took the newspaper out of its traditional place to locate it everywhere where someone was 'in need'. At the same time, it also revealed a new role for the newspaper, by assuming other responsibilities beyond the ones of informing and opinion making, as we can see in how this particular story evolved. The following day, the paper reported with this title: 'The little woman has found a good mother. Yesterday Guillermina was adopted by a married couple'. The opening paragraph is remarkable in the paper's attempt of building up a self-identification among its readers.

> The truth is that our house, at times, more than a newspaper looked like a *procession*, with women coming in and out who wanted to become mothers . . . while others remained seated for long hours waiting to be assisted by the editorial staff, since the editorial office couldn't cope with all the people that turned up. In the meanwhile, Guillermina remained safeguarded.[31]

Here, again, a religious act is evoked by the word 'procession', with its characteristic female component, and the demonstration of compelling maternal feelings, i.e. the 'sacrifice' of long hours waiting. This recreation of a religious ritual into a secularised practice that took place in a newspaper's editorial office was evidently pointing to the absence/void of Catholic commitment, an absence that the newspaper seemed ready to fulfil. The article also remarked on the large number of women, predominantly of 'modest position', who brought 'the newspaper in their hands', thus demonstrating the public (middle to lower-classes) whom the paper was aiming to represent.[32] Class considerations, however, operated more as a way of giving common people a moral recognition for their acts than to instigate in them social or political claims for their deprived condition. Another important aspect in this inaugural article was the paper's role as welfare provider, which was described as follows,

> As far as *we* were concerned, we made sure, since choosing a mother was what it was all about, that she would gather all the required condi-

145

tions for the girl's care . . .After a long detailed examination done over
the applicants, like if [we] were the mother that seeks the best for her
daughter, . . . we *chose* a young married couple, of good appearance
and impeccable behaviour, to whom we handed over the little woman,
by the Orphan House.[33]

The paper was assuming the responsibility of a decision maker. The message
also seems to convey disagreement regarding the child-abandonment system.
Notably, the Orphan House, to which the newspaper should have resorted in
the first instance, is mentioned as playing a merely formal role. This reveals
the paper's desire of placing children in family-type settings rather than in the
existing system of orphanages run by female charities. As we have seen, this
position was vigorously defended by feminists and represented a key source
of conflict between them and male specialists involved in the Pan American
Child Congresses. As far as the moral aspects of child abandonment is concerned, the paper adopted a comprehensive stance towards mothers while
drawing attention to men's attitudes instead, asserting that 'most of the time'
men 'instigated' women to abandon their child.[34]

In 1924, another case was announced in large headlines, ' "I want to
work to feed my children" a poor woman tells us', while in the sub headline
it reads: 'Doña Pabla Palacio, 35 years-old, has three children, the oldest is
10 years-old. She would prefer a family house in the city or in the countryside'.[35] The large photograph accompanying the article left indicates innovation in the layout through the incorporation of sensationalist techniques that
photography was facilitating. In fact much was left to be deduced from the
photographs themselves, as we will see in Chapter 6, while the core of the
message was concentrated in the headlines. Such a technique denotes a readership more likely to read in brief intervals such as middle-class professionals
and the working classes, than the format used by *Los Principios* whose layout
and content implied a more reflexive and time-consuming reading style. The
above-mentioned headline also anticipated the mediation of *us,* the paper,
who gave the afflicted mother 'a voice', who later in the text assured, 'I came
to this newspaper, *La Voz del Interior,* the newspaper of the poor, so my children won't be hungry'.[36] If the catchphrase 'the newspaper of the poor' was
indeed pronounced by this woman, it is less important than the use that the
paper extensively made of it. The sentimental and poignant images that pervaded this type of dialogue were strategically set up in two directions, first,
to enhance the paper's welfare attitude, and second, to encourage readers to

participate and feel part of it, 'imagine the reader the tears that this woman has shed through all her travails'.[37]

The impression given by such brief stories, beyond the paper's political remit and its strategies of representation, is that the spheres of productive work and reproduction were at the time so mutually exclusive, except of course for those who could manage sewing jobs from home or as a wet nurse, while employment in domestic service became difficult to find as maids were often employed as resident servants and their children were rarely welcomed. Nothing suggests, however, that the paper's exposition of these distressing cases was attempting to seek in the readers any further social action or to politically influence them in electoral terms. More generally, the cynical commentaries targeted Catholics' conventional interpretations of human fate and misfortune, and their moral prejudice, which in the paper's view also informed the assistance provided by the charitable system,

> Our Lord gave her a husband', 'Later, Our Lord, always disinterested, added to her three children, abiding by the fact that the offspring, when more than one, is of the exclusive patrimony of the poor. But there is the reprehensible: he forgot to provide them with 'our daily bread'. The reader would be with us in that the Lord has ridiculous ideas and that He has a very fragile memory.[38]

La Voz del Interior's interest in highlighting its own participation and accomplishments as a provider of maternal welfare suggests the permeability of the maternal at the time and its credentials to spur political uses. Under the heading 'Doña Pabla Palacio has secured her children's bread. She and her three children have been taken in by a family that will provide housing, food and salary. Our desires are accomplished';[39] the article detailed at length the way in which the case was duly resolved.[40]

Another article of the 'maternal campaign' was presented under the sensationalist caption, 'In the twentieth-century the tribute of her children is imposed on a mother!'[41] Using an expression that resonated widely in wartime, 'the tribute of her children' is, however, applied here to denounce a long-standing, colonial practice whereby wealthy families informally adopted children of poor single mothers, who were raised as *criados* and formed part of the household mainly as domestics. The figure that embodied that backward past is one of 'the ladies of beneficent institutions' who, according to the paper, asked the mother to give her little daughter in exchange for aid.

147

Another article revolved around the same problem and was presented under the headlines,

> A mother is needed!!! A poor woman gives away her daughter, for she can't maintain her as due to the baby, she is admitted nowhere. The cruelty of being a mother and poor, leads this unfortunate woman to this enormous sacrifice![42]

Here the dignifying attributes of motherhood so much extolled by clerics, Catholics and their press, is used in a sensationalist way to flesh out the challenges for indigent single mothers who sought paid employment instead of charitable aid. In this sense, the maternal campaign helped to disclose to the public eye the mothering experiences of destitute and working-class women as did no other discourse at that time.

In most of the cases that formed part of the campaign, civil society, families or individuals were depicted as the successful providers of welfare to the poor, while statutory institutions and authorities were rarely made accountable for mothers' conditions. The campaign was instrumental in showing that, despite the large number of female charities acting in Córdoba, welfare provision was deficient in a system that largely relied on them. However, this evidence did not immediately persuade the paper that state action was required to solve the situation of mother and child assistance. State welfare legislation such as maternity leave, maternity insurance, maternal services such as the 'maternal home' had been proposed by feminists during the 1920s. Although some of these ideas were discussed elsewhere in the paper, they were done so outside the articles of the campaign, thus depriving it from better grounded ideas for state reforms. As mentioned at the beginning of this chapter, welfare ideas were articulated in ambiguous, sometimes contradictory ways. The fact that the paper proposed to its readers to resort to fundraising, the same method by which charity was sustained, is very telling of the paradoxical visions that the problem of welfare was able to induce. In much the same way, reporters committed themselves to 'visiting rounds' to the homes of the poor in order to assess their needs, as the charitable ladies of Saint Vincent de Paul did at the time. By 1930 the newspaper's maternal campaign came to an end, and although the anguish of poor single or widowed mothers and their children continued being portrayed, their coverage was less systematic. At the same time, the paper started to address the state as the most responsible for the provision of welfare, as we shall see in the next section.

Medical ideas and the paper's own representation of motherhood

The extent to which the press has been influenced by medical ideas and, at the same time, how newspapers have contributed to the spread of them during the first half of the twentieth century is a topic that has received little attention by historians of medicine, who have concentrated on specific aspects of the media such as sanitary campaigns or the advertisements for medicinal products for specific diseases.[43] Here I will tackle the dynamics of press-medicine relationships from the prism of the representations of motherhood that we have seen circulating in other registers, in order to explore how the liberal press has made sense of them while – as I interrogate – it has also created one of its own.

In broad outline, *La Voz del Interior* like other papers of the period was instrumental in the legitimating process of the medical field that started at the end of the nineteenth century, particularly in the promotion of doctors as the only specialists that should be involved in 'the art of delivery' to the detriment of what had previously been the natural territory of *comadronas* and female healers. This, however, did not necessarily imply that the paper was equally instrumental in promoting or disseminating medical knowledge amongst its readers as, for example, the lack of a dedicated health column would indicate. Raising awareness of the importance of medical care was not so much an attempt to culturally influence society or individual practices in their consumption of medical services *per se*, but in an attempt to politically influence public opinion on initiatives and ideas that became identified or associated with political views.

Arguably, the press, and this includes the Catholic press and the national papers, politicised medical discourses in that newspapers circulated and informed the public on medical proposals and debates in a segmented and partisan way. As earlier discussed, in a press where politics and opinion-making loomed large in newspapers' remits, medical ideas were hardly separated from ideological contests, either party forces or the broader 'clerical' and 'anticlerical' divide, that individual doctors represented. Certain medical debates and propositions, especially those related to reproduction and sexuality and its range of related topics, from illegitimacy and child abandonment to birth-control practices and the racial and physical endowments of the population, were introduced to the reader initially by articles written by university doctors, in most cases to spread a liberal, secular view on these matters. Yet as the decades progressed, *La Voz del Interior* introduced a more critical assessment

149

of medical issues in featured articles and through comments in informative pieces that somehow reflect the views of an editorial policy independent from both doctors' thinking, and from mainstream medical theories.

This perspective contributed to build a different representation of the maternal, whose emphasis was not exclusively posed in biological aspects (to give birth to healthy children), but in social, economic and cultural ones that instead contemplated mothers as such. I would argue that the representation of maternity that the paper articulated was built upon a sort of displacement from the medical binomial mother-child to the social mother-as-subject. This was particularly clear in the articles that appeared from the 1930s onwards where medical concepts on maternity were resignified by the paper.

Let's see in more detail these three aspects separately, starting with the support given by the paper to the medical intervention in the assistance of childbirth. In the course of obstetricians' continuing struggles against midwives to ascertain their scientific status over untrained women, *La Voz del Interior* played an outstanding role in the battle against 'illegal midwives' when in 1915 the paper launched a fierce journalistic campaign to denounce the practice of quacks and *comadronas* whose presence were particularly prevalent in rural areas. The campaign was addressed against the provincial Council of Hygiene, and signalled the corruption of its functionaries who received money in exchange for the protection of illegal pharmacists and 'false midwives'. As I have commented in Chapter 1, the campaign reached a climax when the Governor was forced to put forward a bill that led to the reorganisation of the provincial Council of Hygiene in 1916, which included the examination of midwives' skills. The paper celebrated this law as an accomplishment of its own.[44] Ever since, *La Voz del Interior* remained as a sort of law overseer, by publishing the names of proscribed midwives, a list provided by the Council of Hygiene, and a list of graduated ones, as well as by informing readers of any changes in the regulation of their practice.[45]

Equally important for the consolidating process of male specialists was the paper's condemnatory attitude against professional and unprofessional midwives who practiced abortions. In the struggle over women's assistance, the practice of abortion and the social condemnation it met at the time, gave obstetricians a powerful instrument to socially discredit midwives. Arguably, the criminal pages of the paper contributed to shape a feeling of mistrust towards *parteras* by presenting, in a sensationalistic way, cases that had them as protagonists. Some of the headlines that appeared in 1929 and 1930, which notably involved professional midwives, denounced, 'A woman with guts.

150

She devoted herself to activities punished by law. She hid by criminal means someone else's sins'.[46] Another one asserted, 'A midwife from the Public Assistance has committed a grave crime. She attempted to provoke an abortion in a woman and, as a result, an infection has arisen. The state of the patient is alarming'.[47]

The second aspect on which I would like to shed some light in this section concerns the dissemination of medical ideas and concepts by the paper that would have facilitated the spread and penetration of medical knowledge into the reading public. This topic seems to be informed by different layers which altogether reveal certain characteristics of the earlier relationship of medicine and journalism more broadly. In the sampled issues for the period, a type of medical content appeared under the form of news information, whereby the paper emphasised the novelty or therapeutic breakthroughs while seeking to bridge advances in medical knowledge with their human application. A good example of this type of article was the attention devoted to the test of 'partoanalgia', a drug introduced by obstetrician Cantón from Buenos Aires with the aim of reducing pain during delivery. Letters between Dr Cantón and Cordoban obstetricians were published, while the medical results were greeted by the paper as 'an event for our scientific world' and as 'a swift success for innovative medicine [that should be] promptly introduced and applied'.[48]

Another feature that characterised the relationship of medicine and the press during this period is that medical pieces in the female 'social section' advising mothers on childrearing practices, on healthy feeding, or during pregnancy were rare. The paper did not take as its responsibility the task of educating women in how to improve their child care tasks, a fact that could not be attributed to the paper's assumption that its middle-working class readership was not in need of instruction. Broadly speaking the press in Córdoba seems not to have been instrumental in spreading obstetric or paediatric notions in their female readerships, and in the absence of historical surveys in other provincial contexts or in the national press it is difficult to assert if the case of Córdoba was indeed an exception. One possible answer to this phenomenon could be that doctors did not consider press education, at least in its daily format, as a valuable pedagogic source, preferring instead other types of printed materials of varied styles and addressed to different publics, such as manuals, school texts, magazines, and leaflets distributed in hospitals. In the mid-1930s doctors, mainly paediatricians, featured in specialised Buenos Aires's health magazines like *Viva Cien Años* (live a hundred

151

years), which held a column devoted to 'maternity and puericulture', and the ones specifically committed to childrearing such as *Hijo Mío…!* (my child) and *Madre y Niño* (mother and child). Medical columns in magazines of mass circulation in the country such as, *El Hogar* (the household), also appeared in the 1930s, as the one written by paediatrician Florencio Escardó that addressed child health issues with an eugenic perspective. Through his column Escardó also focussed on children's behaviour, whereby he introduced elements of modern psychology and psychoanalysis into paediatrics.[49] It was only in 1958 when this new tendency in childrearing materialised in Buenos Aires in a column written by psychologist Eva Giberti in the newspaper *La Razón*. Following Escardó's psychologically-oriented ideas, Giberti managed to convey in the media the principles of the new Parenting School that reformulated child-rearing methods in Argentina.[50]

But if child-rearing advice and education seems not to have regularly featured in daily newspapers, the latter were instrumental in giving support to the ideas of some prominent doctors that were active in the political arena provided their allegiances were shared by the editorial staff. Physicians, like other men of science, found there an opportunity to publish specialist papers that they had delivered at important congresses. Usually these types of publications referred to topics that received considerable scholarly discussion in their respective specialties, but at the same time, conveyed relevant social implications. Evidence of a selective, anti-Catholic-driven editorial policy was the large space dedicated to a paper discussed by Dr Félix Garzón Maceda at the Third Pan-American Scientific Congress gathered in Peru in 1924. The article spanned over two days under the big headline 'Eugenics, Puericulture and Sexual Education'.[51] Garzón Maceda was a well-known hygienist and politician, generally identified as a man of Catholicism, although his medical ideas evidenced a more complex set of theoretical influences including a positivist, secular vision of medicine. And while it is hard to find his articles in *La Voz del Interior*, it is evident that a concession was made in this case because of the anti-clerical ideas that his paper was posing. The article starts by considering that, 'Eugenics, Puericulture and Sexual education constitute the universal motor by means of which the causes of racial and human degeneration should be removed'.[52] Controversially, he proposed the compulsory study of eugenics in primary, secondary and professional schools; as well as legislation to grant a prenuptial certificate, and sexual education. Undoubtedly, his ideas on sexual education were most challenging for a society like Córdoba where public education managed to avoid the exigencies of a national law (N°1420, sanctioned in 1884) that had granted secular education in all public schools.

Concern about race, degeneration and eugenics occupied much of the medical literature and debates in the 1930s, and discussions occasionally appeared in the paper with articles that alerted readers about the threat posed by social diseases like syphilis, alcoholism, and tuberculosis.[53] In 1934, on the occasion of the II Argentine Congress of Obstetrics and Gynaecology gathered in Buenos Aires, *La Voz del Interior* published the conclusions of the paper, 'Tuberculosis and Pregnancy', presented by Cordoban doctors Lascano and Sayago that I have discussed in Chapter 2. Tuberculosis was the most important cause of death in the province, while the pregnancy of a tubercular woman was thought to complicate the prospect of both mother and child. This confronted physicians with the complicated and sensitive topic of 'therapeutic abortion', which was proposed in these cases to preserve the mother's life, but was a resort that Catholic physicians strongly opposed. From this perspective, the communication of this controversial topic in the press had the importance of informing the public that different medical perspectives were offered, beyond the religious one. The article stated, 'Pre-existent tuberculosis or TB that appeared after pregnancy poses, firstly, a therapeutic problem, and only after the failure of treatments, does it raise discussion on the interruption of gestation'.[54]

In much the same vein, support was also given by the paper to the prophylactic campaign on venereal diseases launched in 1936 by the radical government of A. Sabattini, which received wide coverage, positive commentaries, and the reproduction of speeches delivered by specialists.[55]

Articles concerned with the provision of maternal services, especially those that demanded its improvement, often appeared during the period, and they were mostly written by the paper's journalists. The inauguration of services by the state and by the three beneficent societies above mentioned was received with encouraging and approving articles like the one that reported on the creation of 'maternal canteens' in 1919,[56] or the one that commented on the approval by the national government of the building plans for the Maternity Institute also in that year. In the latter, the heading revealed the two aspects that synthesise the paper's stance on this matter, it reads, 'The protection of mothers. The construction of a maternity hospital'. Here, the social component 'the protection of mothers' preceded and in fact grounded the news-information of the medical one, 'the construction of a maternity'. The text commented,

Helping mothers is one of the noblest initiatives that could be encouraged. The mother in her august mission deserves all the consideration, all the respect, all the help. . . . A woman can be bad, can make mistakes, can be hated, but when she carries her son, when she lets her tenderness shine over this piece of her own flesh, when she is sanctified with this sublime love, then all rancour disappears, to give rise to the purest goodness. The University youth of Córdoba thus understands it, and for long has been claiming from the Ministry the building of a maternity institute.[57]

Here the tone of the first lines of the paragraph satirically resembled the spiritual, ethereal style of *Los Principios*, a strategy deliberately used to emphasise the antithesis between church and university by casting the spiritual motherhood as a fruitless message that could at its best be 'truly materialised' through the initiatives of the University youth. Yet the questioning of Catholic ideas that this perspective entailed was not the only aim of the liberal paper. When, in the following two decades, increasing concern about children's welfare – high infant mortality rates and degenerative diseases – concentrated much of the public attention, a new perspective started to be articulated by the paper that seems to offer balance to a medical discourse that was becoming more and more biologically grounded. This introduces us to the third aspect that I would like to explore in the remainder of this chapter, that is, the way in which the paper resignified the medical discourse on maternity.

With the backdrop of the child welfare movement that, in the 1920s and 1930s, informed much of the debates of the Pan American Child Congresses, as discussed in Chapter 1, the mother and child focus was promoted by different actors (feminist doctors and male medical specialists) with rather competing welfare views. These perceived conflicting tendencies were reflected in *La Voz del Interior*, which often gave space for a perspective in sympathy with feminist thought which contrasted with other segments of the press that proved to be less receptive. This in turn allowed for a more critical elaboration of medical ideas and initiatives related to motherhood. In an article that appeared in 1924, the increasing rates of infant mortality were addressed with an alarmist tone.[58] It is interesting to note, in this case, how the paper resignified the redundant question of mother's ignorance posed by male specialists in the following terms,

What is taught to the young woman? ... "When she gets married she will learn". This is the answer of those who lead women astray. They use the pretext of keeping a candour that doesn't actually exist – because nature is more powerful than conventionalism – thus exposing women to the dangerous dishonour produced by a hypocrite and false education. . . .

To raise girls to live in a bell jar, to neglect the problems of the sexes . . . is to keep the fiction and to be determined to remain ignorant of an essential biological question.[59]

Although the article proposed teaching puericulture in primary schools, its frankness on sexual education alerted the readers that something more urgent should be taught to girls prior to the proper instruction on breast feeding and the healthy care of babies. In reproving those who confused 'innocence with ignorance', it challenged not only the religious conception of womanhood, but also the medical one as the construct 'mother's education' meant something more than childrearing. Indeed, with the backdrop of the 'maternal campaign' taking place in these years, the paper received childrearing educational proposals with less buoyant commentaries. When in 1925, for example, the Mother's Club from Buenos Aires[60] – an upper-class women's group – asked the Governor of Córdoba to support their puericulture campaign, named the 'Child's Week', the paper sceptically commented,

As long as unfair economic inequality persists . . . as along as lower-class women conceive, spent [sic] and lactate under the rule of men and a weak state, and finally, as long as the woman of the lower classes is a slave, a thing, . . . the intentions of the Mothers' Club would be only temporary and accidental solutions . . . even if there would be created as many Mothers' Clubs as mothers exist, the problem won't be efficiently solved.[61]

If for school-girls sexual education should precede or come side by side with 'mother's education', here, it was proposed that the economic situation of working-class women should be prioritised before any puericulture campaign could render a visible benefit. Here, again, this criticism resembled feminist claims more than the one posed by physicians. Another illustrative example can be found when Dr Soria organised in Córdoba a conference-festival in 1927 to launch a welfare organisation he had created, the 'Committee for

155

the Defence of Infancy'. *La Voz del Interior* extensively supported the event through three articles, however, the paper pointed out its own expectations regarding Soria's ideas,

> the distinguished paediatrician should tackle, *it is hoped*, the *true aspects* of the question that is, in our understanding, essentially *economic* ... a question that demands, firstly, to put an end to the social injustice that weighs down our people.[62]

The article also remarked on the social aspects of motherhood as a necessary component to improve the child's assistance, 'by sanctioning the *respect of the woman-mother*, as the best title that society could bestow upon those who gave life to other beings'.[63] Other pieces published in these years also emphasised the fact that mother's problems could not be reduced to education in puericulture notions. Commenting on the entrenched prejudices against single mothers, an article addressed Soria's child-focused campaign and its disregard of mother's social problems.

> In Córdoba, where a campaign is being promoted in favour of the child, we say it would be useless to predicate the child's protection if a mother is abandoned because of love's impulses, inexperience or whatever. Society should dwell not on the causes but instead accept the results for humanity's sake. [64]

In addition, in commenting on cases of infanticide, child abandonment and mothers' suicide reported in the years 1929-1930, the paper articulated a perspective closer to core feminist demands, although feminism as such was rarely explicitly acknowledged. Besides the paper's proverbial criticism of religious and moral values, legal reform of the Civil Code was also suggested. For example, an article was critical of the fact that, 'the instinct of maternity [is only] idealised and praised when it is sanctioned by *law* and religion', to conclude, 'it should be recognised for women the *inalienable right* to maternity, without the child stupidly being distinguished as 'legitimate' or 'illegitimate'.[65]

As the paper's pressure for the provision of maternity services started to grow in the thirties, due to the temporary closure of services[66] and a few cases of babies dying in childbirth,[67] on the editorial pages, the topic was raised with varying degrees of irony, denunciation, and concern. An example that illustrates a shift in relation to the former endorsement of the medical profession is the following piece under the heading, 'The tragic nobility of the maternal function. In the city of Doctors and virtuous ladies'. The connections the paper drew between 'doctors' and 'ladies' were not merely rhetorical, and in the relentless criticism to which charitable ladies were subject to on its pages, we may assume this association was rather offensive. 'Maternity, it has been said, is the sublime function of life *par excellence*', 'very nice things, fitting for topics of sermons and conferences but that are not practiced'. Commenting on a case where a woman had to give birth in the ambulance of the Public Assistance due to the lack of maternity beds, the article scoldingly concluded 'this happened in a doctoral city full of wise people, of gynaecologists, of virtuous ladies and blessed gentlemen', 'what an irony and a shame!'[68]

Towards the mid-1930s, other articles pointed to the state as the most responsible for what it was referred to as the 'tragedies of the mother-woman'. This perspective markedly differed from the one sustained during the 'maternal campaign' of the 1920s. One piece commented that the national press was full of daily dramas staged by poor single mothers who were 'driven mad by the hostility of the environment', mothers who, beset by poverty, ended up tragically throwing themselves and their children into the sea or under a train. The paper advocated for the need of welfare legislation and the provision of services, including a maternity shelter for those 'women sanctified by maternity and tormented by the duty of raising their children', which, according to the article, left mothers only two paths: infanticide or prostitution.[69] This type of article seems to have been inspired by feminist doctor, Elvira Rawson de Dellepiane, whose preoccupation with the destiny of single mothers became an 'obsession', as Dora Barrancos has noted.[70] She championed the creation of sheltered institutions such as the 'maternal home' – as a way of preventing infanticide and suicide – and advocated a secular and human welfare system that relied on the state rather than on the charitable structure. At the same time, during this period, the paper's increasing claims from the state were in tune with Parliamentary debates that led to the sanction of legislation protecting working mothers, such as nursing breaks and paid maternity leave (1934) and maternity insurance (1936). Support for working mothers was also provided in the form of denouncement when employers (or the insurance system more broadly) failed to accomplish the exigencies contemplated in the law, which, as historians have argued, soon revealed its many drawbacks.[71] In this sense, it asserted,

These mothers claim from the public powers and authorities, and from every soul, a reaction that allows them – not to live from alms because it humiliates and corrupts – but to have a honest and decorous job, that today is unattainable because no one employs a domestic servant with children, and there are no workshops with an annexed room for lactation. Maternity [it concluded] should be more than a fact, a right.[72]

During the ensuing years, *La Voz del Interior* continued stressing state responsibility in the provision of welfare services, while it abandoned the scornful style that for decades took charitable ladies and Catholic social action as the main focus of welfare problems. The shift in the philosophy of social provision was described by the paper in 1944 in the following terms,

The democratic spirit and principle that informs and is imposed upon our institutions has, in a gradual and progressive way, absorbed all the circles, even those that had resisted it with recalcitrant obstinacy. . . . With it, the concept of welfare was losing its hallmark of humiliating charity to gain its true character of inexcusable duty by the state, as a way of rewarding taxpayers.[73]

It was this vision, which the paper started to articulate towards the mid-1930s, what paved the way for a different perspective regarding the 'maternal question'. In doing so, it distanced itself from the narrowing perspective of medical specialists who were initially motivated by the desire to help children, relegating the mothers' needs to a merely educational problem, and later in the 1930s by their biological aspirations of protecting mothers' reproductive qualities. Even when the paper was instrumental in the legitimisation of the medical field and in communicating medical ideas that focussed on the dangers of reproduction according to eugenic concerns, its emphasis on social aspects gave the dissemination of medical ideas a different framework. In this sense, one of the paper's major contributions to the circulating representations of motherhood was that it helped to articulate a different perspective, one that focused on the economic, social and cultural aspects rather than on the fragmented versions of a biological and a spiritual maternity. It did so by revealing, most notably through the 'maternal campaign', the mother's material conditions as a key factor to attend to when referring to maternity, since class considerations confronted women with different experiences of motherhood. However, overdoing the dependency of motherhood on economic position led to the interpretation of poor mothers as the 'other', with all the connotations that such representation entailed in terms of an objectivised identity. In Chapter 6, 1 will dwell on this other side of the maternal campaign from a visual point of view.

For the greater part of the period, the paper stubbornly challenged Catholic discourses on motherhood by exposing how their proclaimed spiritual values were socially inconsistent, especially in relation to single motherhood. At the same time, its articles continually stressed the need for a proper education for women, especially a sexual one, and a respect for mothers regardless of their civil status. In doing so, *La Voz del Interior* showed that unless economic and entrenched cultural, social values were challenged, Córdoba's society could improve mother *and* child welfare very little.

On a more general note, what the Córdoba press have shown us is that motherhood acted as a hub for other discourses on sexuality, family, population, gender relationships and politics. This became clearer in a society where the competing visions of Catholics and liberals were relentlessly disputing hegemony over those transcendental issues. Here the press showcased extreme, divergent visions in a profoundly local articulation. How much, for example, was left out of the political uses of motherhood in the case of the liberal press is difficult to discern. But we can at least argue that its representation of the maternal was largely contingent upon representations taking place elsewhere in medical, religious, and political registers.

Notes

1   J. Habermas, *The Structural Transformation of the Public Sphere: An Inquiry into a Category of Bourgeois Society* (Cambridge: MIT Press, 1991).

2   J. Ramos, *Divergent Modernities: Culture and Politics in Nineteenth-century Latin America* (Durham: Duke University Press, 2001), 95.

3   Habermas, *The Structural Transformation of the Public Sphere*, 184.

4   See, for example, K. Williams, *Read All about It!: A History of the British Newspaper* (London: Routledge, 2010).

5   S. Romano, 'Los Fotógrafos y la Fotografía en la Prensa, 1920-1955: Una Mirada Sobre el Fotoperiodismo en La Voz del Interior', in C. Boixadós, M. Palacios and S. Romano (eds.), *Fragmentos de una Historia:*

Córdoba 1920-1955. Fotografías Periodísticas de la Colección Antonio Novello (Córdoba: Pugliese Siena, 2005), 11-17: 13.

6   *La Voz del Interior* (15 March 1929), 4.

7   María Eugenia Echenique was the first feminist writer of Córdoba and among the first in Argentina during the second half of the nineteenth century. She belonged to a small group of elite women, journalists and writers, who contributed to both women's and men's magazines. During the time of nation-building (after the Constitution of 1853), these women decided to enter in the public debate by foregrounding the problems that they envisioned as priorities for women's future: women's education, women's contribution to science and arts, patriotism and a contested vision to the prevailing values of domesticity and feminine beauty. *La Ondina del Plata*, a women's literary and fashion magazine (1875-79), published Echenique's most important works, although she also published articles in newspapers from Córdoba and Buenos Aires. In 1900, the Cordoban editorial Biffignandi published many of her journalistic writings and a series of literary letters known as '*Cartas a Elena*' (1874), an edition that was prepared by her sister and also writer, Rosario, under the title *Colección Literaria*.

8   *La Voz del Interior* (24 November 1904), 3.

9   Ibid.

10   Leonor Allende was the first woman writer and journalist in twentieth-century Córdoba. Coming from an elite, traditional family, she had, however, to earn a living as a journalist when her father committed suicide after going into bankruptcy during the economic crisis of 1890. She worked in the newspapers *La Libertad* and *La Voz del Interior*, and it is very likely that she was the author of some of the feminist articles that appeared between 1904 and the 1920s in *La Voz del Interior*. According to her friend, the Cordoban writer Arturo Capdevila, she published three novels, *Flavio Solari* (1907), *Juan Ramón Zavallos* (1912) and *El Misterio de Ur*, and she also wrote at least three unpublished literary works. A. Capdevila, *Cronicones Dolientes de Córdoba* (Buenos Aires: Emecé, 1963). For an analysis of Allende's novel *Flavio Solari*, see Y. Eraso, *Medical Discourse and Social Representations of Motherhood in the City of Córdoba (Argentina), 1900-1946*. PhD thesis. Oxford Brookes University, 2006.

11   *La Voz del Interior* (11 December 1904), 3.

12 Ibid.

13 *La Voz del Interior* (1 September 1904), 3.

14 María Eugenia Echenique, asserted in her famous essay, 'The Emancipation of Women' that, '[t]he sciences are a sacred patrimony of humankind, which have civilised the world with freedom, and constitute a source of richness that woman must exploit', in *Colección Literaria* (Córdoba: Biffignandi, 1900), 93.

15 *La Voz del Interior* (4 December 1904), 3.

16 One of these articles explained, in 1917, the importance of female work beyond the well-known munitions factories: 'If tomorrow the industrialists or the craftsmen, who complain about the lack of arms, would ask themselves – without prejudice – if women are indeed useful, they would have to recognise it'. *La Voz del Interior* (10 April 1917), 8.

17 Ibid.

18 In 1917, an obituary dedicated to Mrs Casiana Oronel, who played a political role in the foundation of the provincial branch of the Radical Civic Union, stated, 'genius among the women of her time, this province largely owes her the resurrection of the constitutional guarantees, because her persuasive word inside and outside of her modest household, knew how to temper the spirits so as to keep them in a tension of fervent patriotism, always looking forward to a no distant victory'. *La Voz del Interior* (5 April 1917), 4.

19 The article thus celebrated the suffrage bill: 'Step by step, we are ascending uphill in all modern conquests that tend to revolutionise society, turning toward new ideas that eradicate all our ancient mores, so conflicting and retrograde'. *La Voz del Interior* (26 July 1919), 4.

20 *La Voz del Interior* (3 May 1921), 4.

21 According to reports of *La Voz del Interior* and *Los Principios,* which often publicised the names of the members of female organisations, the Patriotic League had enrolled around 550 women in 1919, the majority of whom actively participated in different charitable organisations. *La Voz del Interior* (23 October 1919).

22 The Union was spearheaded by prominent Argentinian writer Victoria Ocampo, and organised a fierce public campaign against the proposed reform that attempted to re-introduce husband's authorisation as a requisite for married women to work out of the home, to administer personal money and belongings, and to get involved in trade

associations. Finally, the bill foundered.

23   *La Voz del Interior* (14 August 1936), 11.

24   *La Voz del Interior* (30 May 1934), 6.

25   *La Voz del Interior* (31 August 1946), 6.

26   I use the expression 'politics of motherhood' first coined by Jane
Lewis in her book *The Politics of Motherhood. Child and Maternal Welfare
in England, 1900-1939* (London: Croom Helm, 1980), although with a
different meaning of the one Lewis has developed to refer to British
welfare policy. In my case, I use the expression to refer to a political
or strategic use of the discourse of motherhood, which could serve to
different interests. I prefer to use 'politics of motherhood' instead of
'maternalist discourse' because of the two connotations with which the
latter has been traditionally associated: women's suffrage and women's
welfare claims.

27   *La Voz del Interior* (7 July 1925), 9.

28   For an analysis of the activities of the Saint Vincent de Paul Society
and especially, on vicentians' relationship with the Argentinian Church
see Y. Eraso, 'Maternalismo, Religión y Asistencia: La Sociedad de
Señoras de San Vicente de Paul en Córdoba, Argentina', in Y. Eraso
(ed.), *Mujeres y Asistencia Social en Latinoamérica*, 199-239.

29   *La Voz del Interior* (14 December 1922), 6.

30   Ibid.

31   *La Voz del Interior* (15 December 1922), 6.

32   Ibid.

33   Ibid.

34   Ibid.

35   *La Voz del Interior* (25 July 1924), 6.

36   Ibid.

37   Ibid.

38   Ibid.

39   *La Voz del Interior* (29 July 1924), 6.

40   The article explained, '[o]ur desire of finding them [mother and
children] the most convenient home, and because we didn't want to
give them up to the first one that came along . . . we *decided* to put them
into a family that demonstrated great interest in protecting them'. Ibid.
My emphasis.

41   *La Voz del Interior* (18 March 1927), 8.

42   *La Voz del Interior* (31 March 1927), 12.

43 For the Argentinian case Cfr. D. Armus, *La Ciudad Impura: Salud, Tuberculosis y Cultura en Buenos Aires, 1870–1950* (Buenos Aires: Edhasa, 2007) in particular Ch. 8; and K. Ramacciotti, 'Las Sombras de la Política Sanitaria durante el Peronismo: Los Brotes Epidémicos en Buenos Aires', *Asclepio*, 58, 2 (2006), 115-38.

44 The headings that announced the Governor's bill read: 'Against quacks. The campaign of *La Voz del Interior*. Two important bills. The urgency of its sanction'. *La Voz del Interior* (9 April 1915), 4.

45 For example, the change in the rules introduced in 1925 that authorised midwives to assist women in normal deliveries (see on p.26). The item was entitled, 'Midwives.' Faculty of prescribing', *La Voz del Interior* (13 August 1925), 9.

46 *La Voz del Interior* (22 April 1929), 9.

47 *La Voz del Interior* (11 February 1930), 14.

48 *La Voz del Interior* (30 April 1915), 4.

49 M. Borinsky, "Todo Reside en Saber Qué es Un Niño". Aportes Para una Historia de la Divulgación de las Prácticas de Crianza en la Argentina', *Anuario de Investigaciones. Facultad de Psicología UBA,* 13 (2005), 117-26. According to Cecilia Rustoyburu, psychoanalytic ideas were used to both interpret and advice on parent-child relationships and they were first introduced through Escardó's column, in 'Padres Extremosos y Niños con Derechos de Beligerancia. Los Consejos sobre Crianza del Dr. Escardó: Pediatría, Psicoanálisis y Escuela Nueva (Argentina, Fines de la Década del 30)'. Paper presented at *Jornadas Historia de la Infancia en Argentina, 1880-1960*, (Prov. Buenos Aires, November 2008).

50 I. Cosse, 'Argentine Mothers and Fathers and the New Psychological Paradigm of Child-Rearing (1958-1973)', *Journal of Family History* 35, 2 (2010), 180–202.

51 *La Voz del Interior* (13 January 1925), 2.

52 Ibid.

53 In 1930, an article was entitled, '[t]his is the painful truth: the race degenerates', and commented on the disappointing results of the medical examination to join the army in that year, whereby 70 per cent of men had been rejected. 'We know that alcoholism and syphilis in the North of the Republic impose a heavy burden on the population.' The article ended with a plea to the Government to find an urgent solution, 'to delay a solution, it would constitute a crime against homeland'. *La*

Voz del Interior (7 February 1930), 8.

54 *La Voz del Interior* (4 August 1934), 8.

55 The conference speech was delivered by Dr Fernandez Verano, President of the Argentine League of Social Prophylaxis, an organisation that was informed by eugenic ideas.

56 The article on the creation of maternal canteens, said: 'We are happy to have to comment with some frequency, the good initiatives that tend to improve the social condition of the people, and to raise the moral level of the poor classes. Now [the initiative] is intended to benefit the mothers, and therefore, their children', *La Voz del Interior* (30 December 1919), 5.

57 *La Voz del Interior* (20 July 1919), 4.

58 'A terrifying social problem. Children die in alarming proportions', stated the headline, *La Voz del Interior* (15 August 1924), 6.

59 Ibid.

60 On this and other women's group that emerged to promote puericulture in the first decades of the twentieth century, see A. Lavrin, *Women, Feminism and Social Change in Argentina, Chile, and Uruguay, 1890-1940* (Lincoln: University of Nebraska Press, 1995), especially Ch. 3.

61 *La Voz del Interior* (22 August 1925), 9.

62 *La Voz del Interior* (5 July 1927), 8. My emphasis.

63 Ibid. My emphasis.

64 *La Voz del Interior* (10 October 1927), 8.

65 *La Voz del Interior* (4 March 1929), 6. My emphasis.

66 In 1930, the two existing maternity wards in the general hospitals were closed down due to the deplorable conditions of the buildings. This situation led to overcrowding the small maternity service of the Public Assistance. The paper demanded from the authorities the immediate provision of a maternity ward, 'we handed in the case to the provincial and municipal authorities, with the aim that they face up as soon as possible its solution'. *La Voz del Interior* (11 February 1930), 11.

67 One of the cases that occurred in 1930 featured in the paper with a sensationalistic style. The headline was entitled, 'The existent chaos in the Public Assistance ends up in a crime of *lessa humanidad*. For not assisting a woman in labour, a life is sacrificed. The culprits'. It was also 'illustrated' with ghastly photographs of the dead baby and the mother lying in a hospital bed. *La Voz del Interior* (18 January 1930), 13.

68 *La Voz del Interior* (10 January 1930), 9.

69 *La Voz del Interior* (15 June 1934), 7.

70 Barrancos, *Inclusión/Exclusión*, 94.

71 For a discussion on maternity legislation during the period 1930-1940, see C. Biernat and K. Ramacciotti, 'Maternity Protection for Working Women in Argentina', *História, Ciências, Saúde – Manguinhos*, 18, 1 (2011), 153-77; and S. Novick, 'Población y Estado en Argentina de 1930 a 1943. Análisis de los Discursos de Algunos Actores Sociales: Industriales, Militares, Obreros y Profesionales de la Salud', *Estudios Demográficos y Urbanos*, 23, 2 (2008), 333-73.

72 *La Voz del Interior* (15 June 1934), 7.

73 *La Voz del Interior* (26 June 1944), 6.

5

Fictionalised Mothers: Absence, Fear, and Rebellion in Literary Representations

The representation of motherhood in fiction is a topic that has produced a considerable amount of scholarly work, especially within gender studies, and from perspectives that have encompassed literary criticism, psychoanalysis, and a combination of both. Psychoanalysis, in particular, has provided the framework for exploring maternal imagery for scholars such as Mary Jacobus, Ann Kaplan, Marianne Hirsch and Jo Malin.[1] In the case of Kaplan, for example, she has attempted 'to demonstrate how fictional mother-representations are produced through the tensions between historical and psychoanalytic spheres'.[2] In exploring maternal subjectivity, most of the materials on which these surveys have been concentrated have resulted in both a narrative and an analysis structured under the premises of a critique of the patriarchal domain. In addition to the psychoanalytic framework, during the last four decades and within the field of literary criticism the topic of motherhood has defined a highly developed area of studies, tackling the fictional representations of the maternal from a myriad of perspectives with contributions that will be beyond the scope of this study to discuss.[3] But just an overview of those literary explorations that have engaged with a historical reconstruction, suggests that the fictional representations of the maternal has substantially predicated the construction of other socio-cultural notions as it became intermingled with forms of political government or mainstream literary movements. An example of the latter is the work of Marylu Hill, whose study of English novels around the 1910s has connected the emergence of a new type of woman, which brought about a new representation of the mother, with one of literary creativity, in that fictional portraits of modern women 'heralded a transition in literature that soon would be recognised as Modernist'.[4] Tracing the mother's representations in a variety of texts written in Augustan England (roughly 1700-1745), Toni Bowers has provided useful insights by revising historical assumptions of maternal behaviours, while reading the maternal against society's struggle over political agency and authority.[5] Overall, these literary analyses have shown first, that motherhood has constituted a complex object of literary plots, and secondly, that its treatment has been intricately linked with particular political, socio-cultural and historical contexts.

Compared to Anglo-Saxon academic production, literary scholars in Argentina have paid scant attention to the topic of motherhood, and, when they have done so, they have focused primarily on contemporary texts. The recent study of Nora Domínguez, *De Donde Vienen los Niños. Maternidad y Escritura en la Literatura Argentina*, constitutes a clear exception to this trend, contributing a path-breaking survey for the period between 1950s and the beginning of this century. There, Domínguez rightly notices that the topic of motherhood, 'constitutes a zone of little interest for literary or cultural criticism',[6] a neglect that she attributes to the more general disregard or marginal place that mothers, as literary figures, have occupied in Argentinian literature. It is also important to note that rather than an exception, this confirms a trend commonly observed in contemporary Western literature, as Elizabeth Podnieks and Andrea O'Reilly have argued, 'The fact that so much attention of late has been so fully directed at locating literary mothers underscores the obvious: they have been missing'.[7] Indeed, as we will see throughout this chapter, representations of motherhood in literature are rather scarce, and mothers certainly did not constitute a privileged topic or a central character of fictional representation. However, as Domínguez's chosen period confirms, since the second half of the twentieth century, this absence, at least within acclaimed writers or within the 'high literature', becomes less evident. My literary search traces back the representations of the maternal in texts that circulated in the decades immediately before those explored by Domínguez, where scholarly studies, with the exception of a few that concentrate on prominent female writers (Nora Lange, Silvina and Victoria Ocampo),[8] are virtually absent. If we look at provincial contexts, as my study will showcase through the case of Córdoba, we can observe the effects of yet another neglect, the one complicated by the impositions of a literary canon operating from Buenos Aires, where both ideological and gender exclusions have traditionally operated.

In my study, the search for provincial literary works was primarily oriented by a perspective that has privileged the circulation over the search of specific literary works or authors of renowned literary aesthetic or stylistic value. I am particularly interested in how motherhood was represented in fiction during this largely overlooked period, rather than in a pre-selection of

167

texts based on gender, styles, or writers' position within the literary field, although references to all these aspects will be integrated into the analysis. The search resulted in a corpus of six novels, whose treatment of the maternal sometimes is tackled explicitly and directly, and at others remains implicit under a more general vision of the 'feminine question'. One characteristic that the selected works share with the broader Argentinian literary field is that most of the authors were to a great extent aiming at defining subjects, social roles and moral characters. More broadly, this literary attitude is known as *realism*, which according to Teresa Gramuglio, has largely affected the Argentinian novel, 'The referential aspects and criticism of the present (and also of moments of the past that somehow assert themselves over the present) have a strong incidence in the new novel that emerges from Mallea to Sábato, . . . as well as years later in Cortázar's *Rayuela* (1963)'.[9] In the present selection, the chosen texts establish a permanent dialogue with the context and time at which they were produced, each of them reflecting the anxieties that most concerned authors in relation to motherhood.

Observed in perspective, the six novels I will be concentrating on offer insight into different aspects of motherhood, as they were emerging and unfolding at a moment of unprecedented social, economic and cultural change. As we have seen in previous chapters, the period corresponds to an active phase in women's public history (feminism, charitable work, enfranchisement discussions, and waged labour) as well as to changes in their legal, civic status. Alongside the process, and between the traditional forms of representation and the new, modern emerging ones, women as social subjects were acquiring a fragmented identity.

I have organised the novels as belonging to two axes or thematic series that, throughout the previous chapters, have appeared as framing discussion on the maternal while largely disputing over its social imaginary: the one that focuses on the materiality of the body, and the one that emphasises its sentimental, spiritual side. In doing so, it is possible to trace their influence over the literary field while enquiring about the re-presentations that fiction itself has forged on the maternal. The fictional mothers whose stories will be considered here exemplify strategies of both modes of compromise and resistance to the main maternal imagery shaped by the medical and journalistic fields: the *illegitimate* mother, the maternal *biotypes*, the *poor* mother, the *Catholic mother*, and the *matron* figure of the charitable lady.

Spiritual motherhood: Sins, neglects, and sacrifices

The maternity of sin

Flor de Durazno (*Peach Blossom* in the English translation) is the most famous novel of the prolific and acclaimed Catholic writer Gustavo Martínez Zuviría (1883-1962), best known by his pen name Hugo Wast. Published in 1911, it became an Argentinian bestseller that was reprinted many times and translated into many languages. It was also made into a movie in 1917 by Francisco Defilippis Novoa, starring Carlos Gardel, Argentina's immortal voice of tango. In 1921 when the movie was shown in Córdoba, the newspaper *La Voz del Interior* mocked the success of the novel among the provincial public, especially the female populace, when it commented, 'it could be assured that there is no lady left who has not read this little novel, recommended by the fathers of the Church'.[10] Indeed, Wast was able to accomplish a profuse literary career and a sales success due to the sustained support received by the Church. A fervent Catholic militant, Martínez Zuviría since his youth had participated in some of the most active branches of the Catholic organisations, like the Catholic Working Circles and the Catholic Youth. When extreme right-wing groups of militaries and Catholic nationalists took power in the decades of 1930 and 1940, Martínez Zuviría was appointed to strategic, cultural offices in the national government, including Director of the National Library and Minister of Justice and Public Education. His *oeuvre* and ideology forms an inextricable part of the cultural project of the Church, whose activities and impact over Argentinian culture, as Gramuglio and Rapalo have pointed out,[11] remains largely unexplored. Although usually discredited by Buenos Aires's literary circles, with the exception of Julio Cortázar, who is reported to have signalled Wast amongst his literary sources of inspiration, the Catholic writer was the most widely read novelist of the first half of the twentieth-century.

The topics that Wast elaborated in *Flor de Durazno* could be read as the anticipation of topics that he elaborated later in *La Novela del Día* (Novel of the Day), the serial penny novel with 331 numbers that appeared in Buenos Aires between 1918 and 1924. *La Novela del Día* was the Catholic version of the sentimental novel, especially *La Novela Semanal* (Weekly Novel), whose liberal treatment of feelings and interpersonal relationships the Catholic version aimed to counteract. Unlike *La Novela Semanal, La Novela del Día* offered platonic love, vivid realism, and a strong Catholic moral message.

Flor de Durazno embodies two scenarios that have been ideologically in dispute since the nineteenth century, the country and the city. Traditionally, for most liberal intellectuals, the dichotomy was represented as 'civilisation' (culture-city) and 'barbarism' (nature-country). In *Flor de Durazno* this dichotomy is kept, but inverted, so the country is the place of nature, that is, pureness, light, simplicity, and noble feelings, whilst the city is the one of obscurity, frivolity, sensuality and perdition. The dichotomy highlights the corruption of the city to the nature-country, where the latter represents tradition, sense of community, united families, and moral guidance by the parish priest. More importantly, here nature also embodies the representation of woman in her natural condition: a weak being, innocent, with good feelings, but with a fragile nature (body).

Rina, the protagonist, is a poor farmer who lives in a far-away rural village in Córdoba province, who is seduced by the 'city', embodied in an aristocratic young man from Buenos Aires. Wast composed his plot from many representations of real life events, like the scenario of Villa Dolores, the home of Córdoba's most famous parish priest, Gabriel Brochero, unmistakably called 'Rochero' in the novel, whose presence in the story serves to enhance the moral authority of the Catholic message. The priest functions as a central/paternal figure, working for the morality of the village, and more significantly, playing the authority of the father, whom mothers consulted to decide the lot of their daughters. The burial of Rina's mother, which opens the story of *Flor de Durazno*, however, indicates that the close relationship between the priest and the mother is broken early, and therefore, anticipates the challenges that her absence poses for her daughter's morality.

Rina falls in love with the rich boy with whom she had grown up every summer, when he comes to the village to spend holidays with his family. Her love appears as something natural, pure, innocent, and true; in contrast with the 'impure' love of the boy, who 'by habit he started the conquest of Rina'.[12] Seduced by his false promises, she surrenders to him, 'one day she closed her eyes',[13] sealing in this act her own destiny. The female figure that Rina embodies is completely asexual, made up of pure spiritual love. More importantly, she is not the owner of her body; she is only responsible for it. As a predestined consequence, 'her sin took form' and pregnancy became the materialised punishment.[14] Unable to hide herself from the view of her father and her villagers, she escapes to the city in search of shelter. She arrives in Buenos Aires, the city of her lover, which receives 'sinner' Rina in the most ruthless and merciless way.

There are some significant medical aspects that Wast made explicit to female readers in order to emphasise the moral and social sanctions that women faced on becoming single mothers. Although the novel tells us nothing about the circumstances of Rina's childbearing in Buenos Aires, Wast seemed interested in conveying some aspects of the social side of medicine. Rina's childbirth takes place in a hospital where she can remain for three months after her daughter's birth, employed in some minor tasks. This sort of 'oasis' in the middle of so much misfortune that the protagonist had previously undergone in Buenos Aires, is, however, designed by the author to guarantee that the baby be born. Mainly, to put options away from the midwife's hands, who might offer, among other solutions, an abortion, an option that never crosses Rina's mind. But also because in Wast's view, medical or charitable welfare should not protect or provide any lasting solution to single mothers, who in the long term should be punished for their moral failure. Once Rina is asked to leave the hospital 'to give room to other more needy girls than her',[15] she experiences the misfortune of being a poor single mother in a big pitiless city: men's sexual harassment, unhealthy rooms, lack of work, a disheartened encounter with her lover who doubts her story of his paternity, and finally, his aristocratic mother refusing any help to her. Wast warns us that a single mother was trapped in a social order that would always decide for her. When a bewildered Rina decides to stop for a moment to think, he questioned, 'to think of what? Everything was already thought! The entire world thought for her'.[16] Left without options, the protagonist returns to her village to later marry a farmer who had always loved her, but could never forgive her for bearing a love child. The final tragedy is unleashed when Rina's husband tries to give the baby-girl to her real father, and as he rejects her, the husband ends up killing the father and then committing suicide in prison. Rina, for her part, dies of a heart attack when her husband snatches her daughter. *Flor de Durazno* thus taught that pure, true feelings were not enough when they sprang up in socially and morally inadequate places. Not even an attempt of reparation – when Rina returned to her village and marries a man of her own social standing – is enough to restore the transgressed moral order. A transgression that also includes that of the class system. As Beatriz Sarlo has observed for *La Novela del Día*, love was never stronger than social barriers.[17]

I would like to interpret Rina's maternal attributes within the context in which the novel was written and along with the propositions of another novel of the time. In doing so, I will return to Rina's options, when she tries to 'stop and think', to ask specifically what other possibilities a single mother had at that time. As it was then very well known, the options were abandonment or infanticide. These possibilities connect us with the ones dramatically existing in Buenos Aires at this time and to which *Flor de Durazno* attempts to respond. In 1913, an interesting article in the prestigious medical journal *La Semana Médica* alerted its readers to the alarming increase of infanticide in Buenos Aires, for which the author, Dr D'Alessandro, advocated the re-installation of the *torno* (turning wheel, see p. 41). The article refers to a play titled *El Torno Libre* ('The free turning wheel') which was staged at a Buenos Aires theatre in 1910, at the time that *Flor de Durazno* was being written. Dr Faustino Trongé, one of the *torno*'s supporters, wrote the script from the perspective of the medical point of view. Dr D'Alessandro, who saw the stage version, commented extensively on the teachings of the play in the above-mentioned medical journal, considering it as 'truly therapeutic against infanticide'.[18] The plot of the play reveals that it was built with the same key elements that informed Wast's novel. In the drama of Dr Trongé, the protagonist is a naive, poor girl, abandoned by her rich lover, who becomes a single mother. The story describes the same tortuous experience as that of Rina. However, when the distressing point arrives, Rina is 'unable to think', while the protagonist of Dr Trongé's play, is able to choose a different solution: she asks a friend if there is a place to leave the baby. The answer came that the *torno* had long been eliminated, but she still had the option of putting the baby into the Orphanage's care. As the baby was rejected there, only then, as the protagonist later tells the judge, she felt she had no choice and became 'unable to think' and so ends by committing infanticide. Here, the options of abandonment/infanticide are converted into a sequence where the latter results in an undesirable consequence arising from the impossibility of achieving the child's abandonment. Contrary to those doctors who supported the reinstallation of the *torno*, Catholics made of the *torno*'s potential double solution, i.e. life for the baby and honour for the mother, an irreconcilable one. In Wast's novel, Rina's daughter is the only 'survivor' of the tragedy, and ends up surrounded by the love of her grandfather (who had previously rejected her) and the love of her wealthy grandmother, who secures her a promising future. From the medical point of view, novels like *Flor de Durazno* must have satisfied many doctors, not only Catholic ones, for the emphasis on the mother and child bond, and also for the unwavering maternal responsibility and self-denial, which, in the end, excessively consumes the maternal self. The following two novels offer insight into other Catholic concerns on mother's role, which in turn, resulted in the reinforcement of their representative moral images.

Mothers not matrons

Los Dos Polos ('The two poles') is a novel written by Juan José Vélez, a well-known Catholic journalist and writer from Córdoba, around the years 1921-1923. The story draws on several topics that reveal the concerns of the time regarding matrimony, economic crisis, children's education, and new habits in society, and to which a moral lesson will be attached. Significantly, the treatment of all these problems in the novel converged on a central topic: the mother's role in a changing society. In this sense, the elements of reality that Vélez extensively made use of, by setting the story in Córdoba and using the real names of clubs, societies, places, etc. served, as with most Catholic authors, to emphasise the conduct that they aimed to instil through their maternal characters. The authoritative presence of a narrator organises the elements in conflict, remarking on the attitudes behind maternal failure and the social conditions that made these motherly failings possible.

The novel is set in a period of economic crisis in the province, a situation that Vélez envisioned as in need of advice, especially for women entering into the labour market to whom the proper way of earning a living merited moral reassurance: girls 'submissive to the paternal order of living, with honesty in scarcity and poverty', and not 'in dishonour with abundance and luxury, but immorally loved and discredited'.[19] The topic of the 'beautiful poor girl', for whom beauty compensated for economic misfortune, serves here to confirm moral values. The main character, Claudina is a poor girl who wanders on the street selling flowers, whose beauty allows her to bridge the 'other pole', by attracting the looks of many elite men, handsome and rich, to whom she approaches with her wares. In this challenging moral universe, she refuses to fall into the easy temptations of trying for a better future. Thus, the plot distances itself from the cliché of the 'seduced and abandoned' poor, beautiful girl that largely filled the pages of the *Novela Semanal* and featured in Wast's *Flor de Durazno*. Confirming Catholic and moral expectations, Claudina's resigned attitude towards adversity and social inequalities, operates as a consolation and an example for a female readership probably under similar economic adversities.

Poverty also unfolded other values. Claudina's honesty and moral stand was also 'proved' when she rejected an 'Award for Virtue', a prize that honoured the working or moral achievements of deprived women, that were distributed in a pompous ceremony by Argentina's most prestigious female charitable organisation, the Society of Beneficence. The protagonist's rejection signals the moral resignation of those who should feel 'already rewarded by God', as Vélez claimed, as if the awards for female virtue should be celebrated in the austerity of pious phrases. However, that act of rejection also indicates something else: it served Vélez to dismiss the attempts of elite beneficent ladies to bridge the divide between social classes, something that is incisively criticised throughout the novel. In this imposed economy of gestures Claudina's resignation is finally rewarded, but with a prize appropriate to her position. She marries a businessman, honourable and hardworking. Yet the novel carefully signals that social elevation is accomplished by two respectable institutions, work in the case of the husband, and matrimony in the case of Claudina. It also demonstrates that social mobility was not easily attained, and in a time of changing women's roles, can prove to be dangerously unstable. In this sense, the protagonist commits three main sins that synthesise her maternal failure: she pretends she is from a higher social status than the one her cradle indicates, she becomes a *matron*, and she behaves as a condescending mother to her son. Strikingly, out of the three, her involvement in charitable activities is the one that truly precipitates the ruin of her family.

Like many middle and upper-class women of the time, charitable work is the place where Claudina spends most of her time out of the home. Signalled as the main cause of family misfortune, the author targets female voluntary work with ruthless criticism, and in doing so, he depoliticises ladies' maternal discourse in a double way: by divesting it of its contribution in the provision of welfare, and by signalling the negligence of maternal duties at home. In this sense, it is instructive to connect the appearance of this novel with a moment when the largest female charity in Argentina, *La Sociedad de Señoras de San Vicente de Paul,* was at its peak of members' recruitment in Córdoba.[20] It is also instructive to link *Los Dos Polos* with the Church's unresolved conflict regarding women's participation in charitable activities as previously discussed. In this sense, Vélez, who was a Catholic militant, sent a clear condemnatory message to mother's welfare role (political maternalism), trivialising *matrons* as subjects, and undermining their input into the welfare system. In a scene where three elite women are 'gossiping' on their way to Claudina's home, each of the ladies is introduced to the reader as follows, the first one, as 'a lady apparently discrete, but vain, in reality'; the second one, as 'the most sly one', and the third one, as 'less gossipy, uptight and with light brain'.[21] These ladies approach Claudina to ask her 'to accept the presidency of the bazaar's commission of the Maternal Asylum'.[22] The choice of Vincentians' most praised institution, the Maternal Asylum - devoted to the assistance of children while their mothers were working out of home - gives the message an undeniably didactic character. The scene ends with Claudina – who has already been involved in many philanthropic organisations – accepting the appointment for 'pure vanity', in a picture where charitable aim is replaced by frivolity and gossip. The same elements are repeated while the bazaar takes place, where the fund-raising aims are absent and substituted for scenes of gossiping, treachery and lack of commitment.

The story has as its turning point, its 'divine punishment', from the two people that Claudina has 'neglected' the most. Her son, who lives a dissipated life, and her husband, who becomes involved in the 'delirium of gambling', losing all the fortune that he had patiently built through honesty and hard work. The story thus 'rewards' the arrogance and snobbishness of Claudina with poverty and family disunity. The negligent spouse and mother is criticised by the husband, who recriminates her for 'pusillanimous ways in maternal duties'. He scolded her, 'public beneficence has distanced you from home, from my side, from your duties'.[23] Mothering in public, the novel warns, was performed to the detriment of mothering in private; consequently there was no possible bridge between them, hence 'the two poles' retained their natural stance as separated positions/spheres. The epilogue of the story anticipates the return to family unity, which is synthesised by a very telling reconciliatory scene where Claudina mends her husband's coat, and he 'discovers' the beauty behind his wife's fingers 'admirably moving whilst using the needle'.[24] This last image embodies a response to the challenge that women's charitable work posed to traditional gender boundaries, and the maternal role. *Los dos Polos* thus illustrates the deep anxieties that were aroused in Cordoban Catholics when women increasingly moved from private motherhood to public forms of political maternalism.

The spiritual mother

The novel I will consider next is entirely devoted to revising women's role in Córdoba society, yet its treatment of maternity, female charity and medicine reveal new insights into the Catholic perspective, somewhat different from the one we have seen in Wast and Vélez. The author is Amalia Beltrán Posse who along with Juan José Vélez, is amongst the most important referents of what can be considered as a 'Catholic literature' in Córdoba. In their works they combined realism, as a platform from which to convey a moral message, with a simple narrative structure and scarce literary or aesthetic resources, thus making their novels easy to read for the young, female public to whom they were intended.

Desde mi Rincón ('From my corner') tells the story of Milagros, an old-fashioned, thirty year-old spinster, with a strong faith in God, who lives in a boarding house where the core of the plot takes place. This house allows her to establish relationships with other lodgers which are otherwise improbable for her morally upright personality and outmoded behaviour, and serves Beltrán Posse as a micro-society where different characters stereotype men's and women's conduct of the society of the time. There, Milagros meets the nephew of the landlady, who after falling very ill comes to the boarding house to be cared for. After Milagros attentively looks after him, they fall in love and the story ends up with their marriage. Thus, the unattractive, pious, old-fashioned but kind and caring spinster ends up with the passionate love of a handsome man. This is not, however, a literary treatment of the 'spinster' as a problematic figure that reduces her to an 'anomaly' of sexual or intellectual aspirations that prevents conformity to social expectations. It is rather a treatment of two confronting figures, the New Woman or the infamous 'girls of the period' characterised by Margarita, the young teacher who 'likes short dresses', is a party goer, graceful and independent, and Milagros the old-maid almost 'redundant' woman, who clarifies 'I do not use make up' and has made of a prolonged celibacy not an anomaly but a virtue.[25]

Beyond this very schematic characterisation of old/new social values that the author reads through the transformation of gender roles, especially those of women, there are some interesting elements to analyse. Remarkably, maternity is represented by its spiritual presence. Milagros' mother had died when she was eighteen, leaving her nothing material but only the spiritual.

> I am now tranquil, my daughter; I am not leaving you a penny, so poor
> I have been! but I leave you the inheritance of faith and dignity that
> since your childhood we managed to inculcate in you, the priest and I.
> You can go quietly in the world. I fear nothing for you.[26]

The biological father, who is never mentioned in the novel, is replaced by the spiritual father, the priest, who is also her uncle. This spiritual father pays

176

for Milagros' education, and also leaves her a pension, thus reproducing the Catholic familial roles that positioned mothers and daughters not in need of earning a living to make them dependant on the 'father's earnings'. This ideal Catholic version of family – composed by a biological mother, who provided spiritual advice as her best capital, and a priest-father who provided moral authority and economic wellbeing – was however, far from the mainstream of medical ideas. In a time when doctors were concerned with raising awareness of mother's biological capital, and in improving the mother-child physical bond, the maternal 'spiritual inheritance' seemed completely useless. On the contrary, in *Desde mi Rincón* the educator role assigned to the mother figure becomes so self-sufficient that not only is her material bequest rendered irrelevant, but so too is her corporal existence.

At the same time, the perspective that the novel set from the female world of welfare and beneficence is similar to that in *Los Dos Polos*, in that charitable ladies are trenchantly criticised by Beltrán Posse. In a very telling passage, Milagros visits a very poor friend, who is pregnant, and has three children and an alcoholic husband. During the visit, a charitable lady comes to offer the poor woman some money. She is depicted as, the 'ex-president of one society of charity, over dressed, full of necklaces, she looked like a rich gipsy. She was driven in a very luxurious car'.[27] Beltrán Posse not only shares the view of matrons as frivolous, rich and false beings that we have seen in Catholic authors or in *La Voz del Interior*, but she takes it a step further to draw attention to the disruptive ideas that matrons were introducing while doing their home visits to the needy. The dialogue reproduced below between the poor mother and the matron, attempts to warn readers about matron's unsettling presence amongst the poor,

> [matron]: - Separate yourself from this swain spouse!, who is filling you up with children and under such situation!
> [woman]: - I can't abandon him; who is going to cook for him, poor thing? His father was the same, why blame him for having inherited this vice?
> [woman]: - What can I do?, he is the father of my children. May the Lord help us according to his will, but to abandon him, never! . . .
> [matron]: - You're stupid! You deserve all that happens to you for being silly![28]

It is also interesting to note the attention to eugenics that this dialogue entails. Alcoholism along with tuberculosis and venereal disease had been in the 1920s at the core of medical debate, and were considered as a 'racial poison' that destroyed health and weakened progeny. In the novel, alcoholism is interpreted as a (moral) vice, rather than a (physical) disease. Moreover, while some obstetricians recommended the need to avoid reproduction until those diseases were controlled, Beltrán Posse asserts that nothing should be done to prevent the reproduction of unfit persons. In her view, as much as in the official Catholic discourse, reproductive problems should be addressed and resolved in a different domain, one that was not medical (biological) or charitable (social), but in the sphere of Catholicism (moral).

Beltrán Posse's clear discomfort with a definition of a maternal virtue led her to place positive maternal attributes in an absent mother who operates from evocation, while the other (live) mothers represented in the novel are rendered either depoliticised (matron) or debiologicised in their reproductive functions (pregnant woman). In this way, the didactic use of the elements of reality with which this novel elaborates its plot, provides us with a hint of competing formulations of motherhood that were simmering at the time. This perceived malaise crystallised just few years later in two main tendencies: the first one was the biologisation of the maternal body that stemmed from the radicalisation of eugenic ideas. The second one refers to the advances of political maternalism, where *matrons*, along with the support of some Catholic groups, actively campaigned for a women's suffrage bill in 1932, which was nearly approved by the Parliament.

Corporal motherhood: Absences and rebellions

Which Motherhood? Just Fatherhood

Throughout his historical novels, Rodolfo Juárez Núñez reinterpreted all the unsolved conflicts of the 1930s – race, nation, and family disintegration – into the post-independence era, when the Argentinian state started to be defined. Set in the anarchic period of 1820, *Sombra del Tejar* ('The shadow of the tile') narrates the story of a Spanish military man who, after marrying a *criolla* (creole), receives the Governor's authorisation to settle lands in the south of Córdoba. Ten men, including a mulatto and a Spaniard – ex captive of Indians – and a little orphan boy (the woman's nephew), accompany the married couple to establish a new life in an inhospitable land.

The woman soon becomes pregnant and this fact will constitute a de-

178

cisive element of the plot, although she is not going to be part of it. At the moment when she is about to deliver her child, she is forced to interrupt labour to hide herself during an Indian raid. Once discovered, she is cruelly murdered by an Indian who stabs her in the forehead. Her husband arrives just in time to 'deliver' the baby by opening the dead mother's womb with his knife. Dispossessed from the act of delivery, this eloquent vision of 'birth without woman' is complemented in the plot through abject representations of the mother, who is evoked in a masculine world that grows confident in the possibilities opened up by the maternal absence. After such an outrageous death, the absence of the mother is replaced by the care of the father, his two rustic, close friends – a mulatto and a Spaniard – and the orphan child who is just five years-old. I will contend that the topic of the mother's absence throughout the novel constitutes one of the most striking treatments of maternity in this period. In what follows I will examine the main elements with which the author elaborates this absence, to later reflect on underlying ideas of fatherhood that the novel posed for the 1930s. In doing so, the imprint of medical and Catholic ideas will also be evaluated.

When the baby-girl is two months-old her life is placed at risk, for she is debilitated because of the lack of milk. One of the father's friends suggests that he find a woman to breast feed the baby. But the father emphatically rejects any sort of mother figure, 'like she was born, she will be raised',[29] he replies. The rejection of a wet nurse that the story conveys surely did nothing to help contemporary medical efforts to combat infant mortality, and its alleged two main causes, deficient alimentation and lack of hygiene. Moreover, such a message contradicted doctors' stress on the irreplaceable attributes of maternal milk for children's health. In the novel, the woman's breast is replaced by a goat, an unhygienic decision in a time when cow and goat's milk were deemed as dangerous carriers of tuberculosis.

More strikingly, the mother-child bond is reconfigured by Juárez Núñez into a 'goat-child' one, thus completely emptying its 'natural' content to resignify another message. The 'goat-mother' receives the baby by 'tenderly licking her cheeks', and ever since it/she becomes an important member of this anomalous family. She is given a name, 'Mora', and is 'maternally' close to the baby, whom she breast-feeds without trouble. Yet the most significant passage of this warped maternal message is conveyed through language. When the baby (called Ñaña) starts to stammer out her first words in front of her father, what she expresses for the very first time is: 'Mora'. The father, who is completely astonished with his daughter's first word, tries in vain to teach her the much more simple word *mamá*, a word that the little girl can never pronounce. Thus, the emptiness left by the mother does not give an idea of her irreplaceable presence (something that the difficult-to-pronounce word 'Mora' belies), but on the contrary, it gives an idea of her complete non-existence, an idea powerfully conveyed by her non-existence in language. As Nora Domínguez has argued, 'mothers' representations can be nearly abject and the representations of her children [reveals] the impossibility for the word, that is, for a narrative'.[30] A maternal tongue thus, evidently interrupted in the narrative, is a representation of the mother that is lost for the reader but not for the fictional character (the daughter), for it is she who naturally finds (and indicates to the father) a substitute for maternal language and for the mother's representation. The scene finishes by the father accepting this surrogate maternal figure: 'Mora, old Mora! Wasn't she the mother of the Ñaña too?'[31]

Denied in language, the mother is also disembodied, for her body suffered pitiless disintegration and despicable cruelty. When she was murdered, a broody hen and its chicks ate her scattered brains. But not only that: After being buried on a hill, the family dog is fed with her body. In this sense, the author accomplishes a complete deconstruction of the maternal, both in language and body, at the time that he also indicates the possibility of her replacement, when the daughter gets fully assimilated into the paternal project. Both ideas were evidently contrary to the physical presence spurred on by doctors, but also, by Catholics, if we consider that mother's representations were built upon her natural, divine and therefore, irreplaceable presence.

I will argue that this novel proposes a resolute defence of the paternal rather than the maternal role. Firstly, the girl is successfully raised by her father, or, as it is stressed in the novel, in the 'father's way'. Secondly, the girl also awakens paternal feelings in the father's male friends, who also claim 'parental rights' over the girl when at some point the father decides to leave them in search for a better place. Fatherhood was not legally at risk by the time the novel was written, but it was evident that, with the enlargement of women's civil rights in 1926, the mother's condition was improved. The law conceded to single mothers the right to custody over their children and to married women to keep the custody of the children of a former marriage, even when they later remarried.

From the Catholic point of view, mothers were responsible for raising their children and educating them in moral values, an education whose content was ruled by the 'spiritual fathers', the priests. While biological fathers

participated in childrearing in a secular way, mothers enjoyed a more powerful position since they mediated with both 'fathers', as Luisa Accati has
argued, 'The mother's strategic position in both families, allowing her to me-
diate between temporal and spiritual authority, gave her great influence with
her children in the development of both their secular and spiritual values'.[32]
It is evident that from both a medical and a Catholic point of view, compared
to the fathers' role, mothers were subjects of more importance for childrearing. Arguably this novel seems to have been written to counteract that perception. However, looked at from the perspective of family disintegration, a
topic that preoccupied Juárez Núñez in many of his novels, *Sombra del Tejar*
can be read as an attempt to socially reinforce the paternal figure, arousing
awareness of his familial value, and irreplaceable authority. In a time when
maternal instinct was somehow proving to be less natural and more cultural,
the father's role could well have represented a substitute, also irreplaceable,
to ensure family preservation.

Women not mothers

Before addressing issues of motherhood as they appeared represented in
the next novel, I should first provide some information on the author as this
will help frame the discussion on his literary stance. Raúl Barón Biza (1899-
1964) was a legendary figure in Córdoba social circles, with a reputation as
a millionaire, a dandy, a writer *provocateur*, a political revolutionary, and an
eccentric figure. His scandalous affairs brought him a great deal of public
notoriety, stories that have been recently contextualised and interpreted in
two publications.[33] He was a duellist many times over, a political prisoner under the military regime of 1930, and had tragic marital relationships – his last
one ended dreadfully when he threw acid at his second wife and then committed suicide. Literature was an inalienable part of his unconventional and
flamboyant life-style, fuelling the inspiration for his irreverent stories – many
of them proscribed for being considered 'obscene' – but also because family wealth allowed him to publish his own books and thus sustain his literary
aspirations with a degree of autonomy. Although writers and critics seem to
have ignored his works and pay scant attention to his contributions to the
literary field, he enjoyed a considerable readership, undoubtedly propelled by
his scandals, as indicated by the many editions of his two best-selling novels,
El Derecho de Matar with an initial edition of 5,000 copies and *El Punto Final*
(1941) with 30,000 copies, an impressive print run for the time.

Like many other writers of the 1930s, Barón Biza's novels addressed the topic of gender roles, although in his case this purpose carried a somewhat anarchic attempt of deconstructing their conventional meaning. Here, I would like to concentrate on his most controversial novel, *El Derecho de Matar* ('The right to kill') published in Buenos Aires in 1933, and immediately seized for being pornographic, resulting in its author's trial and imprisonment. Not only were the language and the description of sexual scenes highly controversial for the time, but the whole provocative tone of the novel made it particularly disturbing, especially the many offensive references explicitly addressed to the Church. Provocatively, the novel was dedicated to Pope Pius XI in the preface, thus fuelling the outrage with which it was received.

El Derecho de Matar is written in a biographical style and narrates the story of Jorge, the main character, and his tortuous relationship with a foreign woman. The plot attempts to draw together three main pressing topics of the time: politics, social values, and gender relationships. My intention here is to focus on the third of these topics, especially on the characterisation of the independent, liberal woman. As mentioned before, the Church's social values are particularly targeted in the novel, and they are especially interrogated through its conceptions about woman and motherhood. As we have seen in previous chapters, Catholic doctrine and the clergy have always tried to equate woman with mother, an identification that, in the 1930s, was vigorously stressed through the figure of the Virgin Mary. Against this pervasive and deeply-entrenched conception, Barón Biza attempts to dissociate and split this one-ideal-being into two, woman *and* mother, leaving the first one in an worldly rather than virginal existence; and the second one on a spiritual level. In what follows we can read this singular dissociation in a passage where Jorge's father is reflecting about woman,

> The mother and the woman haven't got any link between them ...
> the mother is sanctity ... the woman is crime....
> the mother is spirit .... the woman is matter...
> the mother is virtue .... the woman is sin...[34]

The dissociation of the woman-mother ideal is a constant in the novel and it flows through different meanings. Arguably, the most significant way that Barón Biza chose to accomplish it was by empowering women's eroticism and sexuality. The female figures of this, as well as his other novels, were most of the time beautiful, sensual, independent women who, unlike other literary representations of the time, were not characterised as prostitutes.[35] More importantly, they were women who owned their bodies and fully commanded their sexuality. In the novel, Cleo, a foreigner who embodies this type of *femme fatale*, comes to Jorge's village in search of healthy air to cure herself of cocaine addiction. Through the description of her active sexual life, including a lesbian relationship with Jorge's sister, Barón Biza not only ascribes to women's sexuality the power of transgressing the pact that linked motherhood with national interests, but he also signals it as a positive subversion of the moral order. In this way, the treatment of women's sexuality would be instrumental in splitting the woman-mother idea, by separating pleasure from both money (prostitution) and reproduction (family). I think it is instructive to place this treatment of female sexuality in the mainstream of Argentinian literature of the time. In his analysis of sexual discourse in Buenos Aires, Hugo Vezzetti, proposes that for the first three decades of the twentieth century, writer and psychiatrist José Ingenieros and writer Roberto Arlt were the only two voices that 'challenged the common sense', by placing sexuality, pleasure and eroticism against eugenic and Catholic discourses.[36] Indeed, whilst passion was rather absent from the mainstream of literary discourse, sexuality was – especially through the recurrent treatment of the figure of the prostitute[37] – a topic dominated and limited by the two main existing discourses of the time. For eugenists, sexuality was restricted to the couple's awareness of their genetic capital, and for Catholics it was restricted to the reproductive aims of sexual union. Against this backdrop, Arlt's literary treatment of passion[38] has been singled out as a referent, as a counter discourse of sexuality. I suggest that within this emerging, embryonic counter discourse, Córdoba's authors Barón Biza and Juan Filloy, whom I will analyse next, should also be included as part of these new associations of sexuality, especially with happiness, that were pushing forward for more visibility. Besides the different literary projects of Barón Biza and Arlt, the ways in which they expressed ideas of sexuality and passion differed. We may argue that Arlt resorted to placing passion under no regulation, in the anomy of the brothel. Barón Biza, on the contrary, inscribed it in the social domain, instigating women to experience passion as a 'right' and without moral regrets. As he questions in the novel, 'has woman no strength to rebel and shout to the world her sexual right, the most powerful, fair, and legal of all rights?'[39]

The conventionalisms that surround the attributes of a national motherhood are exposed through the double moral standards of women of the privileged classes. Their sexual behaviour signals that respectable ladies could not represent their proclaimed moral support of the Argentinian family. To illustrate this, the author resorts to the most traditional of feminine figures, the charitable *matron*. In the story, Jorge explicitly narrates sconces of a sexual intercourse that he has with 'Mrs X... lady of beneficence', 'one of the most respected surnames of the republic'.[40] In this way, the novel openly challenges bourgeois women, especially Catholic ladies, for their dubious morality in supporting social values and status at the cost of repressing passion and true feelings.

> In exchange for your poor title of Mrs, you have had stolen the right
> to live, and if you want to rebel there is no other way than the shadows
> of the night and the appalling simulation, that exhausts and infuriates
> the nerves during the day.[41]

Another way of disaggregating the woman-mother ideal is by showing women who are aware of and resist the conventions that shaped and constrained their role in society. For example, when Jorge's sister, Irma, rejects marriage with an elite lawyer, she responds with a sarcastic portrayal of Córdoba's society and women's duties. It is also important to bear in mind that for contemporary readers aware of Barón Biza's upper-class social status, the behaviours of the characters in his novels must have enjoyed a degree of credibility that fiction by itself would not have hindered. Irma explains her decision for not getting married as follows,

> Life by his side would be awful. This capital of a province, with its
> churches, its society, its smell of 'sacristy', vulgar and hypocrital. The
> children that he would demand of me, even at the expense of my
> suffering and the deformity of my body, the monotony of these days,
> where all my obligation would be to feed him well and look after his
> clothes. Nights of loneliness in which, after the carnal desire had fin-
> ished, he would spend nights in the Club, pub or brothel. . . . No, little
> brother, you can't demand of me such a sacrifice![42]

In this deconstructive vision of matrimonial life and 'maternal sacrifice', it is not surprising that motherhood suggests in Jorge's mind other representations than the one doctors, Catholics and journalists had publicly construct-ed. Against moral and state regulations, motherhood is delightedly rejected and female sterility is celebrated in a response where hedonistic, aesthetic and ethical reasons play a relevant part. In a passage where Jorge admires Cleo's body, he considers it,

> Sacred twice for satisfying my sensuality and for being sterile, for giving us an interminable pleasure while avoiding the pain of perpetuation, for not letting the body of my female become deformed, avoiding the pain for her, for denying to give life to a being to whom we couldn't assure happiness.[43]

Maternity represents 'suffering' and corporal 'deformity', the latter an expression that it was used by obstetricians, such as Bas (see p. 126), to convey the exact opposite meaning as physical 'decadence' was associated with women's birth control practices. Here the interpretation of bodily deformity is subjective (individual) rather than dictated by a frivolous social concern; it is literally as well as figuratively on a different scale. In the dénouement, Jorge discovers the lesbian affair between Cleo and Irma, and he ends up in an unarticulated ranting, whisky and a gun in hand, about capitalism, communism, beneficence and women's instinct. Despite the increasing tension revealed by Jorge's speech and state after he realises he has been cheated, and contrary to the literary conventions where a crime (here suggested by a character armed and drunk) often closes the fiction, there is no tragic ending, no 'right to kill', just the disorder of a situation that the literary narrative does not attempt to solve.

Whatever the reasons women may have had for limiting their maternity, such a decision, this novel emphasises, belonged to the private rather than the public sphere. It also conveys the idea that medical concerns and moral conventions can be combined to perpetuate female delusional representations. As I mentioned earlier, Barón Biza was not the only writer that tackled passion and sexuality against the predominant principles informed by eugenics and Catholicism. In the final novel I will briefly comment in this section, Juan Filloy appears as another prolific novelist, who in the 1930s fictionalised sexuality to impugn, with ironic exaggeration, reproduction and maternity under the eugenic enterprise.

Women's biotype

> Op Oloop was method personified ... method made word; all his hopes, desires feelings channelled into the vessel of method. . . . Each

wall displayed a profusion of synoptic tables, statistical maps, and polychromatic diagrams. Each piece of furniture was a warehouse of data, of old reports, of studies and experiences. Each drawer, a file folder safeguarding the reliability of Op Oloop's memory.[44]

With this peculiar character, an obsessive statistician, Juan Filloy (1894-2000) built an original and dense plot of 300 pages to narrate the intense events of the last twenty hours of the protagonist's life. To facilitate the understanding of the plot, I shall briefly summarise it as follows: in the morning, Op Oloop goes to the swimming pool and sauna; then he visits his girlfriend (Franziska) to formalise their engagement with her family. On his way, however, he suffers an insignificant traffic delay (a road accident), an unforeseen interruption on his sacred timetable, 'his life – always lived by clock'.[45] This trivial fact triggers his mental collapse at his girlfriend's house, and his subsequent wandering around Buenos Aires's streets in the afternoon. At night he organises a banquet in a hotel with his male friends after which he visits a brothel. Finally, he returns to his apartment and commits suicide.

With these one-day's events Filloy accomplished a fascinating novel, a work much admired by Argentinian writers and literary critics alike – also recently translated into English – although its recognition only came decades after the novel was originally published in 1934. It is worth mentioning that in a period of cultural censorship inaugurated by the *coup d'état* of 1930, the novel was denied publication by the Municipality of Buenos Aires, for it was considered as pornographic and morally offensive,[46] although the sexual themes were less explicit and differently treated than the contemporary novel of Barón Biza. Also, this is a time when Hugo Wast (Martínez Zuviría) was appointed as Director of the National Library (1931-55), giving public expression to his fanatic Catholicism, and becoming an infamous figure in the practices of Argentinian censorship, while his rampant anti-Semitism appeared in a highly controversial two-part novel (*El Kahal* and *Oro*) in 1935.

But to return to *Op Oloop*, the novel is written with a strikingly accurate knowledge of the psychiatry of the time, a knowledge that Filloy himself was familiar with as he was a professional Public Prosecutor. Although *Op Oloop* does not explicitly deal with maternity, it is pertinent for my analysis since it conveys a deep criticism of the principles that informed eugenics and bioti-pology and its compulsion for bio-typological measuring, which, surprisingly, has passed unnoticed in most critical analysis of the novel. In this sense, I will concentrate in highlighting sexual ideas, women's representations and,

186

more broadly, in how the novel reflects what I have termed in Chapter 2, the 'taxonomic will' of the 1930s.

When Op Oloop arrives slightly late at Franziska's house to announce their engagement to her parents – something that nobody except him notices as neither the girlfriend nor the father were at that moment in the house - he experiences something like a fit and starts to become delirious, talking nonsense. He comments, 'Method is practically an organic function for me. I have never, never, never been in violation of the system that's guided my life', as he tries to explain the dread that his delay had occasioned him.[47] Two physicians are called to his assistance, who interpret his nervous shock under biotypological variables and speculations: 'the young physician could see no obvious anomalies in the Statistician, with the exception of his stature',[48] while the other doctor considers him as a 'tonic-sympathetic temperament'.[49] The physicians' knowledge, however, does not affect or predict the course of the story; they just appear in the novel as a source of comedy.

While Op Oloop undergoes an increasingly mad state, Franziska starts to experience something similar, which is deliberately attributed by the family to her organic menstrual state. This endocrine female stigma, which, as we have seen in Chapter 2, became paradigmatic in explaining women's behaviour, is used here to explain the social conventions against which Franziska reacts. Thus the delirium of Oloop's girlfriend is the result of the 'familial orthodoxy and the preconception parrying her impulses', 'sinking flesh into penitence instead of sublimating it in the splendour and freedom of gratification'.[50] The physiological upset, in the case of the fiancée, operates as a catalyst to express dissatisfaction with moral and social values. But in the case of Oloop, his entire mental, physiological system is shattered, initially, by a slight disruption of his methodical routine, but more significantly, by the awareness of love. In both characters, passion and instinct prove to be an uncontrollable force. No system, method or order whether moral, medical or political can overcome it. And the protagonist, who is 'method and order personified', will succumb to it by committing suicide; 'sadly, however, method is of no use when one is dealing with the stratagems of chance'.[51] In this way, the collapse of the statistician entails a response to biotypologists' and eugenists' programmes of measuring and controlling sexuality and reproduction. Within one couple (Op Oloop and Franziska) the fecund quality of bodies upon which maternity rests, is not the main decisive factor; it is rather the domain of feelings, potent and untamed, impossible 'to calculate' what ultimately signals its destiny.

The most significant way in which Filloy conveys the impossibility of controlling sexuality is presented in a very ingenious way. As part of Oloop's mathematic behaviour, he had sex 'twice a week: Wednesdays and Sundays'. His obsession for measuring and controlling sexuality leads him, as in the case of biotypologists, to elaborate a complex statistical system of index cards, taxonomies and records of the prostitutes to whom he visits. This eloquent passage gives an account of that ridiculous obsession,

> So my erotic punctuality became an imperative mathematical desire. I possessed women so that I might possess their statistics [*fichas* (index cards) in the original]. I don't know what strange allure I found by assimilating sex and numbers, whereby the displaced pleasure of copulation was recovered in the joy of computation.[52]

Index cards contain a detailed description of each of the thousand prostitutes he had met, all of them recording information inextricable linked to eugenic issues, such as race, nationality, age, and biological causes: inheritance, traits, degeneration, etc.[53] While explaining his skills as statistician, he comments to his friends the social utility of his findings:

> By speculating philosophically on the figures, one can determine the crisis of modern morality that will be upon us in the near future judging by the rates of divorce, crimes of passion, and the production of bastard children. My thesis on the subject – that a societal organization suitable to the betterment of the individual biotype is prone to eugenic manifestation – was deemed praiseworthy by the London Statistical Society.[54]

In this sense, the entire novel can be read as an attempt to destroy in readers a belief in the objectivity of eugenic theory. As indicated in the tragic outcome (suicide) of Oloop, which brings the story to an end, Filloy repudiates the uses of the body to serve nationalistic causes, and rejects the attempts of the state to regulate sexuality and women's interests. By objecting to biotypological aims his novel ultimately shows that those females bodies, and potential gestating bodies, depended less on the estimate of women's index cards than in the fortuitous, and socially denied, order of female subjectivity.

The two series that make up the literary texts above analysed account for a wide range of topics where representations of the maternal result in competing images and formulations. For some of them, maternity constitutes a defining category of womanhood, while for others it is just one of women's attributes, whose potential rests on female subjectivity rather than in a predetermined natural, social role. Examples of the former are found in the novels of Catholic writers gathered in the series devoted to the 'spiritual mothers', Wast, Vélez and Beltrán Posse. In support of an essentialised maternal figure, they signal and emphasise its deviations with didactic purport. Not least because motherhood, this series reminds us, was not only reduced to a corporal (biological) act, but it was regulated by a series of social, cultural and religious strategies that indicated specific ways of maternal performance: Wast does so through the figure of the illegitimate mother, and Beltrán Posse and Vélez through the figure of the charitable lady (matron) to alert us to the dangers inherent in the politicisation of the maternal figure. As already observed in the discourses of the press, the anxieties and discontent generated by ladies' political use of the maternal found in the literary field another space of contestation.

The series of the 'corporal mother', on the other hand, provides insight into the deep enduring anxieties that followed when eugenics and its concern with the corporal support of maternity came to the fore in the 1930s. This series is composed by novels that, paradoxically, have an elusive – rather than a material – form of representation, one where the maternal body is thought of as pregnancy and in its pre-conceptional stage. Revealingly, Juárez Núñez concedes to mothers their corporal support to pregnancy but not to the act of childbirth. By positioning the mother at this threshold of human gestation, the author revisits traditional literary masculinist appropriations of birth and the correlative abjection of maternal subjects. It also offers a different account to the mother's naturalised role in raising children, proposing that fathers were also able to successfully accomplish that role. In a time when the traditional idea of family was under revision (debates on divorce in 1932, low fertility rate, and illegitimacy) it is not surprising that some voices turned to fatherhood as the role/bond to be reinforced.

Medical obsessions on the pre-conceptional attributes of the maternal body, as well as Catholics' unprecedented extolment of the Virgin Mary and the Catholic mother, were replicated in fiction in plots that transmit a similar exaggeration in the treatment of these topics. While Barón Biza emphasised women's control over their bodies (sexuality) as a way of deconstructing the ideal of the 'Catholic mother' and as a form of eluding a biologically conscious procreation, Filloy shows that the medical effort to eugenically control reproduction was, by principle, an unattainable endeavour. Furthermore, the representations of the anti-maternal *femme fatale* and the debiologised women that both writers present, draws attention to the existence of a female subjectivity not recognised in mainstream maternal discourses. In the next chapters, we shall see how the subjectivity of the mother was perceived in visual culture, and how its erratic presence forged and contributed to other representations of motherhood.

Notes

1   M. Jacobus, *First Things: The Maternal Imaginary in Literature, Art and Psychoanalysis* (London; New York: Routledge, 1995); Ann Kaplan, *Motherhood and Representation: The Mother in Popular Culture and Melodrama* (London: Routledge, 1992). Marianne Hirsch and Jo Malin have analysed the mother and daughter plot in nineteenth and twentieth-century women writers, focussing on women that wrote as daughters autobiographies that represented - and resulted in - biographies of their mothers. J. Malin, *The Voice of the Mother: Embedded Maternal Narratives in Twentieth-century Women's Autobiographies* (Carbondale: Southern Illinois University Press, 2000); M. Hirsch, *The Mother/ Daughter Plot: Narrative, Psychoanalysis, Feminism* (Bloomington: Indiana University Press, 1989).

2   Kaplan, *Motherhood and Representation*, 7.

3   For a comprehensive review of the field see E. Podnieks and A. O'Reilly, 'Introduction: Maternal Literatures in Text and Tradition: Daughter-Centric, Matrilineal, and Matrifocal Perspectives', in E. Podnieks and A. O'Reilly (eds.), *Textual Mothers: Motherhood in Contemporary Women's Literatures* (Ontario: Wilfrid Laurier University Press, 2010), 1-27.

4   M. Hill, *Mothering Modernity: Feminism, Modernism, and the Maternal Muse* (New York; London: Garland Publishing, 1999), 1.

5   T. Bowers, *The Politics of Motherhood. British Writing and Culture 1680-1760* (Cambridge: Cambridge University Press, 1996).

6   Domínguez, *De Donde Vienen los Niños*, 16.

7   Podnieks and O'Reilly, 'Introduction: Maternal Literatures in Text and

Tradition', 5.

8   In my selection, I will not examine the text of Nora Lange, *Cuadernos de Infancia* (1937), whose treatment of motherhood has been sufficiently studied by Francine Masiello and N. Domínguez amongst others. I will instead concentrate in less explored authors, while retaining for my analysis the idea of Lange's 'transgressor' representations as informing a pathway of fictional 'rebellion' against certain maternal constructs.

9   T. Gramuglio, 'El Realismo y sus Destiempos en la Literatura Argentina', in *Historia Crítica de la Literatura Argentina: El Imperio Realista, VI* (Buenos Aires: Emecé Editores, 2002), 15-38: 27. Eduardo Mallea wrote short stories and novels in the decades of 1920 and 1930.

10 *La Voz del Interior*, 3 June 1921, 8.

11 E. Rapalo and T. Gramuglio, 'Pedagogías para la Nación Católica, Criterio y Hugo Wast', in *Historia Crítica de la Literatura Argentina*, 447-75: 470.

12 H. Wast, *Flor de Durazno* (Buenos Aires: Thau Editores, 1944), 127.

13 Wast, *Flor de Durazno*, 143.

14 Ibid., 152.

15 Ibid., 183.

16 Ibid., 209.

17 B. Sarlo, *El Imperio de los Sentimientos* (Buenos Aires: Norma, 2000), 135.

18 A. D'Alessandro, 'El Infanticidio y el Torno Libre', *La Semana Médica*, 1 (1914), 18-28: 24.

19 J. J. Vélez, *Los Dos Polos* (Córdoba: Biffignandi, [s.d.]), 14-15.

20 In the case of the city of Córdoba, membership of the San Vincent de Paul Society reached its highest numbers in the years 1920-1921, with 1,892 female members, which coincided with the highest levels of riots, general strikes, workers militancy and upper-class fear. Cfr. Y. Eraso, 'Maternalismo, Religión y Asistencia', 211.

21 Vélez, *Los Dos Polos*, 43.

22 Ibid., 44.

23 Ibid., 117.

24 Ibid., 119.

25 A. Beltrán Posse, *Desde Mi Rincón* (Córdoba: Biffignandi, 1928), 9-10.

26 Beltrán Posse, *Desde Mi Rincón*, 14.

27 Ibid., 22.

28 Ibid., 23.

29 R. Juárez Núñez, *La Sombra del Tejar* (Buenos Aires: El Ateneo, 1932),

35.

30   Domínguez, *De Donde Vienen los Niños,* 133.

31   Juárez Núñez, *La Sombra del Tejar,* 104.

32   Accati, 'Explicit Meanings', 251.

33   C. Ferrer, *Barón Biza, El Secreto Mejor Guardado de la Historia Argentina* (Buenos Aires: Sudamericana, 2007) and the journalistic work of C. de la Sota, *El Escritor Maldito: Raúl Barón Biza* (Vergara, 2008).

34   R. Barón Biza, *El Derecho de Matar* (Buenos Aires: Editorial Barón Biza, 1933), 32.

35   Male writers in early twentieth-century Buenos Aires often established a link between the traffic of women (prostitutes) and the circulation of money and wealth. While prostitutes threaten the national programme of increasing the population, for being single, childless women; 'the female body acquired a value as a commodity to be exchanged and consumed', as Francine Masiello has observed. Cfr. Masiello, *Entre Civilización y Barbarie. Mujeres, Nación y Cultura Literaria en la Argentina Moderna.* (Rosario: Beatriz Viterbo, 1997), 154.

36   Vezzetti, 'Historia del Freudismo', 216.

37   On the treatment of prostitution in the Argentinian literature of the first decades of the twentieth century, see F. Masiello, *Entre Civilización y Barbarie,* Ch. 4.

38   The most important texts where Arlt tackled women's sexuality as uncontrollable are: *Los Siete Locos* (1929) and *El Amor Brujo* (1932).

39   Barón Biza, *El Derecho de Matar,* 70.

40   Ibid., 65.

41   Ibid., 74.

42   Ibid., 50.

43   Ibid., 148.

44   J. Filloy, *Op Oloop.* Tr. Lisa Dillman (Champaign & London: Dalkey Archive Press, 2009), 6-7.

45   Filloy, *Op Oloop,* 249.

46   See M. Giardinelli, *Don Juan. Antología de Juan Filloy* (Buenos Aires: Ediciones del Instituto Movilizador de Fondos Cooperativos, 1995).

47   Ibid., 35.

48   Ibid., 46.

49   Simpático-Tónico was a classification of temperaments used by biotypologists to refer to a nervous temperament. Ibid., 54.

50   Ibid., 60.

51   Ibid., 22-23.
52   Ibid., 179.
53   Ibid., 180-81.
54   Ibid., 129.

PART III: THE VISUAL RECORD

6

Photojournalism and the Question of Maternal Visualisation before the Technologies of Visualisation

Images. Today we cannot even begin to think about the representation of the body without imagining the unprocessed amount of visual images with which we live every day of our lives. We see more than we can intellectually handle and far more than we request, ever since media and technology have not left a single structure of the body unshown. Moreover, the association of the artistic and scientific fields promise yet more for the delight of our capacity of seeing, by showing us the shape and texture of myriads of unseen organisms that inhabit our bodies. Indeed, the capacity of the electron microscope to magnify up to two million times the actual size of organisms produces astonishing images (photomicrographs), whose social value is at the same time scientific and aesthetic, yet undoubtedly problematic: we can now see beauty in a cancer cell. One can probably argue that revealing or unveiling the body has always been problematic in a moral and a scientific way. I have commented on how, early in the twentieth century, the Pope was concerned with measuring women's dresses to dictate how much cleavage was decorous to be shown, while at the same time, radiologists were trying hard to make the breast translucent, by means of injected fluids and X-rays, to detect cancer tumours. Fashion bears no comparison with medicine, for the latter has enjoyed a sort of free licence to suspend moral scrutiny to render every part of the body visible. Their visual representation in photographic images reached different publics too, one was seen in women's magazines, leaflets, theatre programmes, or the liberal press, the other one was exclusively circulated in medical journals to be analysed by specialists. There was, however, a time when those visual representations of the body left the limited space of medical journals and became public, circulating in a wide range of media, TV, magazines, and the press, and they did so not only because new technologies of visualisation allowed it, but because it became socially acceptable to make parts of the female body transparent. I am referring here to the emergence of prenatal ultrasound screening and endoscopic explorations of the unborn child whose unprecedented photographic images were first revealed to the public in the mid-1960s.

Barbara Duden's historical reconstruction of the unborn child and the way it became a visual, separate entity is an interesting account of the profound political, scientific, religious and social consequences that resulted from rendering a woman's womb transparent. Her starting point is the status of the foetus in contemporary culture, its assimilation with 'life' after the wide range of public debates it generated ('public foetus'), a status that it gained through a process of visualisation when the first pictorial foetus was published in *Life* magazine in April 1965. It is Duden's concern with the visible that interests me here. Of the visualisation of the foetus, she has argued, 'Photographs also broaden their power to give "proof" for the invisible' by placing 'the invisible before the eye'.[1] In this sense, I am interested in a previous stage, one which poses the question of how photographs have rendered real subjects, like mothers, invisible. That is, before our eyes have become accustomed and trained to see the unseen, there was a time in which photography, the same device that now allows us to see 'life' in the womb, was a way of seeing the visible reality. In relation to the maternal, this way of seeing, I would argue, was informed by the same principle that leads Duden – thinking of the unseen unborn – to affirm, 'we have lost the power to discriminate between the seen and the shown'.[2] To explore the tensions that underlie the 'seen' and the 'shown', I will focus my enquiry in photojournalism, as a new photographic genre that appeared in the 1920s with specific, distinctive features. I will integrate its innovative characteristics into my framework of maternal representations, which operates as interrelated objects resulting from specific disciplines. To this aim, I will concentrate on the photographs that were published in the two previously analysed liberal and Catholic papers as they constitute my main documentary source for this investigation.

Photojournalism and the politics of truth

Photojournalism, unlike artistic or familiar photographs produced by a photographic studio, has had a different relation to 'the real'. Photographs in newspapers exist only in relation to the text they are accompanying, sometimes as proof or evidence of news, sometimes as mere illustration of articles. Beyond this setting, they have no meaning. In this relationship to news and information, photography emerged in newspapers as a support to 'truth', or as cultural historian Peter Burke has described it 'as evidence of authentic-

198

ity',[3] in order to make written words visually irrefutable. It is this particular commitment with 'real facts' and the status of 'truth' that photojournalism has ever since enjoyed,[4] that has induced me to seek in newspapers, rather than in any other type of photographic records, images of the maternal.

Before semiotic discourse focused on photographic language to deconstruct what we now call its 'mythical realism',[5] and ordinary people, we may suppose, began to look at photographs with some scepticism about their representative value, photographs were synonyms of 'truth', 'evidence', and the 'real', as they acquired popularity particularly in the press. In this sense, its relationships with Positivism, the scientific paradigm in which photography was born, recalls to us the premises of its status: an external objective reality and a detached observing subject. As Sarah Kember has stated, 'Positivism is regarded as photography's originary and formative way of thinking. It appears to transcend historical and disciplinary boundaries and constitute the stable foundation of realist and documentary practices'.[6] Indeed, the scientific status of criminology and medicine found in photography a way of objectifying 'the normal', as well as certain categories of people, such as the criminal, the insane, the prostitute, the patient, or the poor. For John Tagg, who has studied representations of confined individuals through institutional photographic records, 'what gave photography its power to evoke a truth was not only the privilege attached to mechanical means in industrial societies, but also its mobilisation within the emerging apparatuses of a new and more penetrating form of the state'.[7]

There is still another fundamental perspective to understand the value attached to the photographic record in our period of investigation, which is one that has also induced me to analyse photojournalism as an additional source to explore representations of the maternal. It is its unmistakable distance from painting and other forms of artistic work. In the early twentieth century, as Andy Grundberg has argued,

> Photography was held to be unique, with capabilities of description and a capacity for verisimilitude beyond those of paintings, sculpture, printmaking, or any other medium. ... Modernism required that photography cultivate the photographic – indeed, that it invent the photographic – so that its legitimacy would not be questioned.[8]

Under this Positivist premise of 'truth', with which photography entered in newspapers, what interests me here is not the fact that psychologically what readers saw may have been understood as the 'real' or the 'truth', but the fact that 'the real' may have been understood as that worthy of being visually represented. Secondly, I am interested in pointing to the different politics of representations that each newspaper held, that is, the way in which photography was involved in the social construction of a female identity. In this sense, my first question is, were mothers, whose existence I have explored in various texts produced by medical, religious, journalistic, literary discourses, worthy of being visualised? If so, how were they portrayed? Has photojournalism been a support for those texts that this study has been concentrated on? Or has it developed its own representation of the maternal? I shall start, first, by charting the place of photography in each newspaper in order later to compare their politics of representation of women and motherhood.

La Voz del Interior and *Los Principios*

During the decade of the 1910s photography started to appear both as an illustrative and testimonial complement to various articles related to politics, sports, crime and social reports. The technological advance signalled by the incorporation of a new rotary press, the 'Duplex' (*Los Principios* in 1909; *La Voz del Interior* in 1913), a machine that worked with plaques of zinc and a chemical processing that facilitated the printing of pictures, allowed photography to restructure the appearance of daily news. Yet until the 1920s photographs occupied a rather erratic place throughout the page's design, with very little visual impact. Photographs, along with cartoon advertisements, cut the newspaper's broad sheet into spaces that were not yet hierarchical or differentiated in terms of news' distribution. In Cordoban newspapers, many of the photographs published during the first two decades were in the portrait format or in identity card-like pictures done in photography studios, which were usually provided by the person that made the news in question: politicians, criminals, the person honoured in some social event (birthday, conferences, and weddings) or obituaries.

The 1920s brought about a series of perceived changes in newspapers layout, known as 'new journalism'. Sections became more organised and identifiable, with appealing headlines in bigger and bold typography which were to be found in specific pages, while photographs started to multiply as part of a process that completely transformed newspapers' design. This conspicuous visual change had two main referents, one commercial – the need to make the daily format more appealing to readers and advertisers – and the other one journalistic - the influence and impact that the Buenos Aires' daily *Crítica* (1920) had on the Argentinian press more broadly. *Crítica* incorporated the sensationalist style of American tabloids, where photographs appealed heavily to the emotions, thus creating a different balance in information presentation, where the visual itself narrated the news.[9] This decade, however, marked two different trajectories in the use of photography in Cordoban newspapers.

La Voz del Interior started to use photography as an instrument of political activism and social critique, as the paper accompanied the engagement of larger sectors of society in party politics opened up by the incorporation of new democratic political parties into the electoral battle. Unsurprisingly, the paper's political use of photography also reinforced its combative, anticlerical profile in the provincial scenario. In this sense, as I have discussed in Chapter 4, changes in style were more clearly perceived with the arrival of a new editorial director in 1918, and also with the appointment of Antonio Novello, who was to become the paper's most prominent photoreporter in his long tenure as head of photography until his retirement in 1958.[10] The rapid integration of photoreporters into the newspapers' editorial staff during this period was due to significant technological advances introduced into the photographic equipment, most notably the possibility of carrying the camera in hand, like the legendary 'Spido' popularised amongst reporters in the 1920s, as well as to new developments introduced into the process of picture developing.[11] More importantly, those technological advances were soon translated into a new style of photographic narrative, one that left behind the mere 'ritual of recording', as Paul Vancassel has observed,[12] to become a process of observation, selection, and anticipation of what was worthy to be shown.

In *La Voz del Interior*, photography multiplied its presence with scenes of everyday life, capturing its dynamism with snapshots of town streets and their modernisation, as well as images of the periphery, with its slums and working-class neighbourhoods. The celebration of popular festivities in poorer neighbourhoods was captured as were the exclusive sumptuous parties of the well–to-do families, thus revealing different ways of socialisation amongst classes and sexes. Through its pictures it is possible to sense the thought of liberals in their welcoming attitudes to progress and the advances of modernity as much as their questioning of poverty and social inequalities. Above all, photoreporters made it possible to record the increasing pace of a society that was unmistakably changing.

The Catholic press, on the other hand, recorded an entirely different

201

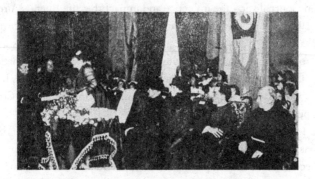

Fig. 6.1 'Los Premios a la Virtud' ['The Awards for Virtue'], *La Voz del Interior* (1 June 1915), 5. Courtesy of *La Voz del Interior*, Córdoba.

picture of Córdoba, primarily, one where the sense of change remained unnoticed. The photographic style of *Los Principios* remarkably differed from the one displayed in the liberal paper, and they did so through various visual strategies. Firstly, during the 1920s, photographs commissioned from photoreporters to cover events in the public space were less important than the photographs of portraits provided by the person referred to in the text. This rendered their visual images static, passive, atemporal and self-referential. The spontaneous photograph, on the contrary, found far less space, thus reflecting the way Catholics were uneasy with the way modernity (speed, progress, and secular time) was taking shape. On the one hand, the newspaper's profile of opinion maker presupposed a readership with a reflective reader more than one that would simply flick through the news. On the other, Catholicism strongly condemned the material aspects of modernity, particularly rejecting all that excited the senses, and so the popularisation of visual images in the printed media became a new source of concern. Accordingly, their engagement with photography had to reflect deep-seated Catholic values such as tradition, order, control, composition where little was left to chance. This also influenced the way photographers performed their work, where it is possible to observe a tendency of photographing people in a standing, or sitting down posture, or in a conventional pose in front of the camera. There is no action in these images, no place for a snapshot. Although many of these aspects were present throughout the period, as the 1930s progressed, the paper started to accommodate in a more dynamic way the powerful value of images to convey Catholic values. Notably, photographs increased in number

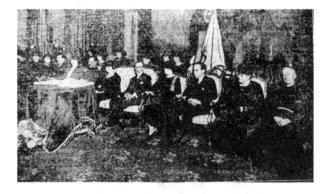

Fig. 6.2 'Los Premios a la Virtud' ['The Awards for Virtue'], *Los Principios*
(11 June 1923), 1.

and size to record the clericalisation of public life experienced in the decade,
as we shall see later.

Concentrating our attention on the politics of representation that informed the portrayal of women in both newspapers, it is not surprising to
observe meaningful differences between them. Female photographs taken by
the newspapers' photographers started portraying what was women's public
activity *par excellence* at the time, their charitable work. The annual distribution
of the Awards for Virtue (*Premios a la Virtud*) organised by the prestigious Society of Beneficence was a social event attended by the representatives of the
most prominent authorities of the society of the time, government, parliament, church and university. The ceremony traditionally included the speech
of the Society's president detailing the year's activities across the many institutions under their administration, a summary of the initiatives ahead, and
the distribution of prizes to poor women for their virtuosity demonstrated
in, what can be called, class consciousness: prizes were given to women's
abnegation, work, altruism, resigned misfortune, and noble poverty amongst
others. The picture of 1915 (Fig.6.1) by *La Voz del Interior* captures the moment in which the president of the Society, standing up, is distributing the
prizes in front of the selected audience that attentively observes her movements. In gender terms, the picture is quite powerful for it shows female
action while the masculine audience, including a priest (first from the right),
is passively sitting down and listening. It is striking to contrast this picture
with the one taken by *Los Principios* of the same event some years later. The

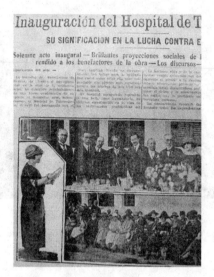

Fig. 6.3 'Inauguración del Hospital de Tuberculosos' ['Inauguration of the Hospital for Tuberculosis'], *La Voz del Interior* (13 November 1922), 6. Courtesy of *La Voz del Interior*, Córdoba.

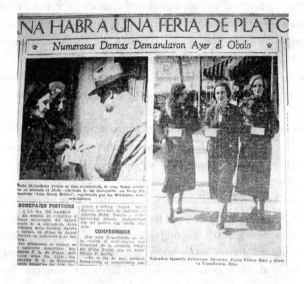

Fig. 6.4 'Numerosas damas demandaron ayer el óbolo' ['Numerous ladies participated in fundraising yesterday'], *La Voz del Interior* (4 August 1934), 8. Courtesy of *La Voz del Interior*, Córdoba.

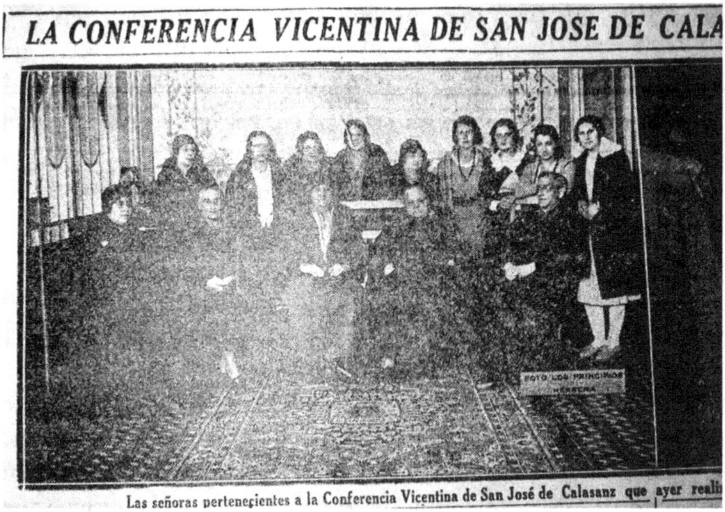

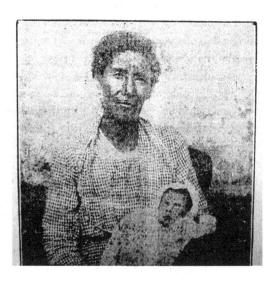

Fig. 6.5 'La Conferencia Vicentina de San José de Calasanz repartió víveres y ropa'
['The Vicentian Conference of San José de Calasanz distributed food and clothing'],
Los Principios (28 August 1930), 12.

Fig. 6.6 'Se necesita una madre' ['A mother is needed'], *La Voz del Interior* (14 December 1922), 6. Courtesy of *La Voz del Interior*, Córdoba.

picture (Fig.6.2) is taken from the same angle and in the same setting (the city's main theatre) as the one of *La Voz del Interior* in 1915. However, in the photograph of 1923, female prominence has been completely erased. Unlike its predecessor, there is no woman standing up, making a speech, distributing the prizes or giving the viewer the idea that ladies were the main organisers and responsible for the event. The photographer chooses to record a moment of quietness and passivity before the action of the Society's president takes place.

Another set of images (Fig.6.3) taken by *La Voz del Interior* provides us with a significant insight into the different politics of female representation that each newspaper pursued. The photographs of the inauguration of the Hospital for Tuberculosis by the ladies of the Society of Beneficence in 1922 arguably emphasise female agency by resorting to a photomontage, a technique that permitted to identify the figures or facts that the paper wanted to highlight at a particular event. In this case, the cropped picture of the Society's president while she delivers her speech is placed on top of another two. At the back of the lady's figure, the relevance of the act is enhanced by the picture of the male authorities posing with the Society's president at the centre. Whilst the picture at the bottom, visualises the female audience, probably members of the Society and other ladies involved in the creation of the hospital. The caption of the photomontage is very telling of the aspects that it aims to visualise.[13] There, the 'authorities' are not properly specified, nor were their names in the report, where we can only read that they were 'provincial and national' representatives. In the picture, however, the Governor of the province is standing beside the Society's president, along with military authorities, members of the Faculty of Medicine, and deputies. The Bishop, on the other hand, is not portrayed in the picture although he was present to bless the hospital opening. Finally, the description of the picture in the bottom points out the large number of women attending the event. Thus the photograph and its caption reflected female authority rather than male authorities, who, in the Catholic press had traditionally been highlighted in the Society's major events.

The pictures of the fundraising campaigns and bazaars also reproduced the same tension towards female activism. While *La Voz del Interior* portrayed snapshots of women walking on the streets, with their collection boxes in hand, talking casually to people (Fig.6.4), *Los Principios* showed them indoors, posing sitting down or standing up, and accompanied by the paternal figure of the priest (Fig. 6.5). In these photographs the depiction of women's fundraising activity offered by the liberal paper strongly contrasted with the stiff posture showed of the charitable ladies as presented by the Catholic press. In addition, in the latter picture (Fig.6.5) we see a group of static ladies posing in their meeting place with the priest at the right, alongside a picture of a group of poor women and children alone, without the presence of the ladies. There is a complete separation of the two groups or social classes; although the description of the photographs indicates that they were 'together' in the act where food and other goods were distributed.[14] In the images of the Catholic paper, priests were frequently accompanying women in different public scenes, as a visualisation of their guarding or protecting role. In photographs representing female charity, the presence of priests mainly served the purpose of showing the Church's social commitment as well as their direction over female charitable activities, a control that, as I have analysed elsewhere, they did not hold.[15] The majority of these photographic images were set in response to the 'maternal campaign' of *La Voz del Interior*, as proof and testimony of, as we read in the headlines of the series, 'Beneficent works of Cordoban Catholicism'. This series of photographic images featured different groups of school children, poor people at a canteen, mothers and children at some of the asylums administered by charitable ladies or by religious Congregations. Yet, none of these pictures allowed readers to *see* the ladies in action, or physically involved in their welfare activities with the poor.

The maternal campaign of *La Voz del Interior*

The first photograph of the campaign in 1922 showed a poorly dressed woman posing for the camera with a baby in her arms (Fig. 6.6). The picture works here as a proof of the story narrated by the woman, where she explains that, due to her lack of economic means, she could not look after the baby, who was in fact an abandoned child, 'given' over to her care (see story on p. 144). The photograph serves to justify the woman's motives, as well as the paper's call for an adoptive mother. This picture and the series it inaugurated of poor mothers and their children, although apparently conveying a 'self-evident' message, framed events that cannot be accepted at face value. Much of its meaning relied on the contingencies of its use by *La Voz del Interior*, where we can read different sub-texts, such as the paper as welfare provider, the ideological battle against Catholics, or broader politics of representation of the maternal as shown through the paper's other sections. As I have argued at the beginning of this chapter, the process of representing certain types of

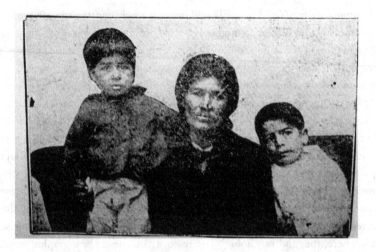

Fig. 6.7 'Quiero trabajar para que puedan comer mis hijos' ['I want to work to feed my children'], *La Voz del Interior* (25 July 1924), 6. Courtesy of *La Voz del Interior*, Córdoba.

images raised alternative readings that may well have diverged from its supposed message. From the campaign's first portrait of a poor woman holding a baby that is not hers and that she offers to someone else, it started a process of objectification of the subject ('poor mother') in what I perceive as a process of 'othering'. To understand this process, it is not enough to see these pictures and their immediate messages, but to see them in relation to other representations of the female that the paper circulated at the time.

The photograph of young ladies fundraising, the ones of beneficent ladies, or the ones under the 'social section' called, the 'brides' gallery' all showed women of upper and middle classes who represented, in their repetition of faces and names, an ideal type of beauty and women's demeanours and gestures. More importantly, in these cases, close-up photographs were provided by the women themselves, who, obviously, could have the chance to show readers their best image. On the other hand, close-up shots taken by the paper's photographers in public spaces were extremely rare and carefully taken. In this sense, the series that visualised poor mothers might perhaps be compared with the photographic style used in the crime section, where close-up photographs taken at the police station had the purpose of exposing the 'true' identity of the person, which worked as a way of case-recognition, official record and instrument of social condemnation. This visual aspect along with others that we will see in the course of this section, render the maternal campaign with an ambivalent message: while the text aimed at denouncing the mothers' conditions (including the politics of motherhood already discussed), their pictures re-presented a stigmatised figure of them.

As it is possible to see in the next story, the 'individualisation' of the mother was accomplished by a combination of graphic resources with a highly visual impact (Fig. 6.7). Headlines of the article, photograph and caption summarise the information for the reader, who can avoid reading the article without missing its compelling social message.[16] The straightforward frontal pose of the photograph, amplified through the eye-contact level between the pictured woman and the reader, attempted to awake in the latter a commiserating attitude towards her. On the surface, the complete name and age of the mother and each of her children along with the close-up picture had the purpose of fleshing out 'real' poor mothers as subjects in need of assistance. But personifying the poor mother and giving her a visibility in this way, did, however, operate as an objectifying way of *seeing* her. Even when some of *La Voz del Interior*'s female readers could have identified themselves at least partly with these stories – of impoverished mothers due to their lost husbands, desertion or their unemployment – the way in which they were shown implied more a 'them' than an 'us' arrangement. As Joan Scott has stated,

> Making visible the experience of a different group exposes the existence of repressive mechanisms, but not their inner workings or logics; we know that difference exists, but we don't understand it as constituted relationally.[17]

In this sense, photography has traditionally been instrumental in identifying people who are not like 'us', people who represent features, qualities and situations that are unfamiliar or alien to the viewer.[18] Not surprisingly, much of the scholarly analysis of photography, especially that grounded in a structuralist approach, has been devoted to illuminate how certain groups, e.g. racial or ethnic minorities, colonial subjects, women, the poor, or diseased people, have been constructed as different through subtle and explicit techniques in their visual representation.

The majority of pictures during the campaign presented a similar close-up format as the first two pictures commented on here. Some of them were taken at the editorial office – where the mother was sitting down surrounded

209

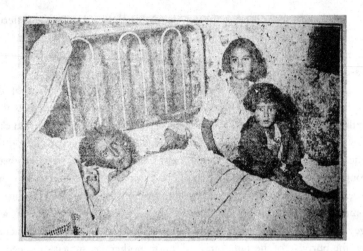

Fig. 6.8 'La pobre madre que murió bacilosa, luego de vivir postrada ante el espanto de la miseria' ['The poor mother that died of tuberculosis after living confined to bed in abject misery'], *La Voz del Interior* (12 March 1929), 13. Courtesy of *La Voz del Interior*, Córdoba.

by her children – to project the idea of the mother's choice when she was searching for help. Others, illustrated the paper's displacement to the mother's home, in a frame where the viewer could see the deprived conditions in which these mothers lived, featuring the protagonist leaning over a ruined wall, or standing in a grim, filthy and cramped room.

Within these pictures, there is one of a mother lying in bed (Fig.6.8) which is striking not so much for the setting of the photograph, but for the title and the caption that accompanies it. Significantly, this picture invites many readings regarding photojournalism itself. It shows its power in arousing poignant feelings, at the same time that it shows its weakness, for without the context provided by an explicative description, the viewer could interpret a complete different story about its content. It also lays bare another attribute of photography itself, the one that indicates its dependence with the subjects represented. As I first saw this picture in a copy of the newspaper from 1929, I had already handled enough information from the maternal campaign to easily contextualise it, as may have happened to regular readers of *La Voz del Interior* at the time. Its location in the last pages, in the section devoted to 'events of the day', its repetition (after seven years of the maternal campaign), and its recognisable features (a close-up, intimate photograph of a mother in bed with many children), all point to the factual representation of the poor mother. Within this context, this picture could have been one more in the series of portraits of poor mothers with children that appeared at the time. However, it is the headline first, and the caption later, that gives us the real content and purpose of the photograph. The headline of the article reads, 'The poor mother that died of tuberculosis after living confined to bed in abject misery. Her children remain in need. One of the many cases of pain'.[19] Once explained, the picture connects us with a different interpretation which, in turn, invites other ways of seeing. As such, there is something highly emotional in it, which belongs to photography itself, and that Roland Barthes has called, 'the defeat of time', '[b]y giving me the absolute past of the pose (aorist), the photograph tells me death in the future'.[20] Arguably, the paper is playing with this feeling of 'the defeat of time', by showing an image of an ill mother 'hours before' a present, which is already past for the readers, since, as they read in the text, 'she died yesterday at 5.00 in the morning'.[21] We may presume that she was worthy of a photoreporter's visit 'hours before' as they must have known this woman was about to die of tuberculosis, thus associating the fatality of the disease with underprivileged sufferers. Photographically, the main reason to photograph this woman dying, beyond the sensationalistic response that the paper was aiming to provoke, is because her absence could not have been represented. When the readers saw this picture, what they saw was no longer there (the mother), but only through her 'absolute past' they can represent/imagine her absence for her still present and needy daughters.

As far as the politics of representation is concerned, it is the calculated publicity of the private that this scene reproachfully transmits, making it visually denigrating for the subjects represented. This contrasts strikingly with the treatment of maternal death in the case of non-poor mothers. In this sense, in the photographs and articles of *La Voz del Interior*, the poor mother became deprived of privacy through a process of being highly individualised, visualised and exposed in the public domain. As a result of this individualisation they became identifiable as unique subjects, as someone who comes to constitute 'the other'. The supposed consensus offered by mothers who turned to the newspaper in search of aid, was exploited by the camera to the extent of effacing their privacy like in the case of the mother dying. The counter-point of this high visibility rested, for the viewer, in the naturalisation of the poor mother as a different, subaltern category.

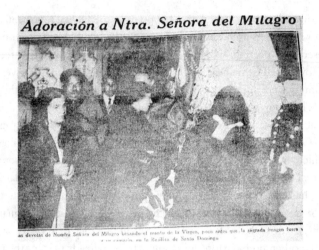

as devotas de Nuestra Señora del Milagro besando el manto de la Virgen, poco antes que la sagrada imagen fuera
... camarín, en la Basílica de Santo Domingo

Fig. 6.9 'Adoración de Nuestra Señora del Milagro' ['The adoration of Our Lady of the Miracle'], *Los Principios* (25 October 1934), 6.

Los Principios and the Catholic mother

In the 1930s when 'Catholic integralism' became an important ideological movement at national and provincial level, the ideal Catholic social order that it endorsed was not only encouraged, in the case of *Los Principios*, by myriads of articles and long editorials, but also through the way images were used in the paper. While the Marian cult was exalted in an unprecedented way, and theatricalised through the parading of the patroness of Córdoba, the Virgin of the Miracle, in the main streets of the city, *Los Principios* started to make use of large photographs to emphasise the magnificence of the events. Pictures showed the figure of the Virgin on high, standing out in white over an interminable multitude of dark heads whose presence escaped the frame of the photograph. Other images, showed in close-up the column of ecclesiastical authorities, with their distinctive dresses, heading the parade with the Virgin at their back and escorted by a column of prominent Catholic men. In these street shots, however, no women were visible close to the Virgin. When women's devotion featured in the paper, these images had, as expected, their own conventions. In one of the few pictures of women in action I found in *Los Principios* (Fig. 6.9) they appear kissing the image of the Virgin. Revealingly, the picture was taken *inside* the church,[22] where women were permitted to show an intimate, physical devotion to the Virgin, while in public, on the

212

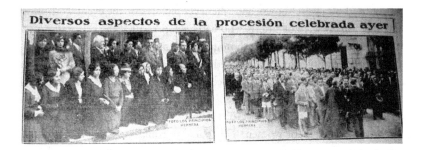

Fig. 6.10 'Diversos Aspectos de la Procesión Celebrada Ayer' ['Different aspects of yesterday's religious festivities'], *Los Principios* (29 October 1934), 7.

street, we can see in another picture (Fig.6.10) the exact moment at which they were photographed. The photograph and its description eloquently inform us about the gendered hierarchies established in the Catholic social order. The submissive pose of women, kneeling on the 'pavement' while the 'street' is occupied by men, who are marching and escorting the Virgin, is instructive.[23] Beyond the graphic divide of the public/private spheres, the street shot also emphasises the guidance of the celibate sons (priests) of the Virgin/mother. They have, as Accati has stated, 'the right to express the most authentic and precious side of their [female] natures, and thus the right to *stand in their place*'.[24] The spiritual authority is followed by the secular one also represented by men (biological fathers/husbands) who thus have the right to stand in women's/mother's places, in their closeness to the Virgin/mother.

The non-representation of mothers in the parades of the Virgin, was due to a separation of groups by sex and age (children/young ladies/ married women) whereby mothers disappear as subjects, either because they were separated from their children or substituted by the ladies group, who, in this way, represented civil status (married women) rather than filiation. The invisibility of mothers in the street parades was also echoed in the absence of photographs of mothers in the newspaper more broadly. The column entitled 'A message to mothers' that appeared in 1945 in the 'society page' to advise mothers on different aspects of their Catholic maternal duties, was not specifically pictured. Instead, other photographs scattered around the column served to illustrate the social page: Portraits of brides, just married women, wedding photographs, but no maternal images. This was also the case in the celebrations of 'the day of the Catholic mother' where no traces

213

of motherhood were shown, and whenever pictures of the event were printed, they usually were of priests who had been present at the celebrations.

The absence of mother's photographic representation thus leaves historians with a complex and interrelated interpretation of variables. In the case
of *Los Principios* and the Catholic ideology that it represented, the first thing
to consider is a theological principle. The figure/symbol of the Virgin-Mother (pregnant since eternity in God's mind) defines maternity as a paradox
or an impossibility for women. This paradox could be traced in Córdoba's
veneration of the Virgin of Miracle, when the Marian cult started to be exalted in the 1920s, as a response to the threat posed by feminism, and in the
1930s to counteract birth-rate control and 'weary' mothers. As we have seen
in Chapter 3, the Virgin-Mother provided inspiration for both particularly
challenging moments, as an exemplary figure of women's social elevation,
and maternal sacrifice. However, the festivities of the virgin, the parades of
the Madonna and child and the 'day of the Catholic mother' remind us that
not every commemoration is held in agreement with an authentic celebration. The worldly mother could not be empowered for its own sake, that is,
by its power of engendering, like maternal feminism was claiming at the time,
but only in a spiritual way. Yet the spiritual was embodied by the figure of
the priest, whose symbolic maternal power is represented – amongst other
things – by the act of giving birth to eternal life in the rite of baptism.[25] As a
result, the newspaper denied the visualisation of the pregnant woman or the
mother and child bond, and systematically showed instead the priest close
to the virgin-mother and to all women who appeared in public, who were
portrayed in a submissive demeanour. Women's essential motherhood, but
always impure maternity, was visually negotiated both by the invisibility of
its referent (pregnancy/mother and child), and the visibility of its potential
redemption (the priest).

No mother

Considering the two newspapers in perspective, the first issue that strikes
us most is the lack of visual representation of *mothers as subjects* understood
as images of pregnant women or/and of mother and child, which together
indicate the way in which we can recognise motherhood in this medium's
culture. Both newspapers predominantly have shown women whose relationship with motherhood rested, sometimes in the text or on occasions,

evocatively or imaginatively, but never visually, not photographed, therefore, no photograph. As Barthes would ask:

This fatality (no photograph without *something* or *someone*) involves photography in the vast disorder of objects – of all the objects in the world: why choose (why photograph) this object, this moment, rather than some other?[26]

The portraits of dead women in obituaries, who although we know they were mothers as we read the text, are not informed from what we see; the 'gallery of brides' or the wedding photographs (mothers-to-be) that filled up newspapers' social sections; or the 'infants gallery' that showed babies and children portrayed alone or with their siblings, none of these pictures visualised mothers.

In this chapter, I have discussed newspapers' different ways of photographing beneficent/charitable ladies as subjects that discursively have quintessentially embodied or articulated maternal values. With the same aim I have drawn special attention to the visualisation of women in *Los Principios*, given the fact that Catholicism has made of motherhood, more than any other circulating discourse at that time, woman's essential role in society. Consequently, from the photographs of charitable ladies, which were frequently published in the Argentinian printed media of the period,[27] one might expect a limited, certainly indirect, or carefully staged representation of the ladies' maternal role, one that was politically disengaged from the values they attached to their presence in the public sphere. But from the Catholic mother one may reasonably expect to see motherhood as the referent, the 'someone' represented. This expectation also applies to *La Voz del Interior*, whose lack of visualisation of mothers, with the exception of the 'poor mother' to whom I return below, also suggests that the mothers' photographic image seems to have been perceived as at odds, or impossible to reconcile with the textual representation supported on its pages. Therefore, considering the status of photography at the time, as the representation of 'the real', and in photojournalism, which has been understood by and large as the representation of 'reality', we may conclude that, except for the 'poor mother' of *La Voz del Interior*, whose otherness made her a different or a particular subject, either that there were no mothers, or that no mother deserved to be visualised.

At the beginning of this chapter, I proposed to trace the visualisation of mothers following the distinction that Duden – analysing the unseen unborn

– has elaborated between the *seen* and the *shown* to enquire into the period before the introduction of the now familiar technologies of visualisation. Since its popularisation in the press in the 1920s, people became used to seeing photographic images. During the same period, maternity became a public concern, whose presence, as analysed throughout this book, has been ubiquitous: maternity institutes, puericulture campaigns, medicalisation of childbirth, and eugenic concerns on reproduction; maternal feminism; the Catholic mother; political uses of the maternal in the press; novels thematising the abandoned, negligent, spiritual, non-reproductive mother. Yet in spite of all these texts, and this panoply of competing discourses, there was no visualisation of mothers. No single pregnant woman and few photographic images, I concede that there were 'few' although I only came across one in my sample featuring a mother and child.

In contrast to this stark invisibility, the only mother who was visualised was the 'poor mother'. In the process, or more specifically, during the years of the maternal campaign, the poor mother became identified as 'the other', in that photographs did not show her as a powerful figure. She was a figure for compassion, in absolute need. None would have liked to be in, or identify with, her maternal experience: haggard and sad faces, badly dressed, ill, living in ruined places, responsible for many children, humiliated by partners, and obliged to beg. The question that really lingered for me was; why were positive experiences of motherhood not shown? Why in the 'soft' social pages was it more important to show picture of brides, weddings, children, women fundraising, but not 'the referent', i.e. mother and child and/or pregnant woman? What was *already* operating in the newspapers was, to use Duden's words again, a discrimination as to what was to be *seen* and what was to be *shown*. The invisibility of the mother allows me to argue that, in terms of what it was shown in media culture more broadly, the pregnant mother became disembodied not 'since' the visibility of the unborn child, but from decades earlier, when she became an invisible subject. In this sense, this case study of photojournalism in Córdoba's press suggests a continuum rather than a disruption. Duden's historical exploration fails to explain this process because she was more interested in highlighting the changes of paradigm in the way that women were able to recognise their own pregnancies. From the eighteenth-century period when pregnancy was a female sensorial experience, primarily oriented by the sense of touch, to the twentieth century when pregnancy became interpreted by medical optical devices that, in turn, had to be explained to mothers by doctors.

The absence of mothers' photographic record beyond the context of poverty induces me to think of their existence as one relegated to two main spheres, one private, and the other medical. Newspapers provide us with hints of both, in the first case, by showing pictures of weddings, babies and children, while in the second one, by photographing the figure of the expert, i.e. obstetricians and paediatricians giving conferences, inaugurating maternities, or attending scientific societies. The authoritative visibility of the medical expert, contrasted in turn with the one of midwives, whose photographs usually appeared in the criminal section accused of having committed abortions or the commitment of malpractice. Both spheres suggest a double process of privatisation of motherhood, whereby on the one hand, the maternal belongs to the private (intimate) sphere of women, whose relevance is visually denied in the press; and on the other, to the private domain of the medical expert whose social value is visually emphasised. As the popularisation of photojournalism in the press and the medicalisation of maternity were parallel processes in Argentina, as it was for most Western countries too, it is difficult to assign to the latter a preceding role in the invisibility of the maternal, despite contributing later to its configuration. According to historians of sciences such as Carolyn Merchant, to answer this question we should go as far back to the Scientific Revolution of the sixteenth and seventeenth centuries when a tradition of modern thought took shape, silencing and making invisible women's engendering qualities by concealing them to her private sphere. Merchant's analysis of what she has termed the 'death of nature', as an event that changed both the perception of nature and of women in Western culture, connects us with a deeper tradition of thought which has had long-term implications. From Greek philosophy to the High Middle Ages, nature was imagined and represented as a pregnant womb, a nurturing mother with an 'inherent creative power'. The Scientific Revolution, however, brought about a different paradigm, one that completely disentangled nature from its organic roots, to replace it by the mechanicist model. As Merchant has noted, 'female imagery became a tool in adapting scientific knowledge and method to a new form of human power over nature'.[28] Hence the domestication of nature/women by scientific knowledge underwent a long period of transformation, but its core principles, I would contend, have been highly iterative, reappearing in the period of my analysis, for example, through the different attitudes towards childbirth (expectant vs. interventionists) discussed in Chapter 1, that for long has divided obstetrics schools. Read in this way, the lack of visualisation of mothers in the photo-

217

graphic record, as I have tried to explain, does not constitute an 'outside' of the circulating texts. Photography's specific intervention in the cultural milieu accounts for the interrelated nature of motherhood and its representations, one that cannot be *developed*, to extend the photography analogy, without first carefully processing its negative.

Notes

1 B. Duden, *Disembodying Women: Perspectives on Pregnancy and the Unborn* (Cambridge, Mass., London: Harvard University Press, 1993), 19-20.
2 Duden, *Disembodying Women*, 19.
3 P. Burke, *Eyewitnessing: The uses of Images as Historical Evidence* (London: Reaktion Books, 2001), 21.
4 However, more recent questions introduced by the advent of digital photography and its numerous possibilities for editing and manipulation of photographs, have sparked debates about the status of photographic realism amongst photojournalists who defend an 'ethical and professional stake in the truth status of the photograph'. This reveals the extent to which the idea of 'truth' has permeated the social understanding of photography until today. In Sarah Kember, '"The Shadow of the Object": Photography and Realism', in L. Wells (ed.), *The Photography Reader* (London: Routledge, 2003), 202-17: 202.
5 From the 1960s the semiotic analysis of photography has convincingly demonstrated that 'the real' is already lost in the act of representation.
6 Kember, "The Shadow of the Object", 209.
7 J. Tagg, 'Evidence, Truth and Order: A Means of Surveillance', in J. Evans and S. Hall (eds.), *Visual Culture: The Reader* (London: Sage Publications and the Open University, 1999), 243-73:245.
8 A. Grundberg, 'The Crisis of the Real, Photography and Postmodernism' in Wells (ed.) *The Photography Reader*, 164-79: 175.
9 S. Saítta, *Regueros de Tinta: El Diario "Crítica" en la Década de 1920* (Buenos Aires: Sudamericana, 1998).
10 Under his direction worked a team of around five or six photographers, including his sons. See 'Presentación', in Boixadós, Palacios and Romano (eds.), *Fragmentos de una Historia*, 7-8.
11 Novello used a camera Spido loaded with a magazine of eleven plaques

218

of glass.

12 P. Vancassel, *Les Regards Photograhiques: Dispositifs Anthropologiques et Processus Transindividuels,* These Doctorale, Université Rennes 2, Haute Bretagne, 2008, 232. Online at: tel.archives-ouvertes.fr/docs/00/29/47/53/PDF/theseVancassel.pdf_(consulted 21.03.2010).

13 The caption of the photomontage reads: '1) The lunch served to the attendant authorities; 2) part of the female audience that filled the galleries of the hospital; 3) the president of the Society of Beneficence, Mrs. Elisa Deheza de Martínez, delivering her speech', in La Voz del Interior (13 November 1922), 6.

14 The description of the photographs reads: 'The ladies members of the Vicentian Conference of San José de Calazans that yesterday distributed food and clothing, and some of the beneficiaries', in *Los Principios* (28 August 1930), 12.

15 Y. Eraso 'Maternalismo, Religión y Asistencia'.

16 The caption of the photograph reads: 'Doña Pabla Palacios and her sons, Carlos and Maria Eustaquio, in our newspaper, after telling us her 'via crucis', in *La Voz del Interior* (25 July 1924), 6. For details of the headlines and the full story see on p. 146.

17 J. Scott, 'Experience', in J. Scott and Judith Butler (eds.), *Feminists Theorize the Political* (New York & London: Routledge, 1992), 22-40: 25.

18 P. Holland, J. Spence and S. Watney, 'Introduction: The Politics and Sexual Politics of Photography', in Spence, Holland and Watney (eds.), *Photography/Politics: Two* (London: Comedia, 1986), 1-7: 7.

19 *La Voz del Interior* (12 March 1929), 13.

20 R. Barthes, *Camera Lucida, Reflections on Photography* (London: Vintage, 2000), 96.

21 'Hours before dying, this poor mother fixed her gaze to the world in a desperate protest. Her children, poor little ones! They don't know yet about pain, but they do know about the most minimum necessities', *La Voz del Interior* (12 March 1929), 13.

22 The caption reads: 'Some devotees of Our Lady of the Miracle, kissing the cloak of the Virgin, soon after the sacred image was returned to its sanctuary in the Basilica of Saint Domingo', *Los Principios* (25 October 1934), 6.

23 The description of the photograph states: 'While the procession was parading in Córdoba's streets, woman adhered to the parade from the pavement, kneeling in order to follow the prayers of Catholic men', *Los*

*Princi*pios (29 October 1934), 7.

24 Accati, 'Explicit Meanings', 253. My emphasis.

25 See Accati, 'Explicit Meanings'.

26 Barthes, *Camera Lucida*, 6.

27 For an analysis of the ladies of the Society of Beneficence of the Capital and their photographic representation in the national press, see M. F. Lorenzo, A. L. Rey and C. Tossounian, 'Images of Virtuous Women: Morality, Gender and Power in Argentina between the World Wars', *Gender & History*, 17, 3 (2005), 567–92.

28 C. Merchant, *The Death of Nature: Women, Ecology, and the Scientific Revolution* (London: Wildwood House, 1982), 165.

7

The Subjectivity of the Mother According to the Artistic Gaze

In the last few decades the visual representation of the maternal body has attracted a wide range of feminist scholars who have selectively explored it from disciplines as diverse as biology, art history, philosophy, cultural studies and psychoanalysis. Outside feminist studies, however, the topic has received less attention, especially in relation to the analysis of the maternal imagery and its connections with other discourses existing at the time. This chapter proposes to analyse the artistic representations of the maternal that circulated during the period, firstly, in relation to prevailing ideas of motherhood analysed in previous chapters (medicine, press, literature and photojournalism), and secondly, in relation to new forms of representations emerging from or formulated within the artistic field. The latter will trace the way in which some artists accorded the mother a subjectivity of her own, while others conveyed one that was moulded from the dominating constructs of the time.

The representations of the maternal in Argentinian fine art will follow, as this chapter proposes, the spaces of circulation of the selected artworks within an artistic field which was itself undergoing a period of institutionalization. The reason to look at the institutional places where these works circulated, the salons where they were accepted to be shown to the public, the prizes that they received and the rationale for their acquisition to integrate a museum's patrimony, is because they tell us about the visibility that these artworks enjoyed at the time, but above all, they inform us about their acceptance in institutional places that attempted to define what represented the 'official art' at local and national levels. From this perspective, the topic of motherhood can be read as a thematic encouraged at a particular moment by the 'official discourse' of the national and provincial salons. Observing the list of first prizes awarded by the National Salon during the period under investigation, it appears that only two works, *Maternidad*, 1930 ('Motherhood') by Ricardo Musso and *Madre Humilde*, 1948 ('The Humble Mother') by Roberto Viola, were awarded prizes, although maternal-related scenes have been represented under different titles. If, as art historian Diana Wechsler points out, 'the jury prizes and signals the desirable tendency'[1] in Argentinian art, I shall argue that the topic of motherhood was not one particularly encouraged by the prevailing national tendencies at least until the 1940s. Thus, the catalogues of the decade of 1920-30, showed an overriding presence of the landscape, specially the rural one, and topics that portrayed a non-conflictive reality, ahistorical and merely evocative; [2] whilst the 1930s signalled the search for 'the native', a topic that stemmed from the cultural, political and biological desire of defining a national identity.[3] As we shall see later, the thematisation of motherhood, especially that of the poor mother, seems to have satisfied the taste in the salons of the Peronist era, inaugurated in 1946, and to which I am going to refer only briefly as they signal a change of paradigm whose implications go beyond the period covered by this volume. In order to examine the artistic productions that have tackled the topic of motherhood, I have organised them according to the specific perspective that they were introducing. In this sense, I have detected artistic expressions that represented the maternal through the act of breastfeeding, the pregnant body, the mother and child relationship, and the mother's subjectivity.

Salons, prizes and tendencies

The process of constitution of a national institutional space for the fine arts in Argentina was initiated in Buenos Aires between the end of the nineteenth and beginning of the twentieth century, a period where far-reaching artistic events took place: the creation of the National Museum of Fine Arts in 1895, the nationalisation in 1905 of the Academy of the *Sociedad Estímulo de Bellas Artes* ('Society to Promote Fine Arts') as the main teaching institution, and finally, the inaugural exhibition of the 'National Salon' in 1911. Other cities rapidly followed suit in the two main provinces of the country, first in Córdoba and later in Santa Fe. In 1896, the government of the province of Córdoba created the 'Provincial Academy of Fine Arts', under the direction of prominent painter Emilio Caraffa. Along with the Academy, Caraffa promoted the creation of the Provincial Museum of Fine Arts (1914), and the organization of the first Provincial Salon of Fine Arts (1916), being the later an important landmark in the promotion of the arts in the region, although its continuity came to a halt in the following years to restart again in the 1930s.[4] Rosario, the city-port of Santa Fe, witnessed the regular exhibitions of the 'Autumn Salon' since 1917, as a result of the initiative of a private group of cultural promoters known as 'The Circle'. In 1920, the Municipal Museum of Fine Arts was created and two years later, the Provincial Museum of Fine Arts was opened thanks to a donation from politician Dr Martín Rodríguez Galisteo to the provincial state. Since 1923, this museum harboured the 'Salon Santa Fe', an annual exhibition that gathered artists of national recognition. Significantly, the creation of these institutions was also accompanied by a system of scholarships that allowed artists to study abroad, mainly in Europe, thus generating a renewal in styles and the emergence of avant-garde movements. By the 1920s, scholarships became more integrated within the teaching spaces and with the official initiatives seeking to promote the artistic field at national and local level. Thus, the provincial Legislature of Córdoba, for example, approved in 1923 a scheme destined to the graduates of the Academy whereby award holders should send their productions back to the province to be assessed by the specialised critic and shared with the society through exhibitions.[5]

All these inaugural gestures showed an unwavering official desire for supporting and boosting the artistic production in a highly contested and hectic intellectual scenario. Yet the relevance of the institutions created during these years was given, as Wechsler[6] has noted, by the operational connection existing among its three main pillars: the Academy, the Museum and the Salon. The Academy worked as a centre of teaching, which also facilitated the connection with the traditional centres of artistic production through scholarships; whilst the Museum, with the acquisition of works, opened up the possibility of engaging with national and international movements; and the Salon functioned as a window that signalled the new national tendencies, through a system of selection and prizes. Once these three institutions started to work, the artistic field became a contested space for aesthetic and political confrontation. On the one hand, it was a space where the avant-garde tendencies and innovative aesthetic expressions disputed the existing artistic order; and on the other, it was a space where left-wing artists in the 1930s, heavily committed to the 'social cause' resisted the cultural politics of the military regime that took power at the beginning of the decade.[7]

From the mid-1920s onwards, a new tendency in Argentinian art sprang from the artists' first European experiences, who struggled to find a place in the National Salon and with it, in the official Argentinian art. The human figure, nudes, still lifes and urban scenes that registered the impact of modernity coupled with a novel treatment of volume and planes, which lead to an 'artistic synthesis, *cubification* of the image, and privilege of the form over the topic represented'.[8] Many of these new tendencies found a space in the 'counter-salons' of Buenos Aires, 'Free Salon' (1924), the 'Salon of the Independents' (1925) and others that year after year purposely harboured the avant-garde aesthetics and worked as spaces at odds with the conventional norms of the National Salon. In Córdoba these modern tendencies were present in what has been called *magic realism, Novecento or retour al'ordre*, characterised by a geometric composition of volumes, in particular of the human figure, and by playing with the perspective (*juegos de perspectiva*) using subtle distortions. The *Novecento* aesthetic would render more enduring reformulations during the second generation of Cordoban painters (of the 1940s and 1950s) who, after exploring the European catalogue, consolidated the Italian one, inspired by the metaphysical painting (*pittura metafisica*) of Carlo Carrà, Mario Sironi and Giorgio Morandi. The decision to strengthen this Italian path has been interpreted amongst art historians,[9] as a strategic and prudent attitude in that it allowed artists to consolidate the modern tendencies already existing in Córdoba, at the time that they eschewed a confrontational attitude in a milieu that was not overly receptive to emerging avant-garde experiences.

As far as the national salons are concerned, as Andrea Giunta has asserted, they 'constitute the most regulated space of the artistic field: the place where the official discourse has the possibility of influence in a direct and almost non-mediated way'.[10] The symbolic importance of the official salons, in what they represented as a field of dispute for aesthetic and ideological (thematic) tendencies, was not, however, a capital-centred affair as indicated by meaningful examples that took place in the provinces. Indeed, in 1931 the provincial Museum of Córdoba opened a salon – the antecedent of the more official one organised from 1933 – set up its rules, and was sponsored by the Provincial Committee of Fine Arts. The salon took place in November, a month after the traditional National Salon of Buenos Aires.[11] In a city where Catholic forces were so inextricably woven into the social fabric it is not surprising that artistic manifestations were part of the agenda of a Catholic culture that in the 1930s became more active thanks to the advances of the Catholic Action league.[12] Revealingly, a couple of months before the provincial salon opened in 1933, the newspaper *Los Principios* organised the 'Autumn Salon' in April, an initiative that attempted to resemble the official one by presenting the salon's rules, a jury elected by the participating artists, and a system of prizes that deliberately displayed the insertion of the Catholics within the network of political power.[13] The 'Autumn Salon' promoted itself as an open place where all schools and tendencies could be represented, as the call anticipated, 'our position, as far as artistic forms is concern, is completely independent',[14] although artists must have been aware of how to interpret this convocation. The salon ran for four years, with very few well-known local artists and supporting many others with an amateur profile. Arguably, the 'Autumn Salon' represented an explicit and competitive intervention by the Catholics in the cultural values of the city, and one that permitted them to venture in the artistic field with their own rules. Like the official state initiative, the Catholics set up a salon and regularly organised exhibitions, distributed prizes, developed a specialised group of art critics, and gathered at the gallery 'Plasman', which remained for many years as they preferred artistic exhibition venue.

The fragmented and divided space of Córdoba, where every cultural or intellectual expression was looked at through the lenses of Catholicism or anti-Catholicism, indicates the extent to which the process of modernity and its related dichotomised values, tradition / change; provincialism / cosmopolitism; religion / science; immutable / transitory; sacred / secular was at stake in the Argentinian provinces. At national level, those conflicting tensions gathered momentum when right-wing Catholic forces gained positions of power in the 1930s. The way in which they have operated in the complex political rhetoric throughout the period provides us with a threshold to interpret how the artistic works that I am going to focus on next, were produced, have circulated, and were received.

Meaningful breasts

In 1925 the first group of artists-scholarship holders sent to Córdoba a selection of the works they had produced during their stay in Europe. The shipment was part of the provincial scholarship program whereby the experience of the beneficiaries could be shown and praised by the Committee of Fine Arts and local critics alike. One of these young artists was Francisco Vidal (1897-1980), who sent a series of paintings that were later analysed by the artist Manuel Coutaret, who was then collaborating as an art critic for the newspaper *La Voz del Interior*. Illustrating Coutaret's laudatory commentary on Vidal's work was *Mujeres de Segovia* (1924) ['Segovia's Women'], which Vidal painted during his first year in Europe, a year that he had spent in Spain before continuing to Italy and France.

The painting represents three Segovian women in close-up with a back-

225

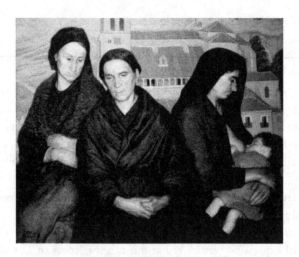

Fig. 7.1 Francisco Vidal, *Mujeres de Segovia* (1924) oil on cardboard, 100 x 119.5 cm
Courtesy of the Museo Provincial de Bellas Artes 'Emilio A. Caraffa',
Córdoba, Argentina

ground composed by a chapel or convent that acts as the setting of the picture. These two plans are fairly differentiated with the use of obscure tones for the women and lighter colours for the background. As a whole, the picture's theme of *Mujeres de Segovia* is a *costumbrista* scene (genre dealing with local customs) of the country which has influenced Córdoba most in its cultural and spiritual traditions. The convent/chapel that dominates the landscape behind the three women confirms the religious setting where these women are placed, as it does so for their circumspect or resigned look, and the care for maternal duties. The three close-up figures compose two groups, the first two on the left and centre share the same attitude as both are looking downwards. Their crossed hands and arms also convey an idea of resignation. Beside these women there is a third one, on the right side, who appears distanced from the unity of the other two, both physically and attitudinally. Unlike the first two women, the third one is in profile, and is concentrating on her baby boy whom she is breastfeeding. This maternal image in profile clearly displays to the viewer her nurturing action in a natural, almost didactic way.

There is a tension in this, at once, separated and in profile image. The tension is given by the religious frame of the back of the painting and the sensuality and eroticism that a 'maternally' swollen naked breast, like this

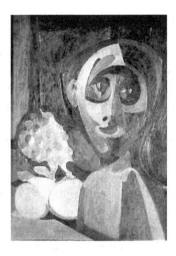

Fig. 7.2 Juan Batlle Planas, *Figura* (1948) oil on canvas, 59,5 x 45 cm
Private collection.

one, conveys. And the history of art confirms that it is not a minor one. It was this tension in particular that decided the disappearance of the *Madonna Lactans* from religious art in the fifteenth century not without first experiencing a very telling transformation. The first representations of the Marian cult through the *Madonna del Latte* in Italy (during the fourteenth and early fifteenth centuries), were images of Mary breastfeeding Jesus. These were soon replaced by images whereby the breast of Mary became disembodied. According to Megan Holmes, the Madonna's bare breast was 'partially covered with the Virgin's veil and drapery; it is [was] displaced to the level of her collarbone, detached from her body, and distorted in size and shape'.[15] Behind this new representation lay a growing concern of theologians about awakening erotic feelings in the devotional gaze of the faithful. When fifteenth century painting turned to a naturalized representation of the human body, stylizing the forms in anatomical precision, as Holmes has argued, the distorted representation of Mary's breast became artistically unsustainable and so came to an end. Ever since, visual images of lactating mothers in Western culture have been beset by religious (moral) and sexual tension, an anxiety that has been artistically reinterpreted by female artists at the end of the twentieth century. Indeed, in analysing the series 'History Portraits' (1989) by the photographer Cindy Sherman, Alison Barlett stated that, 'by picturing the breast as an actual appendage, Sherman highlights the artifice of photography and also satirizes the tradition of depicting the *Madonna Lactans* with a disembodied breast'.[16] This parody along with other provocative views of female issues (childbirth and pregnancy) as we will see later, loomed more radically in the bosom of a group of *fin de siècle* female artists.

In the case of Argentinian art, it was a male rather than a female artist, Juan Batlle Planas (1911-1966), who early and lucidly perceived the 'breast tension' in visual art, in a painting entitled *Figura* (1948) ['Figure']. The canvas meaningfully represents this idea of disembodiment that the nursing female breasts have experienced in visual tradition. It depicts a woman, hidden under a facial mask, with her chest rectangular and flat while her breasts are placed to one side, clearly cut, and emanating bubbles of milk through both nipples. The mask, a resource that Sherman, for example, has extensively used, operates here as a concealment or negation of female identity.

Whilst in the maternal image *par excellence*, the Madonna and Child, the act of breastfeeding conveniently disappeared from religious painting, the representations of breastfeeding arguably inherited this tension which is possible to trace in the conventions used by artists to portray this act. In Argentinian artists, for example, this will be reflected in how much they highlighted the breast, i.e. colours, size, if the mother was in profile or in front, etc. In the case of Vidal's *Mujeres de Segovia*, as stated before, the features of the breast are highlighted by the profile position, light colour – which contrasts with the black dress – and volume. In addition, the context where this painting was produced and received in Córdoba's society give us insight into the extent to which it was altering conventional ideas. In the 1920s women's 'modesty in dress' was a topic that received considerable attention from the Vatican (as we have seen in Chapter 3), which extended precise instructions to bishops on how 'Marylike dresses' should be interpreted. Most memorable were Pius XI's guidelines of a decorous measurement of the cleavage set at 'two fingers breath under the pit of the throat'.[17] Pastoral letters, sermons and the paper *Los Principios* devoted considerable efforts in calling mothers to counteract in their daughters the pernicious influence of women's indecency as portrayed in cinema, clothing and readings. In this sense, the painting of Vidal entered in dialogue with all these speeches of visual correctness and it did so by recurring to the controversial image of the lactating mother. He resorted to the sublime figure of the mother, he dressed her and the rest of the women according to the strict Catholic cannon, but controversially, he filtered a visible breast in the scene. This visibility did not pass unnoticed for the newspaper

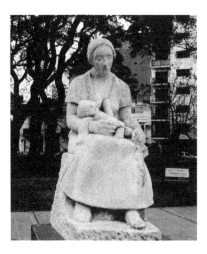

Fig. 7.3 Ricardo Musso, *Maternidad* (1930) stone sculpture located in Plaza 24 de Septiembre, City of Buenos Aires. Photograph courtesy of Gabriela Antonowicz.

La Voz del Interior, which, from the series of paintings sent by Vidal, selected this particular one to show to its readers. The fact that the choice was not random is proved by a clear editorial policy of *La Voz del Interior* in supporting art's nudity both through the publication of images and through scathing editorials written on its defence. On the other hand, and to understand the impact that the visual representation of a woman breastfeeding signified in traditional societies of the country, it is instructive to remember the protest roused by Córdoba's teachers against a puericulture campaign organised by the government in 1927, which used educative posters to show school girls how to breastfeed.[18]

Representations of lactating mothers, however, found in the evocation of the weakness and defenselessness figure of the poor, single mother positive connotations, provided that a clear departure from erotic associations was established. The enthusiastic reception of the sculpture *Maternidad* (1930) ['Motherhood'] by Ricardo Musso (1896-1988), reminds us that this specific figure was at the core of public health debates at the time, which actively encouraged mothers to keep their children as a way of curbing infant mortality rates. After obtaining a scholarship to train in Paris and Italy (1926-1930), Musso became one of the most acclaimed sculptors, winning the second and third prize by the National Salon in 1925, and the first prize in 1941.

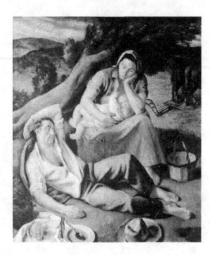

Fig. 7.4 Francisco, Vidal, *Descanso* (1940) oil on canvas, 165.5 x 145 cm Courtesy of the Museo Provincial de Bellas Artes 'Emilio A. Caraffa', Córdoba, Argentina

His work was devoted to the representation of the human figure, especially, the female nude. *Maternidad* became one of his most famous works, after it was awarded a prize at the National Salon in 1930. The sculpture represents a woman sitting and breastfeeding a child. Her simple clothes and bare feet indicate her deprived social condition, which is also emphasized through the afflicted expression on her face. Whatever else could be speculated as the cause of misfortune for this poor woman (partner's abandonment, familiar or social contempt, etc.), it seems that motherhood is a burden for her. This representation seems to be in line with the content and photographs shown in the maternal campaign organised by *La Voz del Interior* analysed in Chapter 4, for its portrayal of poor mothers as passive, needy subjects. In addition, the abstract, spiritual values with which Catholics attempted to associate the maternal here appears to be contested. Not least because class considerations, *Maternidad* seems to suggest, will make of motherhood a 'dignity' to be enjoyed only by comfortably well-off women. Unlike Vidal's painting, where the sacred and erotic were represented as being in tension, here the breast is discretely exposed, although the nursing mother gives room to another type of tensions. One that it is, nonetheless, religious in the sense that it shows that maternity, far from being a 'blessing' could be a heavy burden, a distressing situation for women if they were poor, workers or single mothers. The attributes of class and maternal duties that the sculpture conveys seems to have appealed to the authorities of the Municipality of Buenos Aires, who bought the sculpture in 1934 to place it in the public square '24 de Septiembre', in the working-class neighbourhood of Villa Crespo.

As discussed earlier in Chapter 1, part of the medical discourse of maternity appealed to society and the state to recognise and protect the illegitimate mother. A 'moral of tolerance' implied the understanding that the single mother who cared for her child was a 'weak woman' and therefore 'worthy of consideration', and that contempt, marginalisation and prejudice only instigated 'crime' while annulled in women the sentiment of maternity.[19] This medical perspective gained more support towards the 1930s when the eugenic movement promoted welfare legislation for working mothers, and introduced maternity leave and the right for women to breastfeed during working hours. As eugenist and biotypologist Dr Beruti argued, 'if she [single mother] transgressed for love, she became vindicated through maternity'.[20] In this sense, Musso's *Maternidad* became visually instrumental for the poor passer-by women in Villa Crespo's neighbourhood, in two senses, firstly because it showed that, in spite of her afflicted face, this poor lactating mother did not eschew *maternal responsibility* by resorting to abortion, infanticide or abandonment. Secondly, in a time when the square was normally occupied with laudatory statutes of national heroes, this monument to 'motherhood' operated as a public, artistic recognition of poor mother's social value.

Another painting that meaningfully used the act of breastfeeding to express a perspective on the maternal is Francisco Vidal's canvas *Descanso* (1940) ['Rest']. By the time he painted it he was an acclaimed painter at national level, having won the first prize at the National Salon in 1938, and been appointed director of the Provincial Academy of Fine Arts in Córdoba (1931-1950). Towards the mid-1930s Vidal turned to the Italian Renaissance and post-Renaissance style, which had dazzled him during his formative year in Italy. Paintings of this period showed harmonious compositions with attention to sculptural human figures and the use of luminous tones, as the ones used in *Descanso*. This painting recreates a *costumbrista* scene of rural life. It depicts the tiredness of a couple, taking a rest after the hard work of the morning, along with an empty plate of food and a loaf of bread that seems unable to recover their energies. The scene epitomises the hardship experienced by peasant families, mainly immigrants, who settled in the countryside. The picture draws attention to the central, leading figure of the mother. In doing so it captures, more specifically, the tough times for women who ventured into rural areas in a time when the male farmer was the overriding

231

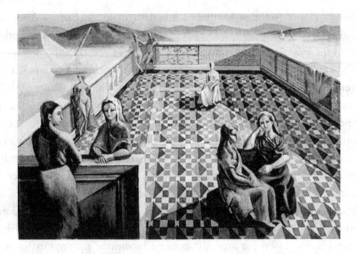

Fig. 7.5 Lino Enea Spilimbergo, *Figuras en la Terraza* (1931) oil on canvas 98 x 142cm
Private Collection. Courtesy of the Fundación Spilimbergo.

figure in rural representations. The body language of the main figures is very telling about who is, in fact, taking a rest. While the man is comfortably lying in the floor, with his arms deployed in a relaxed gesture, the woman is sitting dawn, breastfeeding her baby, and hardly resting her head over her free hand. The obvious uneasiness of the woman's rest conspicuously points to the 'rest without rest' for working mothers in a scenario where they received little recognition for their work. In this sense, the act of breastfeeding becomes a powerful element to communicate motherhood and work as an unrewarding combination in women's life. Another important feature is that the mother is not duly involved in the act of breastfeeding, though not in a negligent manner but in a scenario where what is clearly lacking is 'maternal choice', thus, demystifying the ideal image of tenderness and the mother-child inter-action that the act would spiritually evoke or medically suggest in prevailing discourses.

Mother's subjectivity

In this section I will be considering paintings that offered other ways of entry to the topic of motherhood, one that was done beyond the limited vision of the official discourses whether medical, religious, or journalistic ones. I would contend that their visualisation of motherhood opened up the possibility of

232

an alternative identity that challenged the traditional one, and they did so by representing motherhood from domestic, weak or powerless spaces. The first two paintings belong to Lino Enea Spilimbergo (1896-1964), whose work was widely known beyond Buenos Aires, where he lived until the 1950s before settling in the mountains of Córdoba, a province that exhibited and acquired some of his works for the collection of the provincial and municipal museums. In 1928, having returned from his European stay, where he divided his time between Italy and Paris, he became one of the Argentinian artists whose creative process was influenced by the first and more radical Surrealism. The varied aesthetic resources offered by Surrealism to convey the criticism of the bases of the bourgeois social system were skilfully developed by Spilimbergo to reflect on Argentinian society and women in particular, as demonstrated by the famous series of three canvas called 'terraces'.

In one of these paintings, *Figuras en la Terraza* (1931) ['Figures in the terrace'], the atmosphere resembles the surrealistic and metaphysical Italian style for its dream-like space where the terrace is placed, as well as for the improbable, unrealistic distribution of the figures. The latter constitutes two unities or thematic compositions. In the first one, on the left, two women are placed at a counter, resembling a working scene, whereby the one seen from the back seems to be assisting the woman behind the counter. The second figures, on the right, probably represent a mother with her daughter on a sofa, in an attitude of waiting to be assisted. Thus, these four figures in close-up appear to be thematically connected. Given the way they are dressed, they also seem to represent real women in an everyday scene.

The second thematic composition represents a lonely woman, in a green cape that allows us to see her slender figure in the nude, which she herself seems to enjoy. Her attitude of proudly posing her body – on the side of the terrace – makes her appear like an unconscious, dream-like figure. The last figures in the corner of the terrace represent sexuality, with a woman and a man talking naked in a casual pose. These figures, drawn like mannequins, give a surrealistic representation of the unconscious, where sexual desire resides. The core figure in the centre is a maternal figure (mother and child) which gives to the two already commented upon themes a sort of connection. Spilimbergo has highlighted its centrality both by placing it inside a rectangle with mosaics of different colours, and by casting a circular shadow in the floor. The mother resembles a statue, in white, breastfeeding her baby, which is coloured in a flesh tone. The superposed plan that cuts the mother's left leg, contrasts with the drawing style of the rest of the figures which are

233

represented in a more realistic, natural movement. While this detail could be interpreted as paying homage to Cubism, a movement that had certain influence in Spilimbergo's style, thematically, it seems yet another attempt to engross the viewer's gaze to this figure at the centre. And at the centre there is a mother and child, an inevitable focus for the spectator, and central too for the rest of the women distributed along the picture, although none of them seems to have perceived it. The mother and child figures seem to belong to another type of order, neither the unconscious (in the side and corner), nor the real (figures in the front), but something rather in between. Spilimbergo's painting might well be assessed as conveying the following message: beyond women's everyday life, beyond their desires and sexual life, motherhood stands as an inescapable institution (statue), and one that bestows them with an identity. However, and in spite of its centrality, the maternal figure compared to the naturalism of the others, is the one that has been sculptured (i.e. constructed). And for this reason, and here resides its most significant meaning, it announces to us its weakness.

The surrealistic atmosphere of the composition articulates its message through elements drawn from psychoanalysis. At the beginning of 1930s, psychoanalysis was a non-institutional discipline starting to grow under the auspices of the discourses of intimacy introduced through the sentimental novel along with the magazines intended for a female audience and the so-called 'sexological literature'. The latter, as Hugo Vezzetti has analysed, became popular in the form of an 'epistolary consulting-room' in the newspaper *Jornada* (1931) as well as in a cluster of women's magazines. Its success was linked to its object of study, the sexual and erotic life and dreams' interpretation, and to which it proposed a different response and method of communication (the confession of intimate life) that contrasted with the one offered by the medical expert.[21] In a time when medical science was imbued with eugenic theories, with its concern on sexual reproduction from a *biological* point of view, psychoanalysis gave room to the *sentimental* aspects of the amorous life, its adventures, anxieties and malaises. In this sense, psychoanalysis' status and acknowledgement was resisted and undermined by the prevailing medical and psychiatric discourse and by Catholics alike, although in the latter for moral rather than scientific reasons. Not surprisingly, the new discipline operated over the same subject as biotypologists, the female subject. It would exceed my analysis to explore how the spread of psychoanalysis was coupled with the 'female question'. What I am interested in highlighting here is, first, in the frame of the maternal discourses, the existence/emerging

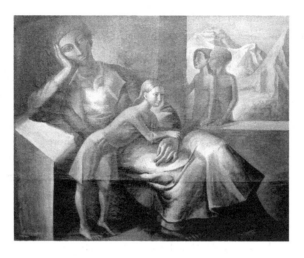

Fig. 7.6 Lino Enea Spilimbergo, *La Espera* (1934) oil on canvas 165 x 210 cm
Courtesy of the Fundación Spilimbergo and the Museo Municipal de Bellas Artes
'Dr. Genaro Pérez' Córdoba, Argentina.

of a discourse attentive to the intimacy of the female subject, to her matrimonial and maternal experiences, at the time that other discourses attempted to draw attention to her biological (medicine) and spiritual role (religion). Secondly, that these discourses had various sociological, ideological, and demographic referents: women's work, a fall in birth-rates, single motherhood, feminism, and a wide range of cultural expressions that informed the visualization of the modern woman through media culture (cinema, photography, magazines, press and advertisements) alongside the sentimental novel. In this sense, and to return to Spilimbergo's painting, it is visualizing something that, although not yet transparent, neither is it invisible, which is the very existence of these competing discourses. By showing the different figures that inhabit the female/maternal subject, i.e. the worldly woman (worker and mother) and the intimate woman (dreams and sexuality), *Figuras en la Terraza* represents motherhood as an institution (central-statute) built on unstable foundations.

Shortly after the series of the terraces, Spilimbergo painted *La Espera* (1934) ['The wait'] a large canvas (165 x 210 cms.) whose size recalls another of his passions, the mural painting, on which he worked just the year before in collaboration with the famous Mexican muralist David Siqueiros in Buenos

Aires. In this painting it is possible to observe the presence of the dream-like atmosphere of the terrace's series, through the two naked children outside the window, although the composition is much more 'realistic' than the above commented painting. In this picture the use of voluminous forms is striking, a peculiarity that constitutes one of Spilimbergo's most recognisable features, along with huge, deep eyes and big hands. Here, all these features are combined to describe the character of the mother. It is well known that Spilimbergo has often portrayed women occupied in daily chores, such as ironing, embroidering, etc. yet most of these paintings were not merely descriptive, they were, on the contrary, loaded with a deeply gendered message.[22] In this sense, *La Espera* forms part of Spilimbergo's exploration of women's subjectivity. In this case what made the topic of this monumental composition is simply a mother waiting, making of this action a sensitive and sensible approach of the maternal time. The spectator is left with the unsolved question of what this woman is waiting for. Psychologically, she conveys a strong concern, to which her daughter, depicted as disproportionately tiny in the picture, does not seemed to relieve. Thus, the painting discloses and endows primacy to that zone of motherhood elsewhere silenced: its subjectivity. The effect that it renders is that it offers, through this aperture to the sentimental, emotional world, a more complex representation of the maternal in relation to the limited one that reduced it to child rearing.

Motherhood as the site of a complex subjectivity also features in the work of Antonio Berni (1905-1981), an artist from Rosario of significant renown in Argentina and Latin America. With Spilimbergo he shared intellectual groups (the 'Florida group' and the 'group of Paris'), political ideas and mural paintings of social content. During his Parisian stay (as grant holder) towards the end of the 1920s, he frequented the philosopher Henri Lefebvre who introduced him to the readings of two authors that had an enduring influence in his pictorial work: Sigmund Freud and Karl Marx.[23] Back in Argentina, he took a militant attitude towards 'the oppressed' where he highlighted the role of urban workers as powerful agents in a time of perceived social conflicts arising from the process of early industrialization. In *Primeros Pasos* (1936) ['First steps'], Berni represented a dressmaker mother – in real life, this was his mother's trade – who pauses in her sewing while her daughter essays some dancing movements. The daughter's 'first steps' in dancing indicates a potential for social aspiration, if not mobility, for working or middle classes. The symbolic 'Singer'-like sewing machine, with the mother's foot on the pedal, contrasts with the flying foot of her daughter, thus providing

236

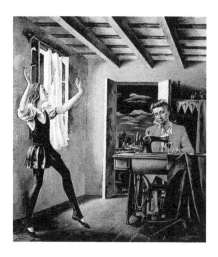

Fig. 7.7 Antonio Berni, *Primeros Pasos* (1936) oil on canvas 200 x 181 cm Courtesy
of the A. Berni Estate and Museo Nacional de Bellas Artes,
Buenos Aires, Argentina.

a connection between two female generations. In this sense, the dressmaker
operates as a condition of possibility for the social aspirations of her offspring, in more than one sense. If the mother's work pays for the dancing
lessons of her daughter, the possibilities offered by the mother as provider,
seems to go beyond the economic one. The depiction of the mother's medi-
tating attitude, pausing in her activity, draws attention, like in Spilimbergo, to
an active female subjectivity yet to be discovered or revealed.

From marginal, assigned and unquestioned female places like domestic
tasks or a home worker, the paintings of Spilimbergo and Berni highlight the
maternal time and mother's concerns and thoughts as unrecognised virtues,
while mothers became subjects of artistic creation and cultural critique. In
doing so, these artists distanced themselves from other painters of everyday
life, who have depicted female or maternal subjects through homogeneous
and comforting representations built upon places regarded as weak and subaltern. Both painters dwelled on canonised female languages, namely, mys-
tery, hands, silence, passiveness, or the domestic sphere (ironing, sewing, etc.)
as metaphoric ways of saying, or of constructing a different identity. These
distinctive representations of the maternal can also be traced in other artists
and writers with whom Spilimbergo and Berni integrated artistic and intellectual groups in Buenos Aires. In analysing South American male avant-garde

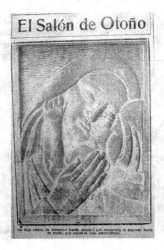

Fig. 7.8 Primitivo Icardi, [no title] c. 1933. Photograph *Los Principios*
(27 March 1934), 2.

poets, contemporary to those painters, literary critic Tamara Kamenszain has
interpreted how a group of male poets have redeemed the maternal figure to
the extent of linking the origin of modern literature to the maternal space.
This poetic masculine rescue of the maternal, that Carmen Perilli has termed
the 'domestic avant-garde',[24] seems to me closely connected to the pictorial
representations here analysed. As Kamenszain has proposed,

> Since no one has demanded that women write, through the centuries,
> many women incubated the symptom, channelling it through talk or
> the domestic works. However, the symptom went on to inhabit their
> sons, and as a result, some works emerged, signed by men but co-
> written by women. . . . It is in the millenary school of domestic tasks
> where the rules of modernity are learnt. Old like the world, only the
> futile and silent [domestic] work can achieve new links.[25]

Mother and child

The following paintings have represented maternal scenes where the mother
and child relationship has been the main feature. By the time Spilimbergo
was working on 'The wait', *Los Principios* was organizing in Córdoba the II

238

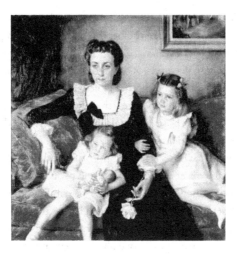

Fig. 7.9 Francisco Vidal, *La Señora de Roca y sus Hijas* (1943) oil on canvas,
110 x 110 cm Courtesy of the Museo Provincial de Bellas Artes 'Emilio A. Caraffa',
Córdoba, Argentina.

'Autumn Salon' in April of 1934. One of the works of sculptor Primitivo
Icardi (1910-1950), then a young artist, was used for the promotion of the
event in the newspaper. It is a bas-relief of a mother with her two children,
inspired by the religious art, probably the late fifteenth-century Madonnas
of Leonardo, particularly in the virginal features of the mother's face. Notably, while the mother clearly resembles Mary, both in image and gesture, the
baby and girl are depicted as real children of the time. The bas-relief is all
the more eloquent of the type of artistic work that the 'Autumn Salon' was
convoking: Catholic topics, a virginal, lovely mother confused in a tender
embrace with her baby and daughter, along with a traditional figurative style
alien to avant-garde influences. In Icardi's work, the mother and child relationship embodies the visual representation of women's pleasure. Although
this was the case for artists exhibiting in salons and galleries organised by
Catholics across the country, the National and Provincial Salons were not
exempt from this representational practice although in a less morally restrictive pictorial way. In the National Salon of 1939, for example, it is possible
to observe in the paintings *Composición* (Composition) by Ernesto Scotti and
Desnudo (Nudity) by Bernardo Goldestein, the links between maternal scenes
and sexually assertive, nude female bodies. If the maternal here, represented
by a mother breastfeeding in *Composición* and a mother and baby in *Desnudo*,

serves to justify the ostensible presence of women's naked bodies is difficult to assert, although judging from the broad cultural censorship of the time, it could well have been the case.

Beyond these visualizations of the mother and child relationship, which framed prevailing ideas of the mother 'solely thinking of her child' whether as virginal-caretakers or child bearers, there were artworks that contributed to the divergence from those national imperatives. A good example is the portrait by Francisco Vidal, *La Señora de Roca y sus Hijas*, 1943 ['Mrs. Roca with her daughters'], whose interpretation of mother and child bounding could be read as the exact reverse of the one proposed by the Marylike image of Icardi. Portrait, as genre, offers the possibility of inquiring into the characters represented in a closer approach, since the person portrayed, as in photography, authenticates the reality of his/her existence. Other conventions 'interfere' in the painting, above all, the inevitable negotiation between the artist and the person to be portrayed about how he/she is going to be represented. When the person to be portrayed, as in this case, is a painter too, we may speculate that the level of that negotiation becomes much more strategic, as the subject is imbued with the languages and conventions of the genre. These negotiations, as I argue, were certainly present in Vidal's portrait. Rosa Ferreyra de Roca was not only one of Córdoba's first professional female painters, but amongst the first artists in introducing avant-garde pictorial tendencies along with controversial, provocative subject matters as showed in her famous painting *La Urna verde*, 1929 ['The green urn'].

In Vidal's portrait some subtle aspects have captured the maternal image of Rosa, an upper-class, liberal, travelled, independent woman who chose Paris when her class turned to Spain and Rome in search of tradition and spiritual values. The portrait reflects the refined posture of Rosa, with her look posed beyond the scene, and a rose in her hand conveying the idea of her sensitivity as artist. The painting in the corner of this portrait gives to the composition a hint of the two elements that conflated in her life, the artist and the mother. The whole image, its elements, the drawing of the figures, even its colours denotes a harmonious, delicate composition. However, there is something that makes this representation of mother and daughters hesitant. The pose of Rosa and the body language of the two topics that the title announces, 'mother' and 'daughters', subvert the theoretical expectations that the theme itself evokes, and this is also evident artistically, if we compare it with Icardi's bas-relief. There is no physical involvement of the mother towards the daughters: she is not embracing, touching, grasping or looking at them. Instead, one of her hands is holding a rose and the other is hanging comfortably on the sofa. The daughters, whose moving legs and bodies are depicted as physically imposing their mother's attention, by being placed literally over her, give the impression of being molesting Rosa who seems to be discretely absent from the scene.

This portrait conveys the idea of a woman who 'shared' her motherhood *with* her profession. A position that in Cordoban society, we may suppose, was one hard to win. Analysing the letters and journals of female German artists, who also were mothers during the early twentieth century, Rosemary Betterton has observed the 'continual process of negotiation between their professional commitment to work and personal expectations of marriage and motherhood'.[26] In the same vain, I consider that this portrait perceptively represents such a negotiation, of a professional artist whose life was neither fulfilled nor exhausted by motherhood. In doing so, it suggests an alternative visual position to represent the maternal whose point of departure seems to reside in the representation of an unrecognised maternal agency, subtly brokered within the inner negotiations of a portrait.

The pregnant woman

In the 1990s feminist scholars drew attention to the visual representation of breastfeeding and pregnant women as controversial, iconic images of Western culture. In this sense, attention has been paid to a growing number of female artists that have focused on maternal issues (pregnancy, childbirth, abortion and lactation) in contemporary art. This is partly explained by the highly controversial work of artists like Cindy Sherman, Susan Hiller, Alison Lapper and Tracey Emin who purposely have 'explored relations between culturally constructed maternal bodies and embodied and imagined differences'.[27] As Betterton has noted about these artists' often disturbing images of the pregnant body, 'they may help us understand cultural anxieties that surround the maternal body and offer different kinds of figurations that acknowledge the agency and potential power of the pregnant subject'.[28] Many contemporary artistic representations have been embedded with debates over the role of the technologies of visualization (prenatal screening), which led to a critical analysis over the historically neglected female agency in the sphere of reproduction, and more specifically, in the act of giving birth. Indeed, as another feminist scholar, Iris Marion-Young, has argued, 'we should not be surprised to learn that discourse on pregnancy omits subjectiv-

241

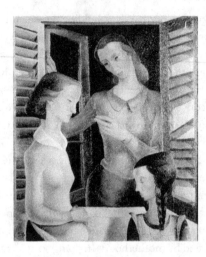

Fig. 7.10 Roberto Viola, *Mujeres en la Ventana* (1939) oil on canvas, 89.5 x 75 cm
Courtesy of the Museo Provincial de Bellas Artes 'Emilio A. Caraffa', Córdoba,
Argentina.

ity, for the specific experience of women is absent from our history'.[29] Much
of feminist analysis dedicated to highlight that absence has been stimulated
by the discourses on the foetus as an independent being, which as we have
seen in the former Chapter, since the 1960s have been visually promoted by
screening technologies. From this perspective, Imogen Tyler has stated, 'I
think that the production of a visual vocabulary of pregnant subjectivity is
necessary to challenge "the visual discourse of foetal autonomy"'.[30]

A somehow broader feminist interpretation has emerged from the si-
lent, absent, non-represented pregnant, female subject, which tended to focus in the works of women artists as the only subjects able of expressing
a female subjectivity. As I have maintained throughout this chapter, a historical interpretation can offer more balance to the existing scholarship by
extending the analysis to male artists and thus offering (male and female)
artists equal coverage in the discussion. By placing visual representations in
historical perspective, we notice that during the first half of the twentieth
century artistic representations of pregnant women in Western culture has
been indeed scarce and sometimes, controversial. Although feminist scholars,
with few exceptions, have tended to consider artistic images of pregnancy, as
Sandra Matthews and Laura Wexler have put it for the case of photography,
as 'the very archetype of the hidden',[31] I consider that representations of the

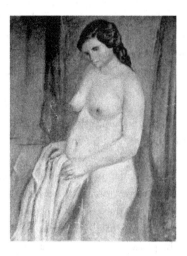

Fig. 7.11 Enrique Borla, *Maternidad* (1946). Photograph XXXVI Salón Nacional de Artes Plásticas. Courtesy of the Archivo Museo Provincial de Bellas Artes 'Emilio A. Caraffa', Córdoba, Argentina.

pregnant body could be less exceptional than an initial view might suggest. Probably the most famous artwork that inaugurates the series of pregnant images in this period is Gustave Klimt's *Hope I* (1903), which depicts a heavily pregnant woman standing nude in profile and looking at the spectator. Behind her, despairing black figures and a skull evoke the female fears (monstrosity, disease or death) that invade the pregnant woman's imagination. The piece was intended for display at the 1903 exhibition of the 'Vienna Secession' artistic movement. However, Klimt was forced to withdraw it, due to the controversy over its explicit content. In 1930, British resident artist Jacob Epstein finished his sculpture in marble *Genesis*, which represents a naked pregnant woman with primitive features, and disproportionate arms and legs. When it was displayed the following year at the Leicester Galleries in London, it prompted, according to Sarah Hyde, 'howls of protest and abuse'.[32] Reflecting on this controversy Hyde has stated that, 'The final insult was not only that this woman appeared to be non-European and unintelligent; she was also not beautiful, and this was if anything the most problematic issue'.[33] In his memories, Epstein himself has recalled his intentions when creating 'Genesis', where it is possible to see how a different representation of the maternal body may collides with culturally constructed ones,

I felt the necessity for giving expression to the profoundly elemental in motherhood, the deep down instinctive female, without the trappings and charm of what is known as feminine . . . How a figure like this contrasts with our coquetries and fanciful erotic nudes of modern sculpture.[34]

In the early 1930s, Frida Kahlo famously painted quite frequently about her own experiences with miscarriages, pregnancy, her own birth and lactation. However, the fact that she only showed her work much later, in 1952, places both the visualization and circulation of it as well as her potential influence and inspiration over other artists, out of the time of its creation, making it difficult to assess in terms of the public's reception. In any case, Kahlo's work accounts for a subject matter (gestating body) that although not common, seems to be in the process of generating a *corpus* in art history. Argentinian art was not an exception in this matter, and only by scrutinising the major spaces of circulation and visibility (in national and provincial salons) in our period, I have found two very telling images of pregnancy, which constitute the topic of analysis for the remainder of this chapter.

The first one, *Mujeres en la Ventana* (1939) ['Women at the window'], is a canvas that represents a dressed pregnant woman by Roberto Viola (1907-1966), an artist whose work Art Historians have placed among the so-called 'generation of the 1940s'. This nationally-acclaimed group of artists that were established in Córdoba, became instrumental in consolidating the Italian aesthetic (*Novecento, pittura metafisica*), and in securing for avant-garde tendencies an enduring experience. *Mujeres en la Ventana* is a good example of that direction, where Viola is experimenting with the geometric style, observable in the women's features, the fragmentation of space, and in a more daring use of colour. 'Women at the window' evokes a typical understated female place, the window and the street; a space where neighbouring women gather to chat or 'gossip', the typical place where female speech takes place or where women's gaze is 'wasted' on trivial curiosities. However, 'the window' here induces a second and more productive way of looking, one that is encouraged by Viola's invitation to look, following a zigzagging imaginary line, at the gaze of these female figures. Starting with the woman at the top, followed by the one on the left, then the girl, and finally, the womb. Notably, Viola wants the spectator to dwell on the womb, by guiding our zigzagging gaze towards it. Unlike the controversial European artwork commented on earlier, the pregnant woman here is dressed, however her clothes do not preclude us from considering this representation of a pregnant body as a clear thematisation and statement on the topic.

I would argue that the most important message that this painting introduces, is the visibility of a pregnant woman *through* the gaze (point of view) of women, thus inducing the spectator to think of the existence of a female subjectivity opposed to or differentiated from the male gaze. Even though the painter is a man, he has deliberately chosen both female figures and their interplay of looks as a way of signalling a female subjectivity over a topic (pregnancy) that was increasingly becoming medically and religiously, a male preserve. The physical sign of maternal origin is another significant insight (or window) that 'women at the window' opens. It seems to convey a didactic message to the observation of the girl. The girl, probably the daughter of one of these women, is noticing the gestating mother's swollen womb. The latter, with her hand on it, is not attempting to hide it from the curious look of the girl; rather she seems to be caressing her womb *in front* of the girl. For a society like Córdoba where, as *La Voz del Interior* criticised, education was to large extent built upon the 'hypocrisy' of Catholic values that taught girls that 'children were brought by a stork from Paris', this picture also seems to have been conceived to shake this belief.

The second artwork I found in my quest for the pregnant body is the painting *Maternidad* ('Motherhood') presented by Enrique Borla (1900-1959) to compete at the National Salon of Fine Arts in 1946. Since the 1940s the National Salon showed an increasing number of works devoted to the subject matter of 'motherhood'. While the majority of them represented it as 'mother and child', the oil on canvas of Borla is remarkable for depicting a fairly large image (140 x 110 cms.) of a naked pregnant woman. In doing so, and by titling it *Maternidad*, Borla was drawing attention to mothers as gestating subjects, and thus cutting a long, pervasive pictorial tradition of the Madonna *and* child stereotype where 'motherhood' was a bond of *two* beings. Visually, motherhood here is one; and only in the imagination could be two. There is no referent of 'the other' as such, nor independence, only the swollen womb of this woman's body, therefore suggesting that self and other, inside and outside becomes a fused or unique entity.

Feminist scholars have frequently resorted to Julia Kristeva's idea of 'motherhood's impossible syllogism', to interpret the impossibility or negation of the representation of the pregnant body from a masculine point of view. In a much-cited paragraph, Kristeva has stated,

245

Cells fuse, split, and proliferate; volumes grow, tissues stretch, and body fluids change rhythm, speeding up or slowing down. Within the body, growing as a graft, indomitable, there is an other. And no one is present within that simultaneously dual and alien space to signify what is going on. 'It happens, but I'm not there.' 'I cannot realise it, but it goes on'.[35]

This assertion attempts to explain the rejection of the far-reaching idea of maternal origin in Western culture, which led, in turn, to the fantasy of self-generation. 'The fantasy of a self freed from connection to the mother', says Betterton has been instrumental, according to a psychoanalytic interpretation, 'for socialization into the symbolic order and the correct assumption of sexual difference'.[36] From a philosophical point of view, this ontological uncertainty of the (doubling) pregnant body, scholars have argued, has been 'repeatedly disavowing maternal origin in its theories and models of subjectivity'.[37] According to prominent feminist psychoanalyst and philosopher Luce Irigaray, the philosophically unrepresentable pregnant body was built upon statements that has been 'covering over the fact that being's unseverable relation to the mother-matter has been buried'.[38] From this perspective we may interpret the visual representation of a pregnant body as introducing a sort of parenthesis into a discourse that has persistently denied its ontological entity and that, not surprisingly, these parentheses have been rare and controversial in Western culture.[39] Influential as it has been, in my interpretation of the artistic representation of the pregnant body I have decided, however, not to use the psychoanalytic framework, firstly for being a different epistemological approach, but above all, for being one that it is ahistorical and auto-referential. The same psychoanalytic methods that, for example, Kristeva uses in her famous work, 'Motherhood According to Giovanni Bellini', are the same that could explain the artistic work of Tracey Emin, or Enrique Borla. What matters to the psychoanalytic perspective it is not the context, but the private, personal biography of the artist. So in order to carry forward my analysis of Borla's painting I will keep it within its historical axis, and thus enquire about the relational configurations (medical, religious, artistic, etc.) that underpin its production, and the space of its circulation, that is, within the particularities of the National Salon of 1946.

By the time *Maternidad* was produced, two medical perspectives had been consolidated. Firstly, the eugenic one, with its taxonomy of the female body divided into three main types (brevilineal, normotype and longuilineal). This classification attempted to train, in the first place, the physician's gaze, and more broadly, society's view in the visual aspects of healthy female proportions. The second medical perspective is the one endorsed by Catholic obstetricians during the early 1940s (discussed early in Chapter 3), and was conceived, like the first one, as a response to perceived demographic problems (*dénatalité*). Its emphasis was on the visual aspects of the feminine body as a source of recognition of pathological signs, whose aetiology lay ultimately in immoral practices (abortions or contraception). Thus, in a time where the medically trained visualization of female fertile body has been so much stirred in the public sphere, it is not surprising to find a range of artistic expressions that would have challenged or redressed those normative standards of corporal maternal virtue.

Borla's rendering of the pregnant body pays no obvious tribute to either perspective, yet by bringing the female body to the fore introduces other possible readings. I would argue that the painting is in line with the visibility of a female subjectivity/intimacy, as it has already been explored by Spilimbergo, Berni, Batlle Planas and Viola. Borla's canvas is of one woman gestating at a moment in which some reflection seems to invade her as she takes off her clothes (culture) or is about to put them on, a moment of self-perception of her gestating body (nature). The painting thematises nothing more (and nothing less) than this. Technically, it is not distracting the viewer with anything new, as Borla had been using monumental figures since the early 1930s.

Maternidad was accepted at the first Peronist National Salon in 1946, which was organised just a few months after Perón's appointment to the Presidency. The painting's exhibition seems to have formed part of an initial aperture observed in the salons of the first years of the Peronist government, which as Andrea Giunta has observed, 'incorporated diverse themes and styles'.[40] Indeed, despite of many excluded artists, the jury of the 1946 Salon accepted the works of artists representative of avant-garde tendencies (such as Berni, Raquel Forner and Emilio Petorutti), who, in addition, were not supporters of the Peronist movement. However, as Giunta herself confirmed later, this policy of accessibility would change shortly afterwards. Within this context it is difficult to know what decided the selective criteria of the jury to accept Borla's *Maternity*. But given the early tendency of Peronist speeches to enhance the mother's figure, it is possible to speculate that this encouraged artists to submit an increasing number of portraits of motherhood — as the salons of these years testify — as a way of raising their chances to compete in the country's main exhibition venue. Borla's portrait

247

of a pregnant woman might also have inspired in the jury the fertility and the nascence of a 'new national era', an idea that the Peronist movement tirelessly sought to install. In any case, the canvas represented the maternal in an unprecedented way and contrasted with other more stereotypical motherhoods showed at the National Salon of that year.

The period ends up with an increasingly politicised representation of motherhood, which, with the exception of the work of Borla, seems to have explored rather less the topic of the female subjectivity and more the one of mothers' public role. Subsequent artistic representations of motherhood in the catalogue of the National Salon bore the imprint of this perceived change in the representational context that led to an increasingly politicised maternal figure. Indeed, the growing prominence of the mother's figure during the Peronist government was shaped by at least three main variables: the eugenic desire of race improvement; the rise of the welfare state, with policies that tended to improve the provision of maternal services; and the consolidation of a moral pattern of familiar organisation. More importantly, the exalted figure of the mother stemmed from a process of negotiation with women's new role as political citizens, after suffrage was granted in 1947. Thus, the emphasis on women's maternal role attempted to limit or adjust their newly acquired political participation with their traditional duties of the home. At the same time, the National Salon of Fine Arts was restructured with rules that sought to set up new premises for the shaping of the 'national taste'. As the first rule of the salon anticipated, the venue was intended to support those works that better represented 'the national life'.[41] Public education also featured prominently amongst the new social functions of the salon, including its aperture to the wider public, especially the working classes. In this scenario, artworks with titles such as 'motherhood' and 'mothers' started to circulate in the salon in an unprecedented way. It is not surprising that the visualisation of the maternal, in particular that of the working-class mother, became a sensitive image that the government sought to integrate into the imagery of the official artistic realm. Notably, the prize awarded to Roberto Viola for his sculpture *Madre Humilde,* 1948 ('The Humble Mother'), featuring a working class mother with a protective son dressed like an urban, industrial worker, suggests that the salons of Peronism stimulated too a new aesthetic that drew inspiration from the working classes, to which many artists, by conviction or opportunity, consented to satisfy.

Notes

1   D. Wechsler, 'Salones y Contra-Salones', in M. Penhos and D. Wechsler (eds.), *Tras los Pasos de la Norma: Salones Nacionales de Bellas Artes (1911-1989)* (Buenos Aires: Ediciones del Jilguero, 1999), 41-98: 55.
2   Wechsler, 'Salones y Contra-Salones', 55-7.
3   M. Penhos, 'Nativos en el Salón. Artes Plásticas e Identidad en la Primera Mitad del Siglo XX', in Penhos and Wechsler (eds.), *Tras los Pasos de la Norma*, 111-52.
4   Between the first Exhibition Hall in 1916 and the one of 1931, the private gallery 'Fasce' (opened in 1920) became the main venue where local artists showed their work.
5   The bill was elaborated by Deodoro Roca, a lawyer and leading figure during the University Reform of 1918, who was then Director of the Provincial Museum, and philosopher Carlos Astrada, in Á. Lo Celso, *50 Años de Arte Plástico en Córdoba* (Córdoba: Banco de la Provincia de Córdoba, 1973), 8.
6   D. Wechsler, 'Un registro Moderno del Arte en Córdoba', in *100 Años de Plástica en Córdoba, 1904-2004: 100 Artistas – 100 Obras en el Centenario de La Voz del Interior* (Córdoba: Pugliese Siena, 2004), 118-24: 19.
7   On the articulation of arts and politics in the 1930s see D. Wechsler 'Imágenes para la Resistencia. Intersecciones entre Arte y Política en la Encrucijada de la Internacional Antifascista. Obras y Textos de Antonio Berni (1930-1936)', in C. Medina (ed.), *La Imagen Política* (México, UNAM, 2006), 385-412.
8   Wechsler, 'Salones y Contra-Salones', 58.
9   See Wechsler 'Un Registro Moderno del Arte en Córdoba', 123. and A. Oviedo, 'Paisajes en la Pintura Cordobesa: (Vaivenes y Fracturas de la Representación)', in *100 Años de Plástica en Córdoba, 1904-2004*, 56-68: 57.
10 A. Giunta, 'Nacionales y Populares: Los Salones del Peronismo', in Penhos and Wechsler (eds.), *Tras los Pasos de la Norma*, 153-88: 154.
11 During the 1940s the Municipality of Córdoba created new exhibition venues: the Municipal Salon of Fine Arts, inaugurated in 1940, and the Municipal Museum of Fine Arts 'Dr Genaro Pérez' in 1943.
12 Amongst the many exhibitions organised by Catholics during this period, the one of 1934 stands out. It was organised by the Catholic Action in the selected salon of the Jockey Club, entitled, 'Artistic

Córdoba, from yesterday until today'.

13 The prizes were denominated as follows; prize 'Governor of the province', 'National Deputy chamber', 'National Senate chamber, 'Municipality of Córdoba', 'University of Córdoba', 'Archbishop of Córdoba', 'President of the nation', '*Los Principios*' along with others that referred to traditional painters. *Los Principios* (9 April 1934), 2.

14 Ibid.

15 M. Holmes, 'Disrobing the Virgin: The Madonna Lactans in Fifteenth-century Florentine Art', in G. Johnson and S. Matthews (eds.), *Picturing Women in Renaissance and Baroque Italy* (Cambridge: Cambridge University Press, 1997), 167-95: 169.

16 A. Bartlett, 'Madonnas, Models and Maternity: Icons of Breastfeeding in Visual Arts', paper delivered at the conference, 'Performing Motherhood: Ideology, Agency and Experience', La Trobe University, 2002. Online at www.usq.edu.au/resources/bartlettpaper.pdf (consulted 27.11.2009)

17 *La Vanguardia,* 10.

18 *La Voz del Interior* (4 November 1927), 8.

19 Nari, 'Las Prácticas Anticonceptivas', 178.

20 Iraeta and Beruti, 'Protección a la Maternidad Ilegítima', 305.

21 Cfr. H. Vezzetti, 'Las Promesas del Psicoanálisis en la Cultura de Masas'.

22 In this sense, the attitude of Spilimbergo could be interpreted as one of criticism and rescue. The famous series 'Brief History of Emma' (1935-36), for example, depicts different moments in the life of a poor girl that was dragged into prostitution through scenes of stark realism and social criticism.

23 A. Anreus, 'Adapting to Argentinian Reality: The New Realism of Antonio Berni', in A. Anreus, D. Linden, and J. Weinberg (eds.), *The Social and the Real: Political Art of the 1930s in the Western Hemisphere* (Pennsylvania State University Press, 2006), 97-114.

24 C. Perilli, 'Los Trabajos de la Araña. Mujeres, Teorías y Literatura', *Espéculo. Revista de Estudios Literarios,* 28 (2004). Online at http://www.ucm.es/info/especulo/numero28/trabaran.html (consulted 25.11.2009)

25 T. Kamenszain, *El Texto Silencioso. Tradición y Vanguardia en la Poesía Sudamericana* (México: UNAM, 1983), 77 and 81.

26 R. Betterton, *An Intimate Distance: Women, Artists and the Body* (London:

Routledge, 1996), 29.

27 R. Betterton, 'Promising Monsters: Pregnant Bodies, Artistic Subjectivity, and Maternal Imagination', *Hypatia*, 21 (2006), 80-100: 97.

28 Ibid., 97.

29 I. Young, *Throwing Like a Girl and Other Essays in Feminist Philosophy and Social Theory* (Bloomington: Indiana University Press, 1990), 160.

30 I. Tyler, 'Reframing Pregnant Embodiment', in S. Ahmed *et al.* (eds.) *Transformations, Thinking Through Feminism* (London: Routledge, 2000), 288-302: 300. Tyler's quotation within her paragraph belongs to Valerie Hartouni.

31 S. Matthews and L. Wexler, *Pregnant Pictures* (New York & London: Routledge, 2000), 1. An exception is Rosemary Betterton's analysis of the German artist Paula Modersohn-Becker and her painting *Self-Portrait on Her Sixth Wedding Day*, 1906, in Betterton, *An Intimate Distance*.

32 S. Hyde, *Exhibiting Gender* (Manchester: Manchester University Press, 1997), 44.

33 Ibid., 45.

34 Ibid.

35 J. Kristeva, *Desire in Language: A Semiotic Approach to Literature and Art,* (edition prepared by Leon Roudiez), (Oxford: Basil Blackwell, 1980), Ch. 9: 'Motherhood According to Giovanni Bellini', 237- 70: 237.

36 Betterton, *An Intimate Distance*, 29.

37 Tyler, 'Reframing Pregnant Embodiment', 291.

38 L. Irigaray, *Speculum of the Other Woman* (Ithaca: Cornell University Press, 1985), 162.

39 Much feminist attention has dwelt on the 1991 front cover of *Vanity Fair* magazine in which a photograph of the actress Demi Moore, naked and pregnant, taken by Annie Leibovitz. The picture aroused a storm of protest amongst the public.

40 Giunta, 'Nacionales y Populares', 162.

41 The National Salon of Fine Arts of 1946 was the first salon of the Peronist era. Prior to its organisation, the rules of the Salon had been changed by Presidential decree (N°5843/46 of 3 August 1946). It was stipulated that, 'it is convenient to concrete in artistic forms the facts and the particularities of the national life'. Amongst other things, it was also established, a) the introduction of prizes that were linked with the ministerial structure of the state ('Ministry of War prize',

'Ministry of Labour prize', etc.); and b) the Ministry's acquisition of the awarded work for display at the Ministry's office. The regulatory power of the state was also perceived through the composition of the jury responsible for the acceptance of works: Four members of the Ministry of Education and Justice and three artists. This disparity in the number of artists to members of the government was questioned by the Association of Artists, but without success. Cfr. Giunta, 'Nacionales y Populares', 159-61.

Epilogue

This book has proposed a different way of looking at the history of motherhood and its representations by bringing together medicine, society and culture in the Argentinian context. In so doing, I have attempted to eschew dichotomous counter-positions between the contents of medicine on the one hand, and ideas, notions, and a range of cultural expressions on the other. I have tried instead to integrate both types of registers in a more complex and, at the same time, concurrent interpretation, whereby 'the medical' started off or initiated a discussion whose continuities and discontinuities were queried in other fields. This approach has also allowed me to elaborate new ways of assessing and testing the penetration of medicine in other relevant and less visited areas further afield; from medical journals, scientific societies and maternity services to Catholic beliefs, novels, paintings, newspapers and their photographic record, mapping a trajectory that has shifted from biological 'maternity' to cultural 'motherhood'. I believe that one of the advantages of enquiring an object of study in this synchronic way is that it enables observation of the transformations experienced by the object of study itself: in my case ('representations of motherhood') from its medical point of departure into other object/objects that constantly rearms its content within the fields that it visits. As we have seen throughout the chapters, in tracing its trajectory, motherhood changes its status, sometimes it is central, at others is contested, sometimes it is re-signified and at other points neglected. A related point that I would like to emphasise here is that these emerging representations have appeared as empirically evident *only* in their connections with these other fields. This implies that if we interrogate motherhood only from the medical field we would not appreciate its implications in society at large, and conversely, if we interrogate it in the artistic field, in isolation from key medical concepts, we might miss some of its most convincing messages. Thus, placing the representations of motherhood in the perspective of the history of ideas, it has returned a more elaborated object, one where, in the inter-crossing of disciplines, records and locales has revealed some distinctive features that I would like to draw out in the pages that follow.

Obstetric literature of the first decades of the twentieth century showed an overriding concern for the techniques of childbirth whose formulations were translated into representations where the female/maternal body became embodied in the uterus. The metaphors that inaugurated the new obstetric language did not differ much from those observed by gender historians for the Europe and the US contexts. However, it is important to retain some of those expressed in our context : the obstetrician called himself 'governor' or 'director' of delivery; the uterus was analogised with a machine that could be 'accelerated', 'des-accelerated' or 'evacuated' at his discretion, whilst female subjectivity was completely erased from the act of delivery. The fragmentation or reduction of the body into the uterus has been interpreted as part of a process of disembodiment of the maternal body, although as we have seen elsewhere, by no means it was the most pervasive one.

On the other hand, the mother's responsibility was called upon when dystocic deliveries, miscarriages or neonatal deaths occurred, due to mother's presumed reluctance to seek obstetrical assistance, or in the case of their children's care due to their negligent behaviour. Mother-blaming culture led doctors to accommodate the idea of mother's natural instinct of caring and nurturing, necessary to naturalise women's maternal role with the need for education on that role. Puericulture campaigns, manuals addressed to mothers, and 'Schools for Mothers' were the main instruments of that educational drive. Yet more controversial were other topics that doctors put forward to society at large in the light of the perceived rise on infanticide, abortions and child abandonment rates. In acknowledging the 'single mother' as a social problem, some doctors envisioned society's reconsideration of its condemnatory attitude towards her but without securing a welfare provision for her protection. Indeed, the rejection of the *torno* (thought to induce 'maternal irresponsibility') was the logic corollary for the very premise of puericulture, whose rationale was built upon the existence of a unique mother-child bond. So for the period pre-1930s, the figure of the single mother was the one that doctors invited society to get involved with. They epitomised the socialised and 'civilised' side of a discourse on maternity that was, otherwise, corporally constructed, as one obstetrician expressed, with 'the boldness of the [obstetric] surgeon in exploring with his scalpel the most hidden fields of the organism, to bring its saving cut'.[1]

Concern about 'illegitimate motherhood', however, did nothing but confirm for the Catholic clergy the dangerous nature of the female body, so that they dwelt on a medically perceived 'social damage' in order to emphasise female sexual purity. Chastity became intensely idealised through the figure of the Immaculate Conception, revitalised during these years by the Catholic press and through the Catholic novel. Catholics shared with doctors the vision that mothers needed to be taught to better accomplish their maternal duties. To the healthy raising of children, the clergy incorporated the transcendental spiritual values that mothers were expected to transmit in the process of rearing. This mutually reinforcing perspective secured mothers' role in the domestic sphere of the family, a perspective that proved to be most challenging. On the one hand, the terms of domesticity were contested in a period of women's entry into the (formal and informal) labour market. On the other, there were feminists and their demands for greater access to citizenship alongside their proposals for maternal and child health reforms. I have argued that Catholics' anxiety about feminism – perceived as a threat to mother's spiritual mission – found in the lofty figure of Mary a powerful referent to contain women's potential attention to other available forms of maternal discourse. It is instructive to observe that the *Madonna della Carità* was not the profile of Mary that the church turned to as an example of maternal virtue. Yet Catholic men failed in deterring women from becoming involved in welfare activities. And against the clergy's ideal role of mothers' devotion to the family, thousands of Catholic women interpreted their natural attributes of caring, nurturing, and consoling in social terms, although not without consequences. Remarkably, the *matron* or the charitable lady became one of the most contested figures throughout our period, as they received the criticism of feminist, liberals and Catholics alike. Such a controversial figure has been largely reflected in the historiography, as studies have tended to over emphasise the development of welfare state initiatives while neglecting female voluntarism as a conservative, Catholic and backward form of assistance. Only recently gender scholars are reassessing the contribution of female charitable groups after being long overshadowed by the analysis of their more progressive feminist peers.

The poor single mother introduced into public discourse by medical specialists was also taken up by the press as a topic on which journalism elaborated its own vision. The eight year-long journalistic campaign of *La Voz del Interior* is a convincing example on how the liberal press took the maternal as political by placing it at the core of its ideological battle against the Catholic forces. This makes Koven and Michel's contention that maternalist discourses could easily 'be harnessed to forge improbable coalitions'[2] a credible claim. The paper's rather progressive stance regarding the 'female question' more broadly, which is variously shown through its support for feminists' initiatives, sexual education, or women's political participation, made its vision on motherhood and the one demonstrated through the maternal campaign in particular difficult to assess. The paradoxes observed during the campaign, including the paper's harsh criticism toward the female charitable groups, its fictionalised position as welfare provider, and its lack of questioning of the state before the 1930s rendered a somewhat restricted impact. However, at its best, we may consider that it added distinctiveness to the circulating discourses on motherhood. By focusing on the concrete situations and needs of poor mothers *La Voz del Interior* challenged at the same time the spiritual, abstract values proclaimed by Catholics, and the alleged mother's ignorance and children-only focus of doctors. On the other hand, in visual terms, its photographic register placed the poor mother in the narrative of 'otherness' whose material needs and emotional suffering probably served more to discourage women from motherhood altogether rather than to foster maternal longing. Criticism towards female welfare along with the paper's campaign against midwives and the invisibility of the mother as subject helped to undermine both maternal agency and the very existence of an independent maternal subjectivity.

Much of my analysis has emphasised the 1930s as a decade in which the consolidation of former prevailing ideologies and also the emergence of new ones dovetailed. The 'biologisation' of medical discourse through eugenic and biotypological theories resulted in medical practices that sought to enhance female fertility through the endocrine treatment of 'unfit' maternal bodies. Such interventions were tested within the larger rhetoric of Argentina's population problems and to which different ideologies concurred: the persistent decline in birth-rates, high indexes of infant mortality and of congenitally weak children produced by hereditary diseases. The arrival of the conservative military forces in 1930 came to signal the crisis of the liberal state, the failure of its modernist project and the crisis of spiritual values that, it was thought, were eroding the social cohesion of the nation. Arguably, nationalism strengthened already existing bonds between the medical field and the state by fusing spiritual and biological values in an unprecedented way, as demonstrated by a chimerical search for the 'Argentinian biotype'.

The influence and coexistence of the two main strands of eugenic thought in the 1930s, the Italian through biotypology and the German through its endorsement of Mendel's laws of heredity (pre-conceptional counselling), gave initiatives and interventions in Argentina and Latin-America more broadly, a different character though, to elucidate what *that* particular character meant requires as much from studies able to hermeneutically unfold the various concepts and 'academic hybrids' that terms such as 'hygiene', 'race', 'white race', 'heredity' were given at the time,[3] as from studies on institutional practices and medical research. To be sure, the transnational nature of eugenic ideas, and the growing literature that focuses on the academic exchanges and inter-connectedness of specific countries help to illuminate certain patterns of the Argentinian case that leave some questions for more detailed investigation. A reading of Maria-Sophia Quine's works on biotypology in Italy, for example, raises many questions as to the alleged similarities with the Argentinian case. In terms of population policies, Quine has argued,

> Talk of any kind of restrictions to reproductive freedoms now became an impossibility, as the regime co-opted eugenics and steered population policy towards an unconditional pronatalist, reformist and environmentalist position.[4]

Also complementing this policy there were strict measures against abortion, birth control and sterilisation that were passed in the new Italian penal code (1931). These along with the rejection of a prenuptial certificate and the enactment of pronatalist welfare measures distanced the, thus conceived, Italian 'Latin' eugenics from what we have seen of the Argentinian case. Likewise, the ambiguities shown at national and international forums by Argentinian specialists regarding sterilisation and the heredity of certain diseases were facilitated by a long-established network of scientific and cultural exchanges with Germany,[5] and in particular with its *Frauenklinik*.

Turning to other aspects of the medical practice that became evident from the 1930s, I have noted the shift in the focus of attention of obstetricians from a concentration on the uterine physiopathology towards the one over the conditions of reproduction. The 'uterus' was overshadowed by the 'ovaries', whose functionality was introduced and explained by endocrinology, thus inaugurating a new 'golden era' of medical knowledge and practice (hormonotherapy). The new perspective was holistic (constitutional) in its interrelation of variables of internal secretion and hereditary factors, but reductionistic in its attempt to classify and correlate different body types with women's fertility. As I have tried to demonstrate in this book, this perspective spurred on a wide range of medical interventions in the female body and women's personal lives, from advice that prevented them from getting married or becoming pregnant (preconception and prenuptial consulting rooms) to endocrine treatments, sterilisations and therapeutic abortions. Further analysis in the way eugenics evolved in the post-1945 period, from the so-called 'new eugenics' – as novel screening technologies and prenatal genetic testing became available – to the US-based efforts of population control in Latin America should explore the connections with the interwar period.

The 'biologisation' of the maternal body so much integrated within the state health policy would find in Catholicism an ideological obstacle, mainly, as it has often been considered, because the church would not easily relinquish its control over reproduction. Yet from my analysis I will argue that Catholicism may have framed discussions in reproductive health, but certainly did not define or determine the scope of eugenic practices in the country. It is instructive to remember that the most negative approach to eugenic initiatives took place precisely at the moment of strongest alliance between church and state, and when integralism positioned Catholicism as the 'true' cultural matrix of the Argentinian nation. Other aspects of the all-encompassing Catholic culture during this period seemed more apparent, notably, in their redefinition of the representation of the virtuous motherhood. The opportune call of Pope Pius XI to 'weary' mothers (*Lux Veritatis*) to seek inspiration in the abnegation and sacrifice of the *Mater Dolorosa*, offered in exchange a series of ritualised dramas mainly, the Virgin's street processions, where maternal bodies were rendered invisible along with their personal expectations. Of all the cultural aspects mobilised by Catholics in these years (novels, art works and the press), photojournalism and the photographic style of *Los Principios* in particular, is the one that better revealed the elements at stake. Above all, the absence of the mother's referent and the visualisation of women with priests or in a submissive position can be understood as a negotiation between two conflicting ideas: mother's essentialised position with that of mother's impure maternal origin. Thus, visualisations had to broker and accommodate motherhood's paradoxical meanings, and photographs did so by, at one and the same time, showing and concealing the elements in dispute. In this sense, the visibility conceded to the 'spiritual son' instead of the biological one, appears as a redemption of the maternal fall, but also as a guarantee of control over the mother's sexual nature.

Among the different representations of motherhood that took shape during this period, there was one in particular that introduced a new perspective centred on the mother's subjectivity. This distinctive form of representation had significant points in common, firstly, the belonging to the artistic field; secondly, the time of appearance (1930s); and finally, the subjects of enunciation. Here the fact that the artists and writers that made up my corpus were mostly men may pose debatable questions to more traditional perspectives on gender and feminist studies. On the one hand, we have seen through the analysis of visual images that feminist perspectives have tended to ontologically deny male subjects the *logos*, that is, the very possibility of expressing a female subjectivity. On the other, Latin American gender studies in particular have been prone to concentrate only on issues related to women, and from a perspective grounded in the existence of a dichotomous construction of female identities in relation to a patriarchal power. This perspective has often emphasised women's discrimination, oppression and subalternisation, and it has also celebrated women's resistance without a detailed reappraisal of the conditions of that resistance, or without acknowledging the possibility that the resistance may have had a masculine origin.

In my research it became apparent that it was in the work of male artists where the gendered malaise was more clearly articulated. This, of course, raises the question of, why was this distinctive representation of the maternal gender specific. In other words, why didn't women, in the sources analysed, voice that discomfort which affected their own representational image? This is a question that invites reassessment of both sources and perspectives, one that future studies might consider in their scrutiny of gender influences on the literary and artistic fields. Firstly, a comprehensive search of literary and artistic sources relies, to a great extent, on the good fortune of the researcher. As it is often the case, many literary texts that have circulated in the past have not been re-edited and various artistic works have not been, for example, photographed for an exhibition catalogue, making their accessibility a random opportunity (i.e. meeting the private owners of these works). To be sure, we should presume the existence of myriads of sources that have circulated during this period, and that have not been unearthed for various reasons. Amongst these reasons are censorship, the impositions of the canon, and the 'politics of memory' of what has been preserved for us in museums, libraries, and archives. Secondly, in an attempt to avoid simplistic or sweeping conceptualisations of female agency, Latin American literary critics have proposed the need of a critical look able to detect 'a surplus in the texts that remains partially obscure if they are not focussed through a gender perspective that would read the message produced by the subject of enunciation'.[6] To this aim they have proposed different terms to account for the strategies use by women writers, thus Francine Masiello refers to 'verbal puns and double-entendres', 'masks', and 'ventriloquism'; Alicia Genovese to

259

'the double voice'; and Josefina Ludmer to the 'tricks of the weak'.[7] Hence, further studies able to concentrate in a wider range of sources (poetry, short stories), or less acclaimed genres (illustrations, letters, diaries), as well as larger spaces of circulation (exhibitions, magazines, literary meetings) are needed to have a deeper response as to whether female resistance was weak, strong or simply absent. In any case, for the sources that I have explored in this book, I shall neither conclude for this period that female artists were completely alien to Ludmer's 'tricks' nor that their lack of engagement in discussions of the maternal, confirms a female status as 'conforming', 'complicit' or 'co-opted' by prevailing discourses.

We have seen a number of outstanding efforts in fiction that have contested, in different ways, the eugenic endeavour of a sexuality controlled by the interests of the state. Filloy's *Op Oloop* masterfully showed that impossibility (by combining the author's deep knowledge in biotypology with his exceptional literary skills) through the story of an obsessive statistician whose classificatory ambition reaches the point of suicidal despair when confronted with the anomie of love. Barón Biza, in *El Derecho de Matar*, emphasised through multiple forms of women's sexuality (pre-marital, adulterous, lesbian, and sterile female bodies), as a way of underlining women's rejection of becoming reproductive beings for the sake of the nation. Part of the pictorial record has also captured the same emerging signs – female sexuality, feminine world, subjectivity – that threatened to erode the structure of motherhood at a time when its ideological components (medical and religious) were most apparent and pressuring. Notably, Spilimbergo and Berni's paintings connected motherhood with a zone of female subjectivity that was thematised from socially-discredited female spaces. In *La Espera* and *Primeros Pasos*, an inscrutable mother's sensitivity seems to be longing to express a subjectivity of her own to the indifference of the defining discourses of maternal identity. In addition, Viola's *Mujeres en la Ventana* and Borla's *Maternidad* have also drawn attention to the existence of a female maternal subjectivity, which they have placed on that 'site of cultural anxiety' represented by the pregnant body. Both paintings contrasted remarkably with the proliferation of 'motherhoods' observed in the early years of the Peronist government, where the figure (and image) of the poor mother served to support state demands on mothers as political citizens.

The period that this book has analysed thus concludes with the symptoms of an emerging maternal subjectivity and a state that seemed ready to capitalise on mothers' newly granted political rights. It seems to me that the raising, iconic figure of a childless Eva Perón to 'mother the nation' was subtended by the competing motherhoods that preceded hers. Yet historians have often associated Evita's political motherhood with the Virgin attributes or with the internalisation of the Marian model, which is arguably an oversimplification of the status of the representations of motherhood at the time. In the same way, I have contended here that medical discourses on maternity did not play an overriding role in defining the representations of motherhood, although it arguably stimulated cultural responses in varied and often contesting ways. In interrelating a series of disciplines and their sources this book has broadened the ground on which representations of motherhood were constructed. From this perspective, motherhood emerged in Argentinian society as an object not *defined* by a unique discourse, but rather as an object that remitted to a diffuse corpus where various, competing, temporal, registers have penetrated it to shape its contours.

Notes

1 Lascano and O'Farrel, 'La Cirugía Obstétrica en la Placenta Previa', 417.

2 S. Koven and S. Michel, 'Introduction: "Mother Worlds" ', in Koven and Michel (eds.), *Mothers of a New World: Maternalist Politics and the Origins of Welfare Sates* (Routledge: London, 1993), 1-10: 5.

3 M. Turda, 'Race, Science and Eugenics in the Twentieth Century', in A. Bashford, P. Levine (eds), *The Oxford Handbook of the History of Eugenics* (New York: Oxford University Press, 2010), 98-127.

4 M.S. Quine, 'The First-Wave Eugenic Revolution in Southern Europe: *Science Sans Frontières*', in A. Bashford and P. Levine, *The Oxford Handbook of the History of Eugenics* (New York: Oxford University Press, 2010), 377-97: 386.

5 About the German-Argentinian medical exchanges see A. Reggiani, 'De Rastacueros a Expertos. Modernización, Diplomacia Cultural y Circuitos Académicos Transnacionales, 1870-1940', in R. Salvatore (ed.), *Los Lugares del Saber. Contextos Locales y Redes Transnacionales en la Formación del Conocimiento Moderno* (Rosario: Beatriz Viterbo Editora, 2007), 159-87; and Y. Eraso, 'A Burden to the State'.

6 A. Genovese, quoted in N. Domínguez, 'Reflexiones Finales. Acerca de

la Crítica', in N. Domínguez and C. Perilli (eds), *Fábulas del Género: Sexo y Escrituras en América Latina* (Rosario: Breatriz Viterbo, 1998), 195-215: 198.

7   J. Ludmer, 'Las Tretas del Débil', in P. González and E. Ortega (eds), *La Sartén por el Mango: Encuentro de Escritoras Latinoamericanas*, (Puerto Rico: El Huracán, 1985), 47-54; and Masiello, *Entre Civilización y Barbarie*.

Sources and Select Bibliography

Primary Sources

Archival Material

Archivo de la Archidiócesis de Córdoba:
 Libro de Autos y Visitas Parroquiales, 1885-1916.
 Libro de Autos y Edictos Episcopales, 1905-1920.
Archivo Museo Municipal de Bellas Artes 'Genaro Pérez', Córdoba.
 Folders: 'Lino Spilimbergo'
   'Roberto Viola'
   'Ricardo Musso'
   'Francisco Vidal'
Archivo Museo Provincial de Bellas Artes 'Emilio A. Caraffa', Córdoba.
 XXXVI Salón Nacional de Artes Plásticas. 1946. Buenos Aires: Ministerio
  de Justicia e Instrucción Pública.
 XXXVIII Salón Nacional de Artes Plásticas. 1948. Buenos Aires: Secretaría
  de Cultura de la Nación.

Periodicals

Archivos de los Hospitales de la Sociedad de Beneficencia de la Capital
Boletín del Instituto de Maternidad de la Sociedad de Beneficencia de la Capital
Boletín de la Oficina Sanitaria Panamericana
Boletín Eclesiástico de la Diócesis de Córdoba
Congreso Nacional: Cámara de Senadores.
Criterio
La Semana Médica
La Voz del Interior
Los Principios
Obstetricia y Ginecología Latino-Americanas
Revista Argentina de Obstetricia y Ginecología
Revista de la Facultad de Ciencias Médicas
Revista de la Asociación Médica Argentina
Revista de la Universidad Nacional de Córdoba
Revista del Círculo Médico de Córdoba
Revista Eclesiástica

Literary sources:

Barón Biza, Raúl. 1933. *El Derecho de Matar.* Buenos Aires: Editorial Barón Biza.

Beltrán Posse, Amalia. 1928. *Desde Mi Rincón.* Córdoba: Biffignandi.

Echenique, María Eugenia. 1900. *Colección Literaria.* Córdoba: Biffignandi.

Filloy, Juan. 2009. *Op Oloop.* (tr. Lisa Dillman) Champaign & London: Dalkey Archive Press.

Filloy, J. 1997. *Op Oloop.* Buenos Aires: Losada.

Juárez Núñez, Rodolfo. 1932. *La Sombra del Tejar.* Buenos Aires: El Ateneo.

Vélez, Juan José. [s.d.] *Los Dos Polos.* Córdoba: Biffignandi.

Wast, Hugo. 1944. *Flor de Durazno.* Buenos Aires: Thau Editores.

Medical sources (see abbreviations):

Actas de la II Conferencia Pan-Americana de Eugenesia y Homicultura de las Repúblicas Americanas. 1934. Buenos Aires: Fascoli y Bindi.

Acuña, Mamerto. 1925. 'Protección a la Mujer Embarazada, a las Madres Solteras y Madres Abandonadas' in *IICNM*, III. Buenos Aires: Casa Editora de A. Guidi Buffarini: 269-75.

Álvarez, José Manuel. 1896. *La Lucha por la Salud. Su Estado Actual en la Ciudad de Córdoba.* Buenos Aires: Biedma.

Baldi, Eduardo. 1940. 'Sobre algunas Observaciones de Fracasos de la Esterilización Quirúrgica' in *IVCAOyG.* Buenos Aires: Guidi Buffarini: 305–9.

Bas, Bernardo. 1942. *Aborto y Denatalidad.* Córdoba: Pereyra.

Bas, B. 1945. 'Porque la Denatalidad es un Peligro para la Nación y el Individuo' in Bas, B. *Artículos Sueltos.* Córdoba: Pereyra: 35-58.

Belbey, José. 1935. 'La Esterilización Humana por el Estado', in *VCNM*, VIII. Rosario: Talleres Gráficos Pomponio: 325-29.

Bello, José. 1940. 'Mortinatalidad y Organización Sanitaria' in *IVCAOyG.* Buenos Aires: Guidi Buffarini: 813-18.

Beruti, Josué. 1916. 'Nuestro Gremio de Parteras. Reformas Necesarias para su Mejoramiento y Dignificación' in *La Semana Médica* 23 (1).

Beruti, J. 1932. 'La Desnutrición Voluntaria en la Mujer Moderna' in *Actas y Trabajos del IVCNM*, VI. Buenos Aires: Spinelli: 340-58.

Beruti, J. León, J. and Diradourian, J. 1935. 'La Abreviación del Parto

Aproximadamente Fisiológico' in *VCNM*, V. Rosario: Talleres Gráficos Pomponio: 395-403.

Beruti, J. León, J. and Diradourian, J. 1935. 'La Inducción del Parto por Medios Puramente Médicos en Embarazadas con Rotura Prematura Espontánea de las Membranas Ovulares' in *VCNM*, V. Rosario: Talleres Gráficos Pomponio: 587-91.

Brandán, Ramón. 1947. 'Patología de la Contracepción. Síndrome de Sedillot' in *Revista de la Facultad de Ciencias Médicas*. Universidad Nacional de Córdoba. 5 (5): 537-75.

Cantón, Eliseo. 1914. 'Protección a la Madre y al Hijo. Puericultura intra y extra-uterina: Profilaxis del Aborto, Parto Prematuro, Abandono e Infanticidio, Maternidad-Refugio' in *La Semana Médica*, 21: 39-44.

Carranza Casares, Carlos. 2008. 'Consorcio de Médicos Católicos' in *Iatría* 78 (189): 6-7.

Carro, Víctor. 1935. 'El Régimen Alimenticio de la Embarazada Obesa' in *RCMC*: 327-47.

Cetrángolo, Antonio. 1935. 'La Crisis de la Profesión Médica' in *RCMC*: 341-52.

Chasín Ida and Schteingart, Mario. 1935. 'Las Inyecciones Endovenosas de Foliculina en las Menorragias' in *VCNM*, V. Rosario: Talleres Gráficos Pomponio: 441-44.

Comas, Juan. 1943. 'La Biotipología de Arturo Rossi' in *Boletín Bibliográfico de Antropología Americana* 7: 99-113.

Coni, Emilio. 1918. *Asistencia y Previsión Social. Buenos Aires Caritativo y Previsor.* Buenos Aires: Ed. Spinelli.

Couvelaire, Alexandre. 1930. *La Nouvelle Maternité Baudelocque. Clinique Obstétricale de la Faculté de Médecine de l'Université de Paris.* Paris: Masson.

'Creación del Departamento Nacional de Maternidad e Higiene Infantil'. 1937. *Congreso Nacional: Cámara de Senadores.* Buenos Aires: Imprenta del Congreso: 10-16 and 284-95.

D'Alessandro, Antonio. 1914. 'El Infanticidio y el Torno Libre' in *La Semana Médica* 1: 18-28.

Del Campillo, Ernesto. 1908. *'La Gota de Leche': Cuatro Años de Funcionamiento del Consultorio Protector de la Infancia.* Córdoba: Imp. Mitre.

Dezeo, Pilades. 1939. 'Demografía Internacional' in *VICNM*, III. Rosario: Est. Gráfico Pomponio: 612-32.

Díaz de Guijarro, Enrique. 1944. *El Impedimento Matrimonial de Enfermedad. Matrimonio y Eugenesia.* Buenos Aires: Kraft.

Dionisi, Humberto. 1940. 'Embarazo Ectópico' in *RCMC*: 2313-29.

Escuder, Carlos. 1940. 'Discusión' in *IVCAOyG*. Buenos Aires: Guidi Buffarini: 325-31.

Fernández, Ubaldo. 1916. 'La Asistencia del Parto' in *La Semana Médica* 23: 312-17.

Franceschi, Gustavo. 1934. 'Dios y la Fisiología' in *Criterio* 317: 295-97.

Galíndez, Benjamín. 1921. 'El Aborto Criminal en Córdoba' in *RCMC* 9: 245-68.

Garzón Maceda, Félix. 1927. *Historia de la Facultad de Ciencias Médicas, I*. Córdoba: Imprenta de la Universidad.

Gordillo, A. *et al.* 1937. 'Esterilización Biológica Temporaria de la Mujer' in *Revista de la Asociación Médica Argentina* 50: 291-96.

Guiroy, Alfredo and González Collazo, Alfredo. 1935. 'La Ruptura Artificial Precoz de la Bolsa de las Aguas' in *VCNM*, V. Rosario: Talleres Gráficos Pomponio: 761-67.

Herrera, Roberto. 1940. 'Consideraciones Acerca de la Esterilización' in *IVCAOyG*. Buenos Aires: Guidi Buffarini: 304-5.

'Infancia'. 1936. *Boletín de la Oficina Sanitaria Panamericana* (Enero): 27-36.

Iraeta, Domingo and Beruti, Josué. 1925. 'Protección a la Maternidad Ilegítima' in *IICNM*, III: 303-16.

Lanza Castelli. 1911. *Mortalidad Infantil*. Córdoba: Imprenta el Comercio.

Lascano, José. 1928. 'La Distocia en Córdoba' in *RCMC*: 173-93.

Lascano, J. 1939. 'Asistencia Pre-natal' in *VICNM*, III. Rosario: Est. Gráfico Pomponio: 528-52.

Lascano, J. 1937. *El Instituto de Maternidad de la Facultad de Ciencias Médicas de la Universidad Nacional de Córdoba*. Córdoba: Imprenta Pereyra.

Lascano, J. 1941. 'Aspecto Social de la Asistencia Obstétrica. Reseña Histórica y Legislación Argentina' in *Revista de la Universidad Nacional de Córdoba* 28: 1449-75.

Lascano, J. 'Vista Panorámica del Estudio de la Obstetricia', *Revista de Facultad de Ciencias Médicas*, 2 (1944), 177-98.

Lascano, J. 1938. 'La Obstetricia en los Últimos 25 años' in *Annaes Brasileiros de Gynecología* 6 (5): 1-19.

Lascano, J. and O'Farrel, Manuel. 1925. 'La Cirugía Obstétrica en la Placenta Previa' in *IICNM*, III. Buenos Aires: Casa Editora de A. Guidi Buffarini: 417-51.

Lascano, J. and Sayago, Gumersindo. 1934. 'Tuberculosis y Embarazo', in *IICAOyG*. Buenos Aires: Caporaletti Hnos.: 38-75.

Lerena, Carlos. 1933. 'Eutanasia y Eugenesia' in *Criterio* 293: 206-7.

Licurzi, Ariosto. 1937. 'La Esterilización Eugénica de los Degenerados y Criminales', *RCMC.* 207-25.

Marramá, Cataldo. 1939. 'Evacuación Extemporánea del Útero: Método de Paul Delmas' in *RCMC*: 1563-90.

Martínez, Gregorio. 1913. 'Introducción al Estudio de la Puericultura' in *RCMC* 3: 404-16.

'Maternidad Modelo'. 1931. *Boletín de la Oficina Sanitaria Panamericana (Agosto): 986-1022.*

Memoria Médico-Administrativa. 1934. Asilo Colonia Regional Mixto de Alienados en Oliva. Córdoba. Archivo del 'Hospital Psiquiátrico Dr Emilio Vidal Abal'.

Navarro, Antonio. 1939. 'Anomalías del Desarrollo Somático y Morfológico' in *RCMC*: 1811-55.

Navarro, A. 1941. 'Semiología de las Facies' in *RCMC*: 273-81.

Pende, Nicola. 1928. *Constitutional Inadequacies. An Introduction to the Study of Abnormal Constitutions.* Philadelphia: Lea and Febiger.

Peralta Ramos, Alberto. 1925. 'La Obstetricia del Médico Práctico' in *IICNM*, III. Buenos Aires: Casa Editora de A. Guidi Buffarini: 645-63.

Peralta Ramos, A. 1939. *Obstetricia, Ginecología y Puericultura, III.* Buenos Aires: Imprenta Mercatali.

Peralta Ramos, A. 'Habilitación Definitiva del Instituto de Maternidad', *Archivos de los Hospitales de la Sociedad de Beneficencia de la Capital. Años 1929-1932*: 9-23.

Peralta Ramos, A. 1944. 'Discurso Homenaje. Informaciones Latino-Americanas' in *Obstetricia y Ginecología Latino-Americanas* 3: 649-59.

Peralta Ramos, A. and Guiroy, Alfredo. 1935. 'Gobierno y Dirección del Parto', in *VCNM*, V. Rosario: Talleres Gráficos Pomponio: 389-94.

Peralta Ramos, A. and Schteingart, M. 1935. 'Los Factores Endocrino-Constitucionales en la Obstetricia y Ginecología' in *VCNM*, V. Rosario: Talleres Gráficos Pomponio: 686-94.

Peralta Ramos, A. and Peralta Ramos, Guillermo. 1940. 'Indicaciones y Técnica de la Esterilización Artificial Definitiva de la Mujer' in *IVCAOyG.* Buenos Aires: Guidi Buffarini: 309-25

Peralta Ramos, G. Schteingart, M. and Chasain, I. 1935. 'Constitución y Esterilidad', *VCNM*, V. Rosario: Talleres Gráficos Pomponio: 432-40.

Peralta Ramos, G. and Schteingart, M. 1935. 'Esterilización Temporaria por Método Biológico' in *VCNM*, V. Rosario: Talleres Gráficos Pomponio:

656-58.

Pérez, Manuel. 1940. 'Esterilización: Definición, Historia, Indicaciones' in *IVCAOyG*. Buenos Aires: Guidi Buffarini: 47-121.

Piantoni, Carlos and Luque, Pedro. 1939. 'Protección Médico-social de la Primera Infancia en Córdoba' in *VICNM*, III. Rosario: Est. Gráfico Pomponio: 574-78.

Pla, Pedro. 1935. 'El Tratamiento de la Insuficiencia Genital en Ambos Sexos con Inyecciones de Orina de Embarazada' in *VCNM*, V. Rosario: Talleres Gráficos Pomponio: 445-50.

Risolía, Arturo. 1940. 'Esterilización en la Mujer' in *IVCAOyG*. Buenos Aires: Guidi Buffarini: 122-299.

Rodríguez, Mercedes. 1943. 'Los Factores Sociales en la Hipoplasia Genital' in *VCAOyG*. Buenos Aires: s.n.: 806-11.

Rossi, Arturo. 1944. *Tratado Teórico Práctico de Biotipología y Ortogénesis, I.* Buenos Aires: Ideas.

Soria, Benito. 1919. 'Obras realizadas en Córdoba en Pro de la Infancia y Escuela de Madres' in *Revista de la Universidad Nacional de Córdoba* 2: 84-98.

Soria, B. 1924. 'Protección a la Infancia' in *Revista de la Universidad Nacional de Córdoba* 2: 30-48.

Torre, Mario. 1958. 'Mortalidad Materna' in *Obstetricia y Ginecología Latino-Americanas* 16 (7-8): 233-39.

Vidal Abal, Emilio. 1937. 'Consideraciones sobre Profilaxis Mental a Propósito del Tema Praxiterapia' in *Boletín del Asilo de Alienados en Oliva* 16: 119-26.

Other

Código Penal de la República Argentina. 1989. Buenos Aires: Zavalía.

Bunge, Alejandro. 1940. *Una Nueva Argentina.* Buenos Aires: G. Kraft Ltda.

Lueza, H.F. 1936. *Breve Reseña Histórica. Congregación de las Hermanas Carmelitas Descalzas de la Tercera Orden: Sus Fundaciones y Obras en las Repúblicas de Argentina y Uruguay (1896-1936).* Buenos Aires: J. Belsolá y Cia.

Mensaje del Gobernador de la Provincia de Córdoba Dr. Eufrasio S. Loza. Leído ante la Asamblea Legislativa al Inaugurarse el Período. 1° de Mayo de 1917 (Córdoba: Imprenta de la Penitenciaría, 1917).

Moreyra, Beatriz, Remedi, Fernando and Roggio, Patricia (eds). 1998. *El Hombre y sus Circunstancias. Discursos, Representaciones y Prácticas Sociales en*

Córdoba, 1900-1935. Córdoba: Centro de Estudios Históricos.
Población 1869-1960 (Córdoba: Dirección General de Estadística, Censos e Investigaciones, 1961).
Sínodo Diocesano Celebrado en Córdoba por el Iltmo. y Rmo. Señor Obispo Don Fray Zenón Bustos y Ferreira el Año del Señor de MCMVI: Resoluciones y Apéndices. Córdoba: Tip. La Industrial, 1907.

Secondary Sources

Accati, Luisa. 1995. 'Explicit Meanings: Catholicism, Matriarchy and the Distinctive Problems of Italian Feminism' in *Gender and History* 7: 241-59.

Agulla, Juan Carlos. 1976. *Eclipse of an Aristocracy: An Investigation of the Ruling Elites of the City of Córdoba.* Alabama and London: University of Alabama Press.

Anreus, Alejandro. 2006. 'Adapting to Argentinian Reality: The New Realism of Antonio Berni' in Anreus, A. Linden, Diana and Weinberg, Jonathan (eds). *The Social and the Real: Political Art of the 1930s in the Western Hemisphere.* Pennsylvania: Pennsylvania State University Press: 97-114.

Armus, Diego. 2007. *La Ciudad Impura: Salud, Tuberculosis y Cultura en Buenos Aires, 1870–1950.* Buenos Aires: Edhasa.

Auza, Néstor. 1988. *Aciertos y Fracasos Sociales del Catolicismo Argentino: Grote y la Estrategia Social, I.* Buenos Aires: Docencia y Don Bosco.

Auza, N. 1988. *Aciertos y Fracasos Sociales del Catolicismo Argentino: Proyecto Episcopal y lo Social, III.* Buenos Aires: Docencia y Don Bosco.

Balsamo, Anne. 1996. *Technologies of the Gendered Body: Reading Cyborg Women.* Durham: Duke University Press.

Barrancos, Dora. 1991. 'Contracepcionalidad y Aborto en la Década de 1920: Problema Privado y Cuestión pública' in *Estudios Sociales* 1:75-86.

Barrancos, D. 2002. *Inclusión/Exclusión. Historia con Mujeres.* Buenos Aires: Fondo de Cultura Económica.

Barrancos, D. 1989. 'Anarquismo y Sexualidad' in Armus, Diego (ed.). *Mundo Urbano y Cultura Popular.* Buenos Aires: Sudamericana: 15-37.

Barrancos, D. 1996. *La Escena Iluminada. Ciencia para Trabajadores 1890-1930.* Buenos Aires: Plus Ultra.

Barthes, Roland. 2000. *Camera Lucida: Reflections on Photography.* London: Vintage.

Bassin, Donna, Honey, Margaret and Kaplan, Meryle (eds). 1994.
Representations of Motherhood. New Haven and London: Yale
University Press.

Benjamin, Marina (ed.). 1991. *Science and Sensibility: Gender and Scientific
Enquiry, 1780-1945*. Oxford: Basil Blackwell.

Betterton, Rosemary. 1996. *An Intimate Distance: Women, Artists and the Body*.
London: Routledge.

Betterton, R. 2006. 'Promising Monsters: Pregnant Bodies, Artistic
Subjectivity, and Maternal Imagination' in *Hypatia* 21: 80-100.

Biernat, Carolina. 2007. *¿Buenos o Útiles?: La Política Inmigratoria del Peronismo*.
Buenos Aires: Editorial Biblos.

Biernat, C. and Ramacciotti, K. 2011. 'Maternity Protection for Working
Women in Argentina' in *História, Ciências, Saúde – Manguinhos* 18 (1):
153-77.

Billorou, María José. 2007. 'Madres y Médicos en Torno a la Cuna. Ideas y
Prácticas sobre el Cuidado Infantil (Buenos Aires, 1930-1945)' in La
Aljaba, Segunda Época 11: 167-92.

Billorou, M. J., Di Liscia, María Silvia and Rodríguez, Ana María. 2007.
'La Disputa en la Construcción de la Cuestión Social en el Interior
Argentino. Tensiones entre el Estado y las Mujeres (1900-1940)' in
Bravo, Celia, Gil Lozano, Fernanda and Pita, Valeria (eds). *Historias de
Luchas, Resistencias y Representaciones. Mujeres en la Argentina, Siglos XIX y
XX*. Tucumán: Universidad Nacional de Tucumán: 123-49.

Birn, Anne-Emanuelle. 2007. 'Child Health in Latin America:
Historiographic Perspectives and Challenges' in *História, Ciências, Saúde
–Manguinhos* 14 (3): 677-708.

Birn, A.E. 2002. "No More Surprising than a Broken Pitcher?": Maternal
and Child Health in the Early Years of the Pan-American Sanitary
Bureau' in *Canadian Bulletin of Medical History* 19 (1): 17-46.

Birn, A.E. 2006. 'The National-International Nexus in Public Health:
Uruguay and the Circulation of Child Health and Welfare Policies,
1890-1940'in *História, Ciências, Saúde – Manguinhos* 13 (3): 33-64.

Boixadós, Cristina, Palacios, Marta and Romano, Silvia (eds). 2005.
*Fragmentos de una Historia, Córdoba 1920-1955: Fotografías Periodísticas de la
Colección Antonio Novello*. Córdoba: Pugliese Siena.

Bonaudo, Marta. 2006. 'Cuando las Tuteladas Tutelan y Participan. La
Sociedad Damas de Caridad (1869-1894)' in *Signos Históricos* 15:70-97.

Borinsky, Marcela. 2005. "Todo Reside en Saber Qué es Un Niño". Aportes

Para una Historia de la Divulgación de las Prácticas de Crianza en la Argentina' in *Anuario de Investigaciones*. Facultad de Psicología UBA 13: 117-26.

Bowers, Toni. 1996. *The Politics of Motherhood. British Writing and Culture 1680-1760*. Cambridge: Cambridge University Press.

Burke, Peter. 2001. *Eyewitnessing: The uses of Images as Historical Evidence*. London: Reaktion Books.

Caldwell, Lesley. 1986. 'Reproducers of the Nation: Women and the Family in Fascist Policy' in Forgacs, David (ed.). *Rethinking Italian Fascism. Capitalism, Populism and Culture*. London: Lawrence and Wishart: 110-41.

Capdevila, Arturo. 1963. *Cronicones Dolientes de Córdoba*. Buenos Aires: Emecé.

Carbonetti, Adrián. 1997. *Enfermedad y Sociedad. La Tuberculosis en la Ciudad de Córdoba, 1906-1947*. Córdoba: Municipalidad de Córdoba.

Chartier, Roger. 1988. *Cultural History*. Oxford: Polity Press.

Cosse, Isabella. 2010. 'Argentine Mothers and Fathers and the New Psychological Paradigm of Child-Rearing (1958-1973)' in *Journal of Family History* 35 (2): 180–202.

Correa, Alejandra. 2000. 'Parir es Morir un Poco. Partos en el siglo XIX' in Gil Lozano, Fernanda, Pita, Valeria and Ini, Gabriela (eds). *Historia de las Mujeres en la Argentina. Tomo I, Colonia y siglo XIX*. Buenos Aires: Taurus: 193-213.

Cueto, Marcos. 1994. 'Laboratory Styles in Argentine Physiology' in *Isis* 85: 228-46.

Dalla Corte, Gabriela and Piacenza, Paola. 2006. *A las Puertas del Hogar: Madres, Niños y Damas de Caridad en el Hogar del Huérfano de Rosario, 1870-1920*. Rosario: Prohistoria Ediciones.

Di Liscia, María Silvia. 2002. 'Hijos Sanos y Legítimos: Sobre Matrimonio y Asistencia Social en Argentina (1935-1948)' in *História, Ciências, Saúde-Manguinhos*, 9 (suppl.): 209-32.

Domínguez, Nora. 1998. 'Reflexiones Finales. Acerca de la Crítica' in Domínguez, N. and Perilli, C. (eds). *Fábulas del Género: Sexo y Escrituras en América Latina*. Rosario: Breatriz Viterbo: 195-215.

Domínguez, N. 2007. *De Donde Vienen los Niños. Maternidad y Escritura en la Cultura Argentina*. Rosario: Beatriz Viterbo.

Duden, Barbara. 1993. *Disembodying Women: Perspectives on Pregnancy and the Unborn*. Massachusetts and London: Harvard University Press.

Eraso, Yolanda. 2001. 'Ni Parteras, ni Médicos: Obstetras. Especialización

Médica y Medicalización del Parto en la Primera Mitad del siglo XX' in
Anuario de Escuela de Historia 1: 109-124.

Eraso, Y. 2003. 'Los Sucesores de Ilitía. La Construcción de la Identidad
Femenina desde el Parto' in Boria, Adriana and Dalmasso, María Teresa
(eds). *Discurso Social y Construcción de Identidades: Mujer y Género.* Córdoba:
Ferreira Editor: 61-70.

Eraso, Y. 2007. 'Biotypology, Endocrinology, and Sterilization: The Practice
of Eugenics in the Treatment of Argentinian Women during the
1930s' in *Bulletin of the History of Medicine* 81(4): 792–822.

Eraso, Y. 2007. 'Género y Eugenesia: Hacia una Taxonomía Médico-Social
de las Mujeres-Madres en la Década de 1930' in Bravo, Gil Lozano,
and Pita (eds). *Historias de Luchas, Resistencias y Representaciones. Mujeres
en la Argentina, siglos XIX y XX.* Tucumán: Editorial de la Universidad
Nacional de Tucumán: 361-90.

Eraso, Y. (ed.). 2009. *Mujeres y Asistencia Social en Latinoamérica, siglos XIX
y XX. Argentina, Colombia, México, Perú y Uruguay.* Córdoba: Alción
Editora.

Eraso, Y. 2010. 'A Burden to the State'. The Reception of the German
'Active Therapy' in an Argentinian Colony-asylum' in Ernst, Waltraud
and Mueller, Thomas (eds). *Transnational Psychiatries. Social and Cultural
Histories of Psychiatry in Comparative Perspective, c. 1800-2000.* Newcastle
upon Tyne: Cambridge Scholars Publishing: 51-79.

Ferrer, Christian. 2007. *Barón Biza, El Secreto Mejor Guardado de la Historia
Argentina.* Buenos Aires: Sudamericana.

Gaudiano, Pedro. 1998. 'El Concilio Plenario Latinoamericano (Roma
1899). Preparación, Celebración y Significación' in *Revista Eclesiástica
Platense,* 101: 1063-78.

Giardinelli, Mempo. 1995. *Don Juan. Antología de Juan Filloy.* Buenos Aires:
Ediciones del Instituto Movilizador de Fondos Cooperativos.

Giunta, Andrea. 1999. 'Nacionales y Populares: Los Salones del Peronismo'
in Penhos and Wechsler (1999): 153-88.

Gramuglio, Teresa. 2002. 'El Realismo y sus Destiempos en la Literatura
Argentina' in *Historia Crítica de la Literatura Argentina: El Imperio Realista,
VI.* Buenos Aires: Emecé Editores: 15-38.

Grundberg, Andy. 2003. 'The Crisis of the Real: Photography and
Postmodernism' in Wells, Liz (ed.). *The Photography Reader.* London:
Routledge: 164-79

Guy, Donna. 1990. 'Public Health, Gender, and Private Morality: Paid

Labour and the Formation of the Body Politic in Buenos Aires' in *Gender and History* 3: 297-317.

Guy, D. 1998. 'The Politics of Pan-American Cooperation: Maternalist Feminism and the Child Rights Movement, 1913-1960' in *Gender and History* 10: 449-69.

Guy, D. 1994. 'Niños Abandonados en Buenos Aires (1880-1914) y el Desarrollo del Concepto de la Madre' in Fletcher, Lea (ed.) *Mujeres y Cultura en la Argentina del siglo XIX*. Buenos Aires: Feminaria: 217-26.

Guy, D. 2009. *Women Build the Welfare State: Performing Charity and Creating Rights in Argentina, 1880–1955*. Durham and London: Duke University Press.

Habermas, Jürgen. 1991. *The Structural Transformation of the Public Sphere: An Inquiry into a Category of Bourgeois Society*. Cambridge: MIT Press.

Halperín Donghi, Tulio. 1998. *El Espejo de la Historia. Problemas Argentinos y Perspectivas Latinoamericanas*. Buenos Aires: Sudamericana.

Hall, Anne and Bishop, Mardia (eds). 2009. *Momy Angst: Mothers in American Popular Culture*. California: Praeger.

Hall, Linda. 2004. *Mary, Mother and Warrior: The Virgin in Spain and the Americas*. Austin: University of Texas Press.

Hill, Marylu. 1999. *Mothering Modernity: Feminism, Modernism, and the Maternal Muse*. New York; London: Garland Publishing.

Hirsch, Marianne. 1989. *The Mother/Daughter Plot: Narrative, Psychoanalysis, Feminism*. Bloomington: Indiana University Press.

Holland, Patricia. 1998. 'The Politics of the Smile: 'Soft News' and the Sexualisation of the Popular Press' in Carter, Cynthia, Branston, Gill and Allan, Stuart (eds). *News, Gender and Power*. London and New York: Routledge: 17-32.

Holland, P., Spence, Jo and Watney, Simon. 1986. 'Introduction: The Politics and Sexual Politics of Photography' in Spence, Holland and Watney (eds). *Photography/Politics: Two*. London: Comedia: 1-7.

Holmes, Megan. 1997. 'Disrobing the Virgin: The Madonna Lactans in Fifteenth-century Florentine Art' in Johnson, Geraldine and Matthews, Sara (eds). *Picturing Women in Renaissance and Baroque Italy*. Cambridge: Cambridge University Press: 167-95.

Hyde, Sarah. 1997. *Exhibiting Gender*. Manchester: Manchester University Press.

Ini, Gabriela. 2000. 'Infanticidios, Construcción de la Verdad y Control de Género en el Discurso Judicial' in Gil Lozano, Fernanda, Pita, Valeria and Ini, Gabriela (eds). *Historia de las Mujeres en la Argentina. Tomo I, Colonia y siglo XIX*. Buenos Aires: Taurus: 235-51.

Irigaray, Luce. 1985. *Speculum of the Other Woman*. Ithaca: Cornell University Press.

Jacobus, Mary. 1995. *First Things: The Maternal Imaginary in Literature, Art and Psychoanalysis*. London; New York: Routledge.

Jordanova, Ludmilla. 1989. *Sexual Visions: Images of Gender in Science and Medicine between the Eighteenth and Twentieth Centuries*. London: Harvester Wheatsheaf.

Kamenszain, Tamara. 1983. *El Texto Silencioso. Tradición y Vanguardia en la Poesía Sudamericana*. México: UNAM.

Kaplan, Ann. 1992. *Motherhood and Representation: The Mother in Popular Culture and Melodrama*. London: Routledge.

Kember, Sarah. 2003. "'The Shadow of the Object'': Photography and Realism' in Liz Wells (ed.). *The Photography Reader*. London: Routledge: 202-17.

Koven, Seth and Michel, Sonya (eds). 1993. *Mothers of a New World: Maternalist Politics and the Origins of Welfare Sates*. Routledge: London.

Kristeva, Julia. 1980. *Desire in Language: A Semiotic Approach to Literature and Art*. Ed. by Leon Roudiez. Oxford: Basil Blackwell.

Lavrin, Asunción. 1995. *Women, Feminism and Social Change in Argentina, Chile and Uruguay 1890-1940*. Lincoln: University of Nebraska Press.

Lawrence, Christopher. 1999. 'A Tale of Two Sciences: Bedside and Bench in Twentieth-century Britain' in *Medical History* 43: 421-50.

Lawrence, C. and Weisz, George (eds). 1998. *Greater Than the Parts: Holism and Biomedicine, 1920-1950*. New York: Oxford University Press.

Levine, Philippa and Bashford, Alison. 2010. 'Introduction: Eugenics and the Modern World' in Bashford, A. and Levine, P. *The Oxford Handbook of the History of Eugenics*. New York: Oxford University Press: 3-24.

Lewis, Jane. 1980. *The Politics of Motherhood: Child and Maternal Welfare in England, 1900-1939*. London: Croom Helm.

Liebscher, Arthur. 1988. 'Towards a Pious Republic: Argentine Social Catholicism in Córdoba, 1895-1930' in *Journal of Church and State* 30: 549-67.

Lo Celso, Ángel. 1973. *50 Años de Arte Plástico en Córdoba*. Córdoba: Banco de la Provincia de Córdoba.

Lobato, Mirta. 2007. *Historia de las Trabajadoras en la Argentina (1869-1960)*. Buenos Aires: Edhasa.

Lobato, M. and Suriano, Juan. 2000. *Atlas Histórico. Nueva Historia Argentina*. Buenos Aires: Editorial Sudamericana.

Lorenzo, María Fernanda, Rey Ana Lía and Tossounian, Cecilia. 2005. 'Images of Virtuous Women: Morality, Gender and Power in Argentina between the World Wars' in *Gender & History* 17 (3): 567–92.

Loudon, Irvine. 1998. 'Maternal Mortality: 1880-1950. Some Regional and International Comparisons' in *Social History of Medicine* 1 (2): 183-228.

Ludmer, Josefina. 1985. 'Las Tretas del Débil', in González, Patricia and Ortega, Eliana (eds), *La Sartén por el Mango: Encuentro de Escritoras Latinoamericanas*. Puerto Rico: El Huracán: 47-54.

MacKenzie, Donald. 1981. Statistics in Britain 1865-1930. The Social Construction of Scientific Knowledge. Edinburgh: Edinburgh University Press.

Malin, Jo. 2000. *The Voice of the Mother: Embedded Maternal Narratives in Twentieth-century Women's Autobiographies*. Carbondale: Southern Illinois University Press.

Marland, Hilary. 2004. *Dangerous Motherhood: Insanity and Childbirth in Victorian Britain*. Basingstoke: Palgrave McMillan.

Marland, H. (ed.). 1993. *The Art of Midwifery: Early Modern Midwives in Europe*. London and New York: Routledge.

Marland, H. and Rafferty, Anne Marie (eds). 1997. *Midwives, Society and Childbirth: Debates and Controversies in the Modern Period*. London and New York: Routledge.

Martin, Emily. 1989. *The Woman in the Body: a Cultural Analysis of Reproduction*. Milton Keynes: Open University Press.

Matthews, Sandra and Wexler, Laura. 2000. *Pregnant Pictures*. New York & London: Routledge.

Masiello, Francine. 1997. *Entre Civilización y Barbarie. Mujeres, Nación y Cultura Literaria en la Argentina Moderna*. Rosario: Beatriz Viterbo.

Mead, Karen. 2000. 'Beneficent Maternalism: Argentine Motherhood in Comparative Perspective, 1880-1920' in *Journal of Women's History* 12: 120-45.

Mead, K. 2001. 'Gender, Welfare and the Catholic Church in Argentina: Conferencias de Señoras de San Vicente de Paul, 1890-1916' in *The Americas* 58: 91-119.

Merchant, Carolyn. 1982. *The Death of Nature: Women, Ecology, and the Scientific Revolution*. London: Wildwood House.

Miranda, Marisa. 2003. 'La Antorcha de Cupido: Eugenesia, Biotipología y

Eugamia en Argentina, 1930-1970' in *Asclepio* 55 (2): 231-55.

Miranda, M. 2005. 'La Biotipología en el Pronatalismo Argentino (1930-1983)' in *Asclepio* 57 (1): 189-218.

Miranda, M. and Vallejo, Gustavo (eds). 2005. *Darwinismo Social y Eugenesia en el Mundo Latino*. Buenos Aires: Siglo XXI Editores.

Miranda, M. and Vallejo, G. 2008. 'Formas de Aislamiento Físico y Simbólico: La Lepra, sus Espacios de Reclusión y el Discurso Médico-legal en Argentina' in *Asclepio* 60 (2): 19-42.

Misner, Paul. 2004. 'Catholic Labor and Catholic Action: The Italian Context of "Quadragesimo Anno" ' in *The Catholic Historical Review* 90 (4): 650-74.

Moreyra, Beatriz. 2000. 'Crecimiento Económico y Desajustes Sociales en Córdoba (1900-1930)' in Moreyra B. et al. *Estado, Mercado y Sociedad: Córdoba, 1820-1950, Tomo I*. Córdoba: Centro de Estudios Históricos: 275-335.

Moreyra, B. 2009. *Cuestión Social y Políticas Sociales en la Argentina. La Modernidad Periférica. Córdoba, 1900-1930*. Bernal: Universidad Nacional de Quilmes.

Moscucci, Ornella. 1990. *The Science of Woman: Gynaecology and Gender in England, 1800-1929*. Cambridge: Cambridge University Press.

Myers, Jorge. 1997. 'Historia de las Ideas e Historia Disciplinares. Comentario a la Ponencia de Hugo Vezzetti' in *Prismas. Revista de Historia Intelectual* 1: 219-26.

Nari, Marcela. 2005. *Políticas de Maternidad y Maternalismo Político en Buenos Aires (1890-1940)*. Buenos Aires: Biblos.

Nari, M. 1995. 'La Educación de la Mujer (o Acerca de Cómo Cocinar y Cambiar los Pañales a su Bebé de Manera Científica)' in *Mora* 1: 31-45.

Nari, M. 1996. 'Las Prácticas Anticonceptivas, la Disminución de la Natalidad y el Debate Médico, 1890-1940' in Lobato, Mirta (ed.). *Política, Médicos y Enfermedades. Lecturas de Historia de la Salud en la Argentina*. Buenos Aires: Biblos: 154-89.

Nari, M. 1999. 'La Eugenesia en Argentina, 1890-1940' in *Quipu* 12: 343-69.

Novick, Susana. 2008. 'Población y Estado en Argentina de 1930 a 1943. Análisis de los Discursos de Algunos Actores Sociales: Industriales, Militares, Obreros y Profesionales de la Salud' in *Estudios Demográficos y Urbanos* 23 (2): 333-73.

Oakley, Ann. 1984. *The Captured Womb: A History of the Medical Care of Pregnant Women*. Oxford: Basil Blackwell.

Otero, Hernán. 2006. *Estadística y Nación: Una Historia Conceptual del Pensamiento Censal de la Argentina Moderna, 1869-1914.* Buenos Aires: Prometeo Libros.

Oudshoorn, Nelly. 1994. *Beyond the Natural Body: An Archaeology of Sex Hormones.* Routledge: New York.

Oviedo, Antonio. 2004. 'Paisajes en la Pintura Cordobesa: (Vaivenes y Fracturas de la Representación) in *100 Años de Plástica en Córdoba*: 56-68.

Paul, Diane. 1991. 'The Rockefeller Foundation and the Origins of Behaviour Genetics' in Benson, Keith, Maienschein, Jane and Rainger, Ronald (eds). *The Expansion of American Biology.* London: Rutgers University Press: 262–83.

Penhos, Marta and Wechsler, Diana (eds). 1999. *Tras los Pasos de la Norma: Salones Nacionales de Bellas Artes (1911-1989).* Buenos Aires: Ediciones del Jilguero.

Penhos, M. 1999. 'Nativos en el Salón. Artes Plásticas e Identidad en la Primera Mitad del Siglo XX', in Penhos and Wechsler (1999): 111-52.

Perry Nicholas and Echeverría Loreto. 1988. *Under the Heel of Mary.* London and New York: Routledge.

Podnieks, Elizabeth and O'Reilly, Andrea. 2010. 'Introduction: Maternal Literatures in Text and Tradition: Daughter-Centric, Matrilineal, and Matrifocal Perspectives' in Podnieks, E. and O'Reilly, A. (eds). *Textual Mothers: Motherhood in Contemporary Women's Literatures.* Ontario: Wilfrid Laurier University Press: 1-27.

Quine, Maria Sophia. 2010. 'The First-Wave Eugenic Revolution in Southern Europe: Science Sans Frontières' in Bashford, A. and Levine, P. *The Oxford Handbook of the History of Eugenics.* New York: Oxford University Press: 377-97.

Ramacciotti, Karina. 2006. 'Las Sombras de la Política Sanitaria durante el Peronismo: Los Brotes Epidémicos en Buenos Aires' in *Asclepio* 58 (2): 115-38.

Ramos, Julio. 2001. *Divergent Modernities: Culture and Politics in Nineteenth-century Latin America.* Durham: Duke University Press.

Rapalo, Ester and Gramuglio, T. 2002. 'Pedagogías para la Nación Católica: Criterio y Hugo Wast' in *Historia Crítica de la Literatura Argentina: El Imperio Realista, VI.* Buenos Aires: Emecé: 447-75.

Recalde Héctor. 1992. 'Transformaciones dentro del Discurso Higienista' in Salvatore, Ricardo (ed.). *Reformadores Sociales en Argentina, 1900-1940: Discurso, Ciencia y Control Social.* DTS 119, Instituto Torcuato Di Tella:

40-45.

Reggiani, Andrés. 2010. 'Depopulation, Fascism, and Eugenics in 1930s Argentina' in *Hispanic American Historical Review* 90 (2): 283-318.

Reggiani, A. 2007. 'De Rastacueros a Expertos. Modernización, Diplomacia Cultural y Circuitos Académicos Transnacionales, 1870-1940' in Salvatore, Ricardo (ed.). *Los Lugares del Saber. Contextos Locales y Redes Transnacionales en la Formación del Conocimiento Moderno.* Rosario: Beatriz Viterbo Editora: 159-87.

Rodriguez, Julia. 2006. *Civilizing Argentina: Science, Medicine, and the Modern State.* Chapel Hill: The University of North Carolina Press.

Rodriguez, J. 2011. 'A Complex Fabric: Intersecting Histories of Race, Gender, and Science in Latin America' in *Hispanic American Historical Review* 91(3): 409-28.

Rodríguez, Ana M. T. 2008. 'La Perspectiva Católica Sobre la Salud y la Práctica Médica en la Argentina de los Años Treinta. La Visión de los Médicos Confesionales' in *Anuario de Estudios Americanos* 65 (1): 257-75.

Romano, Silvia. 2005. 'Los Fotógrafos y la Fotografía en la Prensa, 1920-1955: Una Mirada Sobre el Fotoperiodismo en La Voz del Interior' in Boixadós, Palacios and Romano (2005): 11-7.

Ruggiero, Kristin. 1992. 'Honour, Maternity and the Disciplining of Women: Infanticide in Late Nineteenth-century Buenos Aires' in *Hispanic American Historical Review* 72: 353-73.

Saítta, Sylvia. 1998. *Regueros de Tinta: El Diario "Crítica" en la Década de 1920.* Buenos Aires: Sudamericana.

Sarlo, Beatriz. 2000. *El Imperio de los Sentimientos.* Buenos Aires: Norma.

Scarzanella, Eugenia. 1997. 'Criminología, Eugenesia y Medicina Social en el Debate entre Científicos Argentinos e Italianos, 1912-1941' in Troncoso, Hugo and Sierra, Carmen (eds). *Ideas, Cultura e Historia en la Creación Intelectual Latinoamericana: Siglos XIX y XX.* Quito: Ediciones Abya-Yala: 217-34.

Schiebinger, Londa. 1994. *Nature's Body: Sexual Politics and the Making of Modern Science.* London: Pandora.

Schiebinger, L. 1989. *The Mind has no Sex?: Women in the Origins of Modern Science.* London, Massachusetts: Harvard University Press.

Schneider, William. 1990. *Quality and Quantity: The Quest for Biological Regeneration in Twentieth-century France.* Cambridge: Cambridge University Press.

Schorske, Carl. 1980. *Fin-de-Siècle Vienna: Politics and Culture.* New York:

Knopf.

Scott, Joan, 1988. *Gender and the Politics of History.* New York: Columbia University Press.

Scott, J. 1992. 'Experience' in Scott, J. and Butler, Judith (eds). *Feminists Theorize the Political.* New York & London: Routledge: 22-40.

Stepan, Nancy. 1991. *"The Hour of Eugenics": Race, Gender and Nation in Latin America.* Ithaca and London: Cornwell University Press.

Stern, Alejandra. 2000. 'Mestizofilia, Biotipología y Eugenesia en el México Pos-revolucionario: Hacia una Historia de la Ciencia y el Estado, 1920-60' in *Relaciones* 81: 57-91.

Tagg, John. 1999. 'Evidence, Truth and Order: A Means of Surveillance' in Evans, Jessica and Hall, Stuart (eds.). *Visual Culture: The Reader.* London: Sage Publications and the Open University: 243-73.

Thébaud, Françoise. 2002. 'A Medicalização do Parto e suas Conseqüências: O Exemplo da França no Período entre as duas Guerras' in *Estudos Feministas* 2: 415-27.

Torrado, Susana. 1999. 'Transición de la Familia en la Argentina, 1870-1995' in *Desarrollo Económico* 39: 235-60.

Tracy, Sarah. 1998. 'An Evolving Science of Man: The Transformation and Demise of American Constitutional Medicine, 1920-1950' in Lawrence and Weisz (1998): 161-88.

Treichler, Paula. 1990. 'Feminism, Medicine and the Meaning of Childbirth' in Jacobus, Mary, Fox Keller, Evelyn and Shuttleworth, Sally (eds). *Body/Politic: Women and the Discourses of Science.* New York: Routledge: 113-38.

Treichler, P., Cartwright, Lisa and Penley, Constance (eds). 1998. *The Visible Woman: Imaging Technologies, Gender, and Science.* New York: NYU Press.

Turda, Marius. 2010. 'Race, Science and Eugenics in the Twentieth Century' in Bashford, A. and Levine, P. *The Oxford Handbook of the History of Eugenics.* New York: Oxford University Press: 98-127.

Tyler, Imogen. 2000. 'Reframing Pregnant Embodiment' in Ahmed, Sara *et al.* (eds). *Transformations: Thinking Through Feminism.* London: Routledge: 288-302.

Vagliente, Pablo. 2000. *Indicios de Modernidad. Una Mirada Socio-Cultural desde el Campo Periodístico en Córdoba, 1860-1880.* Córdoba: Alción Editora.

Vezzetti, Hugo. 1999. 'Las Promesas del Psicoanálisis en la Cultura de Masas' in Devoto, Fernando and Madero, Marta. *Historia de la Vida Privada en la Argentina. Tomo III. La Argentina entre Multitudes y Soledades:*

De los Años Treinta a la Actualidad. Buenos Aires: Taurus: 173-97.

Vezzetti, H. 1997. 'Historia del Freudismo e Historia de la Sexualidad: El Género Sexológico en Buenos Aires en los Treinta' in *Prismas. Revista de Historia Intelectual* 1: 211-18.

Vincent, Mary. 2001. 'Gender and Morals in Spanish Catholic Youth Culture. A Case Study of the Marian Congregations 1930-1936' in *Gender & History* 13 (2): 273-97.

Wainerman, Catalina. 1980. 'La Mujer y el Trabajo en la Argentina desde la Perspectiva de la Iglesia Católica' in *Cuadernos del CENEP* 16, Centro de Estudios de Población: 1-30.

Wechsler, Diana, 2004. 'Un registro Moderno del Arte en Córdoba', in *100 Años de Plástica en Córdoba:* 188-24.

Wechsler, D. 1999. 'Salones y Contra-Salones' in Penhos and Wechsler (1999): 41-98.

Wechsler, D. 2006. 'Imágenes Para la Resistencia. Intersecciones entre Arte y Política en la Encrucijada de la Internacional Antifascista. Obras y Textos de Antonio Berni (1930-1936)' in Medina, Cuauhtémoc (ed.). *La Imagen Política.* México: UNAM: 385-412.

White, Hayden. 1969. 'The Task of Intellectual History' in *The Monist* 53: 606-26.

Williams, Kevin. 2010. *Read All about It!: A History of the British Newspaper.* London: Routledge.

Williams, Susan. 1997. *Women and Childbirth in the Twentieth Century: A History of the National Birthday Trust Fund, 1928-93.* Stroud: Sutton.

Young, Iris M. 1990. *Throwing Like a Girl and Other Essays in Feminist Philosophy and Social Theory.* Bloomington: Indiana University Press.

Zimmermann, Eduardo. 1994. *Los Liberales Reformistas. La Cuestión Social en la Argentina, 1890-1916.* Buenos Aires: Sudamericana y Universidad de San Andrés.

100 Años de Plástica en Córdoba, 1904-2004: 100 Artistas – 100 Obras en el Centenario de La Voz del Interior. 2004. Córdoba: Pugliese Siena.

Unpublished sources (thesis and papers)

Eraso, Yolanda. 2006. *Medical Discourse and Social Representations of Motherhood in the City of Córdoba (Argentina), 1900-1946.* PhD thesis. Oxford Brookes University.

Roitemburd, Silvia. 1998. Nacionalismo Católico Cordobés. Educación en los Dogmas para un Proyecto Global. Tesis Doctoral. Universidad Nacional de Córdoba.

Rustoyburu, Cecilia. 2008. 'Padres Extremosos y Niños con Derechos de Beligerancia. Los Consejos sobre Crianza del Dr. Escardó: Pediatría, Psicoanálisis y Escuela Nueva (Argentina, Fines de la Década del 30)'. Paper presented at *Jornadas Historia de la Infancia en Argentina, 1880-1960* (Prov. Buenos Aires, November 2008).

Vidal, Gardenia. 2000. 'El Avance del Poder Clerical y el Conservadorismo Político en Córdoba durante la Década del 20'. Paper presented at the *Latin American Studies Association* (Miami, March 2000).

Internet sources

Acha, Omar. [s.d.] 'El Catolicismo y la Profesión Médica en la Década Peronista' in *Centro Cultural de la Cooperación*. Online at: http://www.centrocultural.coop/descargas/historia/el-catolicismo-y-la-profesion-medica-en-la-decada-peronista.html (consulted 17.08.2010)

Bartlett, Alison. 2002. 'Madonnas, Models and Maternity: Icons of Breastfeeding in Visual Arts'. Paper presented at the conference *Performing Motherhood: Ideology, Agency and Experience* (La Trobe University, 2002). Online at: www.usq.edu.au/resources/bartlettpaper.pdf (consulted 27.11.2009)

'Confederación Médica de la República Argentina'. Online at: http://www.comra.org.ar/ (consulted 6.02.2010).

'El aporte de la migración internacional en el crecimiento de la ciudad de Buenos Aires. Años censales, 1855/2010'. 2011. Buenos Aires: Dirección General de Estadística y Censos, Ministerio de Hacienda. Online at: http://www.estadistica.buenosaires.gov.ar/areas/hacienda/sis_estadistico/ir_2011_471.pdf (consulted 22.08.2011).

Encyclicals have been consulted at the *Vatican Official Website*. Online at: http://www.vatican.va/.

Houssay, Bernardo. 'The Role of the Hypophysis in Carbohydrate Metabolism and in Diabetes', Nobel Lecture, 12 December 1947, in *Nobelprize.org*. Online at: http://nobelprize.org/medicine/laureates/1947/houssay-lecture.html (consulted 25.02.2011).

La Vanguardia, (11 July 1929), 10. Online at http://www.lavanguardia.com/hemeroteca/index.html (consulted 30.04.2011)

'Ley Nacional N° 17132. Ejercicio de la Medicina, Odontología y

Actividades Auxiliares'. *Notivida*. Online at: http://www.notivida.com. ar (consulted 6.02.2010).

Miranda, Lida. 2008. 'Una Modernización en Clave de Cruzada: El Diario Católico de Buenos Aires en la Década de 1920: El Pueblo' in *Revista Escuela de Historia* 7. Online at: http://www.redalyc.org/src/inicio/ ArtPdfRed.jsp?iCve=63818509004 (consulted 20.05.2011).

Perilli, Carmen. 2004. 'Los Trabajos de la Araña. Mujeres, Teorías y Literatura' in *Espéculo. Revista de Estudios Literarios* 28. Online at http:// www.ucm.es/info/especulo/numero28/trabaran.html (consulted 25.11.2009)

Quintana, Luis A. 2009. 'La Constitución del Diario Católico La Mañana, Santa Fe 1934-1937. Aportes Para un Uso Didáctico de la Cultura Católica' in *Clío & Asociados* 13: 13-33. Online at: http://www. fuentesmemoria.fahce.unlp.edu.ar/art_revistas/pr.4623/pr.4623.pdf (consulted 20.05.2011).

Ramella, Susana. 'Ideas Demográficas Argentinas (1930-1950): Una Propuesta Poblacionista, Elitista, Europeizante y Racista' in *Revista Persona*. Online at: http://www.revistapersona.com.ar/ Persona11/11Ramellatesis.htm (consulted 4.03.2009).

Scarzanella, E. 2003. 'Los Pibes en el Palacio de Ginebra: Las Investigaciones de la Sociedad de las Naciones sobre la Infancia Latinoamericana (1925-1939)' in *Estudios Interdisciplinarios de América Latina y el Caribe*, 14 (2). Online at: http://www1.tau.ac.il/eial/index. php (consulted 25.07.2009).

Vancassel, Paul. 2008. *Les Regards Photograhiques: Dispositifs Anthropologiques et Processus Transindividuels*. These Doctorale. Université Rennes 2, HauteBretagne. Online at: tel.archives-ouvertes.fr/docs/00/29/47/53/ PDF/theseVancassel.pdf (consulted 21.03.2010)

Index

Printed in the United States
by Baker & Taylor Publisher Services